CW00696733

MEDICAL
INTELLIGENCE
UNIT

CHEMOKINES IN DISEASE

Alisa E. Koch, M.D.

Nortwestern University Medical School
Chicago, Illinois, U.S.A.

Robert M. Strieter, M.D.

University of Michigan Medical School
Ann Arbor, Michigan, U.S.A

Springer

New York Berlin Heidelberg London Paris
Tokyo Hong Kong Barcelona Budapest

R.G. LANDES COMPANY
AUSTIN

MEDICAL INTELLIGENCE UNIT
CHEMOKINES IN DISEASE

R.G. LANDES COMPANY
Austin, Texas, U.S.A.

International Copyright © 1996 Springer-Verlag, Heidelberg, Germany

All rights reserved.
No part of this book may be reproduced or transmitted in any form or by any means, electronic or mechanical, including photocopy, recording, or any information storage and retrieval system, without permission in writing from the publisher.
Printed in the U.S.A.

Please address all inquiries to the Publishers:
R.G. Landes Company, 909 Pine Street, Georgetown, Texas, U.S.A. 78626
Phone: 512/ 863 7762; FAX: 512/ 863 0081

International distributor (except North America):

Springer-Verlag GmbH & Co. KG
Tiergartenstrasse 17, D-69121 Heidelberg, Germany

 Springer

International ISBN: 3-540-61354-4

While the authors, editors and publisher believe that drug selection and dosage and the specifications and usage of equipment and devices, as set forth in this book, are in accord with current recommendations and practice at the time of publication, they make no warranty, expressed or implied, with respect to material described in this book. In view of the ongoing research, equipment development, changes in governmental regulations and the rapid accumulation of information relating to the biomedical sciences, the reader is urged to carefully review and evaluate the information provided herein.

Library of Congress Cataloging-in-Publication Data

Chemokines in disease / [edited by] Alisa E. Koch, Robert Strieter.
    p. cm. — (Medical intelligence unit)
   Includes bibliographical references and index.
    ISBN 1-57059-365-5 (RGL alk. paper). — ISBN 0-412-11411-9 (CH alk. paper)
    1. Chemokines—Pathology.   I. Koch, Alisa E., 1956–. II. Strieter, Robert, 1952-. III. Series.
    [DNLM: 1. Chemokines—physiology. 2. Chemotaxis, Leukocyte-physiology. 3. Inflammation—immunology. QW 700 C5175 1996]
QR185.8.C45C484   1996
616.07'9—dc20
DNLM/DLC
for Library of Congress

96-22712
                  CIP

PUBLISHER'S NOTE

R.G. Landes Company publishes six book series: *Medical Intelligence Unit, Molecular Biology Intelligence Unit, Neuroscience Intelligence Unit, Tissue Engineering Intelligence Unit, Biotechnology Intelligence Unit* and *Environmental Intelligence Unit.* The authors of our books are acknowledged leaders in their fields and the topics are unique. Almost without exception, no other similar books exist on these topics.

Our goal is to publish books in important and rapidly changing areas of bioscience and environment for sophisticated researchers and clinicians. To achieve this goal, we have accelerated our publishing program to conform to the fast pace in which information grows in bioscience. Most of our books are published within 90 to 120 days of receipt of the manuscript. We would like to thank our readers for their continuing interest and welcome any comments or suggestions they may have for future books.

Shyamali Ghosh
Publications Director
R.G. Landes Company

DEDICATION

I dedicate this book to my husband, Dr. Howard Stein, and my son, Joshua Walter Stein.

—Alisa E. Koch, M.D.

I would like to thank my wife, Marcia, and my children, Eric, Lindsay and Brett, for all their patience with this endeavor.

—Robert M. Strieter, M.D.

CONTENTS

ABBREVIATIONS

MIP-1α	macrophage inflammatory protein-1 alpha
MIP-2	macrophage inflammatory protein-2
MCP-1	monocyte chemoattractant protein-1
IL-8	interleukin-8
ENA-78	epithelial cell-derived neutrophil activating protein-78
LAM	lipoarabinomannan
MBMM	murine bone marrow-derived macrophages
TNF	tumor necrosis factor
IL-1	interleukin-1
IFN-γ	interferon-γ
IL-10	interleukin-10
PMN	polymorphonuclear leukocyte
CFU	colony forming units
hr	human recombinant
mr	murine recombinant
i.p.	intraperitoneal
i.t.	intratracheal

EDITORS

Alisa E. Koch, M.D.
Department of Internal Medicine
Division of Arthritis and Connective Tissue Disease
Northwestern University Medical School
Chicago, Illinois, U.S.A.
Chapters 5, 11

Robert M. Strieter, M.D.
Department of Internal Medicine
Division of Pulmonary and Critical Care Medicine
University of Michigan Medical School
Ann Arbor, Michigan, U.S.A
Chapters 1, 5, 7, 8, 11

CONTRIBUTORS

Sunil K. Ahuja, M.D.
The Laboratory of Host Defenses
National Institute of Allergy
  and Infectious Diseases
National Institutes of Health
Bethesda, Maryland, U.S.A.
Chapter 3

Douglas A. Arenberg, M.D.
Department of Internal Medicine
University of Michigan Medical School
Ann Arbor, Michigan, U.S.A.
Chapter 11

Stephen W. Chensue, M.D., Ph.D.,
Department of Pathology
  and Laboratory Medicine
The Veterans Affairs Medical Center
Ann Arbor, Michigan, U.S.A.
Chapter 9

Lisa M. Colletti, M.D.
Department of Surgery
University of Michigan Medical School
Ann Arbor, Michigan, U.S.A.
Chapter 7

Christophe Combadiere, Ph.D.
The Laboratory of Host Defenses
National Institute of Allergy and
  Infectious Diseases
National Institutes of Health
Bethesda, Maryland, U.S.A.
Chapter 3

Gregory J. Dolecki, Ph.D.
Departments of Medicine
  and Molecular Biology
  and Pharmacology
Washington University
  Medical School
St. Louis, Missouri, U.S.A.
Chapter 6

Kimberly E. Foreman, Ph.D.
Department of Pathology
Skin Disease Research Laboratories
Loyola University Medical Center
Maywood, Illinois, U.S.A.
Chapter 4

Ji-Liang Gao, Ph.D.
The Laboratory of Host Defenses
National Institute of Allergy
  and Infectious Diseases
National Institutes of Health
Bethesda, Maryland, U.S.A.
Chapter 3

Akihisa Harada, M.D.
Department of Hygiene
Kanazawa University School
  of Medicine
Kanazawa, Japan
Chapter 10

Gary B. Huffnagle, M.D.
Departments of Pathology
  and Medicine
Division of Pulmonary and Critical
  Care Medicine
University of Michigan Medical School
Ann Arbor, Michigan, U.S.A.
Chapter 8

Steven L. Kunkel, Ph.D.
Department of Pathology
Division of Pulmonary and Critical
  Care Medicine
University of Michigan Medical School
Ann Arbor, Michigan, U.S.A.
Chapters 1, 5, 7, 8, 11

James B. Lefkowith, M.D.
Departments of Medicine
  and Molecular Biology
  and Pharmacology
Washington University
  Medical School
St. Louis, Missouri, U.S.A.
Chapter 6

Nicholas W. Lukacs, Ph.D.
Department of Pathology
University of Michigan Medical School
Ann Arbor, Michigan, U.S.A.
Chapter 9

Kouji Matsushima, M.D., Ph.D.
Department of Pharmacology
Cancer Research Institute
Kanazawa University
Kanazawa, Japan
Chapter 10

Naofumi Mukaida, M.D., Ph.D.
Department of Pharmacology
Cancer Research Institute
Kanazawa University
Kanazawa, Japan
Chapter 10

Philip M. Murphy, M.D.
The Laboratory of Host Defenses
National Institute of Allergy
  and Infectious Diseases
National Institutes of Health
Bethesda, Maryland, U.S.A.
Chapter 3

Brian J. Nickoloff, M.D., Ph.D.
Department of Pathology
Skin Disease Research Laboratories
Loyola University Medical Center
Maywood, Illinois, U.S.A.
Chapter 4

Peter J. Polverini, D.D.S., DM.Sc.
Department of Molecular
  Pathogenesis
University of Michigan Dental School
Ann Arbor, Michigan, U.S.A.
Chapter 11

Armen B. Shanafelt, Ph.D.
Institute of Molecular Biologicals
  and Institute of Research
  Technologies
Bayer Corporation
West Haven, Connecticut, U.S.A.
Chapter 11

Theodore J. Standiford, M.D.
Department of Internal Medicine
Division of Pulmonary and Critical
  Care Medicine
University of Michigan Medical School
Ann Arbor, Michigan, U.S.A
Chapter 7, 8

Dennis D. Taub, Ph.D.
Clinical Services Program
National Cancer Institute-FCRDC
Frederick, Maryland, U.S.A.
Chapter 2

Galen B. Toews, M.D.
Department of Internal Medicine
Division of Pulmonary and Critical
  Care Medicine
University of Michigan Medical School
Ann Arbor, Michigan, U.S.A.
Chapter 8

Alfred Walz, Ph.D.
Theodor-Kocher Institut
University of Bern
Bern, Switzerland
Chapter 1

Xiaobo Wu, M.D.
Departments of Medicine
  and Molecular Biology
  and Pharmacology
Washington University
  Medical School
St. Louis, Missouri, U.S.A.
Chapter 6

PREFACE

The salient feature of a variety of inflammatory conditions such as infections, allergic disorders, autoimmune diseases, or ischemia/reperfusion injury is the association of infiltrating leukocytes. These extravasating leukocytes often contribute to the pathogenesis of the underlying disease. However, it should be appreciated that leukocyte recruitment is also critical for host defense, leading to clearance of the inciting factor(s), i.e., infection. While the events of leukocyte trafficking may appear intuitive, it has taken over 150 years of research to elucidate the molecular and cellular steps involved in the process of leukocyte migration. The maintenance of leukocyte recruitment during inflammation requires intercellular communication between infiltrating leukocytes and the endothelium, resident stromal and parenchymal cells. These events are mediated via the generation of early response cytokines, e.g., IL-1 and TNF-a, the expression of cell surface adhesion molecules, and the production of chemotactic molecules, such as the chemokines.

The human C-X-C and C-C chemokines family of chemotactic cytokines are two closely related polypeptide families that behave, in general, as potent chemotactic factors for either neutrophils, mononuclear cells, or lymphocytes, respectively. These cytokines in their monomeric form range from 7 to 10 kDa and are characteristically basic heparin-binding proteins. The chemokines display three highly conserved cysteine amino acid residues: the C-X-C chemokine family has the first two NH_2-terminal cysteines separated by one non-conserved amino acid residue, the C-X-C cysteine motif; the C-C chemokine family has the first two NH_2-terminal cysteines in juxtaposition, the C-C cysteine motif. Interestingly, C-X-C chemokines are clustered on human chromosome 4, and exhibit between 20% to 50% homology on the amino acid level, and the C-C chemokines are clustered on human chromosome 17 and exhibit between 28% and 45% homology at the amino acid level. There is approximately 20% to 40% homology between the members of the two chemokine families.

The murine homologues of the human C-X-C chemokines are KC, macrophage inflammatory protein-2 (MIP-2) crg-2, and MIG, and are structurally homologous to human GROα, GROβ/GROγ, IP10, and MIG, respectively. No murine or rat structural homologues exist for human IL-8. The murine C-C chemokines, in general, are known by the same names as their human counterparts, with the exception of T cell activation gene-3 (TCA-3), which is structurally homologous with I-309. Chemokines have been found to be produced by an array of cells including monocytes, alveolar macrophages, neutrophils, platelets, eosinophils, mast cells, T lymphocytes, natural killer cells (NK cells), keratinocytes, mesangial cells, epithelial cells, hepatocytes, fibroblasts, smooth muscle cells, mesothelial cells, and endothelial cells. These cells can produce chemokines in response to a variety of factors, including viruses, bacterial products, IL-1, TNF, C5a, LTB4 and IFNs. The production of chemokines by both immune and non-immune cells supports the contention that these cytokines may play a pivotal role in orchestrating inflammation. To illustrate the importance of chemokines during the pathogenesis of inflammation, this book will focus on the role of C-X-C and C-C chemokines in human disease.

CHAPTER 1

C-X-C CHEMOKINES—
AN OVERVIEW

Alfred Walz, Steven L. Kunkel and Robert M. Strieter

INTRODUCTION

The recruitment of leukocytes during an inflammatory response is the hallmark of a variety of disorders that include trauma, infection, autoimmune diseases, exposure to environmental/occupational noxious agents, cancer, allograft rejection and ischemia-reperfusion injury. Acute inflammation is a condition that is defined by the predominance of neutrophils. However, the histopathology of a number of disorders is associated with a pleomorphic leukocyte infiltration, and the presence of a specific population of leukocyte may not necessarily correlate with the temporal evolution of the inflammatory response.

The resolution of pulmonary inflammation is determined by whether the inciting factor(s) persists. For example, the host's response to a bacterial challenge of *Streptococcus pneumoniae* is associated with an exuberant inflammatory reaction characterized by tissue injury, deposition of fibrin, extravasation of neutrophils and elimination of the offending bacteria, leading to resolution of inflammation and re-establishment of normal lung function. In contrast, chronic lung inflammation, such as idiopathic pulmonary fibrosis (IPF), is manifested by a neutrophilic alveolitis and an intense interstitial mononuclear leukocyte infiltration that is associated with tissue destruction, fibroproliferation and exaggerated extracellular matrix production and deposition. This type of inflammation often fails to resolve and ultimately progresses to end-stage pulmonary fibrosis. While the specific molecular mechanisms that either induce an acute inflammatory reaction or perpetuate chronic inflammation have not been fully elucidated, it is now clear that leukocytes, stroma and parencyhmal cells produce a variety of molecules that regulate leukocyte recruitment during inflammation.

Chemokines in Disease, edited by Alisa E. Koch and Robert M. Strieter.
© 1996 R.G. Landes Company.

The recruitment of specific leukocyte subpopulations in response to injury is a fundamental mechanism of inflammation. The elicitation of leukocytes is dependent upon a complex series of events, including endothelial cell activation and expression of endothelial cell-derived leukocyte adhesion molecules, leukocyte-endothelial cell adhesion, leukocyte activation and expression of leukocyte-derived adhesion molecules, leukocyte transendothelial migration and leukocyte migration beyond the endothelial barrier along established chemotactic gradients. While the events of leukocyte extravasation may appear intuitive, it has taken over 150 years of research to elucidate the molecular and cellular steps involved in the process of leukocyte migration.

Historically, the first observations of leukocyte migration date back to the initial observation of leukocyte adherence followed by transendothelial migration by Augustus Waller in 1846, who described extravasation of leukocytes in a frog tongue.[1] This observation was followed by the first description of leukocyte migration in response to chemotactic signals, reported in the late nineteenth century.[2] These studies demonstrated that leukocytes migrated in response to either products of other leukocytes or killed bacteria. Although these studies were descriptive in nature, they were the first to establish leukocyte extravasation in response to a chemotactic signal.

The development of a chemotactic chamber in 1962 by Boyden was a historical event that allowed the quantitative analysis of leukocyte migration in vitro.[3] This chamber separated leukocytes from a specific chemotactic signal by an interposing filter. Leukocytes that had migrated in response to a specific chemotactic stimulus could then be microscopically quantitated by counting leukocytes at either the "leading front" or adhering to the under surface of the filter. While molecules may in vivo behave as leukocyte chemotaxins, the use of these chambers allowed the assessment in vitro of whether a molecule be-

haves as a direct or indirect leukocyte chemotaxin. Moreover, by modifying this technique, Zigmond and Hirsch could distinguish chemotaxis, a process of leukocyte migration in response to a concentration gradient, from chemokinesis, a property of random leukocyte motion.[4] In the late 1960s, investigators identified the first chemotactic molecules.[5-7] These studies demonstrated that N-formylmethionyl peptides from bacterial cell walls and the anaphylatoxin, C5a, were chemotactic for leukocytes. These findings were followed by the discovery that specific products of arachidonate metabolism were leukocyte chemotaxins. Both platelet activating factor (PAF) and leukotriene B_4 (LTB4) were shown to have significant chemotactic activity for leukocytes at pM to nM concentrations.[8,9] These findings supported the premise that leukocyte recruitment is critical to host defense, and that a number of factors that possess potent and overlapping leukocyte chemotactic activity are necessary to assure continued leukocyte emigration at sites of inflammation (Table 1.1).

While the above leukocyte chemotaxins are important in leukocyte extravasation, they appear to lack specificity for particular subsets of leukocytes. The nonspecificity of these chemotactic factors for subsets of leukocytes is interesting, however, it is apparent that the nature of the stimulus, and the subsequent spectrum of chemotactic factors produced, determines the subpopulation of leukocytes elicited during an

---

Table 1.1. Chemotactic factors

Lipids
　　Leukotriene B_4 (LTB$_4$)
　　Platelet-activating factor (PAF)

Peptides
　　Formylmethionylleucylphenylalanine (fMLP)

Polypeptides
　　Anaphylatoxin C5a
　　Platelet-derived growth factor (PDGF)
　　Fibronectin
　　Collagen fragments
　　Transforming growth factor-beta (TGFβ)

inflammatory response. For example, during neutrophil extravasation associated with acute lung injury, neutrophil chemotaxins predominate over other leukocyte chemotactic factors. In contrast, a different set of leukocyte chemotaxins predominate when a specific antigenic stimulus in the lung leads to cell-mediated immunity, resulting in the production of chemotactic factors that recruit exclusively mononuclear cells leading to granulomatous inflammation. Thus, a diversity of chemotactic factors must exist with specific activity to target subsets of leukocytes and maintain leukocyte migration. Recent advances in understanding leukocyte chemotaxis have revealed two supergene families of chemotactic cytokines, and a consensus group has termed these cytokines the C-X-C and C-C chemokines.[10] These two families have been shown to display unique and specific chemotactic activity for subsets of leukocytes. The purpose of this chapter will provide an overview of the C-X-C chemokine family, whereas in chapter 2 the C-C chemokine family will be reviewed.

THE C-X-C (α) CHEMOKINE FAMILY

ISOLATION OF NEUTROPHIL CHEMOTACTIC ACTIVITY ATTRIBUTABLE TO A NOVEL CYTOKINE FAMILY

A variety of biologically active agents have been proven to elicit a neutrophil chemotactic response, both in vitro and in vivo. For example, the intradermal injection of lipopolysaccharide (LPS) has been shown to cause a local extravasation of neutrophils,[11] whereas systemically administered LPS results in sequestration and activation of neutrophils within the microvasculature and extravascular compartments of the lungs. This latter effect of LPS rapidly peaks within one hour and persists more than 16 hours poststimulation.[12] Interestingly, LPS does not have a direct effect in mediating neutrophil chemotaxis.[13,14] This suggests that LPS must induce neutrophil recruitment indirectly through the genera-

tion of factors that directly act on neutrophils leading to chemotaxis and activation. Although LPS-induced tumor necrosis factor α (TNF) and interleukin-1 (IL-1) were initially felt to be significant monocyte-derived neutrophil chemotactic factors,[15-20] subsequent investigations, using both in vitro or in vivo models of neutrophil elicitation, have shown that recombinant forms of these cytokines lack direct chemotactic activity for neutrophils.[14,21] Confusion in this area was greatly clarified by the isolation, purification, cloning and expression of a novel group of neutrophil chemotactic and activating factors, the C-X-C chemokine family.[22-28]

INTRODUCTION TO THE C-X-C CHEMOKINE FAMILY

The human C-X-C chemokine family of chemotactic cytokines are polypeptide molecules that appear, in general, to have proinflammatory activities.[22-28] These cytokines in their monomeric forms range from 7-10 kDa and are characteristically basic heparin-binding proteins. This family displays four highly conserved cysteine amino acid residues, with the first two cysteines separated by one nonconserved amino acid residue, the C-X-C cysteine motif (Table 1.2). In general, these cytokines appear to have specific chemotactic activity for neutrophils. Because of their *chemo*tactic properties and the presence of the C-X-C cysteine motif, these cyto*kines* have

---

Table 1.2. The C-X-C chemokines

Interleukin-8 (IL-8)
Epithelial neutrophil activating protein-78 (ENA-78)
Growth-related oncogene alpha (GROα)
Growth-related oncogene beta (GROβ)
Growth-related oncogene gamma (GROγ)
Granulocyte chemotactic protein-2 (GCP-2)
Platelet basic protein (PBP)
Connective tissue activating protein-III (CTAP-III)
    Beta-thromboglobulin (βTG)
    Neutrophil activating protein-2 (NAP-2)
Platelet factor-4 (PF4)
Interferon-γ-inducible protein (IP-10)
Monokine induced by interferon-γ (MIG)

been designated the C-X-C chemokine family. Interestingly, these chemokines are all clustered on human chromosome 4 (q12-q21), and exhibit between 20-50% homology on the amino acid level.[22-28] Over the last 2 decades, several C-X-C chemokines have been identified and include platelet factor-4 (PF4), NH_2-terminal truncated forms of platelet basic protein [PBP; connective tissue activating protein-III (CTAP-III), β-thromboglobulin (βTG) and neutrophil activating protein-2 (NAP-2)], interleukin-8 (IL-8), growth-related oncogene (GROα, GROβ, GROγ), interferon-γ-inducible protein (IP-10), monokine induced by interferon-γ (MIG), epithelial neutrophil activating protein-78 (ENA-78) and granulocyte chemotactic protein-2 (GCP-2).[22-31] The murine homologues to the human C-X-C chemokine family include KC, macrophage inflammatory protein-2 (MIP-2), crg-2 and MIG, and are structurally homologous to human GROα, GROβ and GROγ, IP-10, and MIG, respectively.[22-28] No murine or rat structural homologue exists for human IL-8.[22-28] The NH_2-terminal truncated forms of PBP are generated when PBP is released from platelet α-granules and undergoes proteolytic cleavage by monocyte-derived proteases.[32] PF4, the first member of the C-X-C chemokine family to be described, was originally identified for its ability to bind heparin, leading to inactivation of heparin's anticoagulation function.[33] Both IP-10 and MIG are interferon-inducible C-X-C chemokines.[29,34] Although IP-10 appears to be induced by all three interferons (IFN-α, IFN-β and IFN-γ), MIG is unique in that it appears to be expressed only in the presence of IFN-γ.[29] While IFNs induce the production of IP-10 and MIG, these cytokines have been found to attenuate the expression of both IL-8, GROα and ENA-78.[35-39] These findings would suggest that members of the C-X-C chemokine family demonstrate disparate regulation in the presence of IFNs. GROα, GROβ and GROγ are closely related C-X-C chemokines, with GROα originally described for its melanoma growth stimulatory activity.[40-42] IL-8,

ENA-78 and GCP-2 were all initially identified on the basis of their ability to induce neutrophil activation and chemotaxis.[22-28] IL-8 and other C-X-C chemokines have been found to be produced by an array of cells including monocytes, alveolar macrophages, neutrophils, platelets, eosinophils, mast cells, T lymphocytes, natural killer cells (NK cells), keratinocytes, mesangial cells, epithelial cells, hepatocytes, fibroblasts, smooth muscle cells, mesothelial cells and endothelial cells (Fig. 1.1). These cells can produce chemokines in response to a variety of factors, including viruses, bacterial products, IL-1, TNF, C5a, LTB4 and IFNs.[21-28,43-78] The production of C-X-C chemokines by both immune and nonimmune cells within tissue supports the contention that these cytokines may play a pivotal role in orchestrating inflammation.

GENOMIC STRUCTURE, GENE REGULATION AND mRNA TRANSCRIPTS OF THE C-X-C CHEMOKINES

The genes for PF4, PBP, IL-8, GROα, GROβ, GROγ, IP-10 and ENA-78 are clustered on human chromosome 4, q12-21.[41,79-88] While the genes for IL-8, GROα, GROβ, GROγ, IP-10 and ENA-78 have four exons and three introns, PF4 and PBP have three exons and two introns. The first and second introns of all the genes of this chemokine family are highly conserved. The clustering and similarity of the exons and introns of this superfamily suggests that they may have diverged from a common ancestral gene. The 5'-flanking region of IL-8 contains the usual "CCAAT" and "TATA" box-like structures, and in addition, this region has a number of potential binding sites for several nuclear factors.[81,89] The putative essential transcription regulatory elements of the IL-8 promoter binding sites are shown in Table 1.3. The octamer binding sites are dispensable for IL-8 gene activation, whereas the combination of nuclear factor (NF)-κB (p65/RelA) and AP-1 or NF-κB (p65/RelA) and NF-IL-6/cis-regulatory enhancer binding

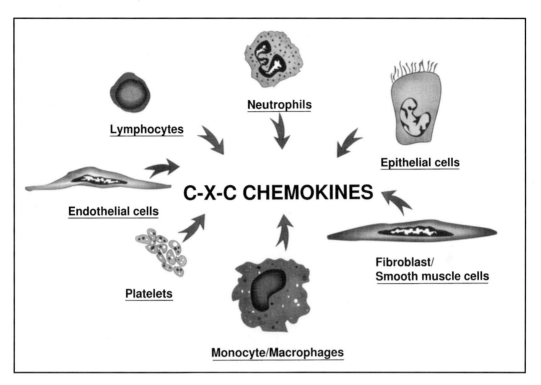

Fig. 1.1. C-X-C chemokines are produced by a variety of cells that include neutrophils, epithelial cells, fibroblasts, smooth muscle cells, monocytes, macrophages, platelets, endothelial cells and lymphocytes.

protein (C/EBPβ) binding results in IL-8 gene transcription in a variety of cells in response to PMA, hepatitis virus X protein, IL-1 and TNF.[89] However, NF-κB (p65/RelA) binding appears to be essential to IL-8 gene expression.[89,90] The NF-IL-6/C/EBPβ and NF-κB (p65/RelA) binding sites are located between nucleotide -94 and -71 of the IL-8 promoter.[89] Kunsch and colleagues, recently examined the functional interaction of these two transcriptional families in the regulation of the expression of the IL-8 gene and found synergistic transcriptional activation of the IL-8 gene.[90] Their studies demonstrated the following: (a) that maximal inducible gene expression of IL-8 was achieved when both NF-IL-6/C/EBPβ and NF-κB (p65/RelA) binding sites were occupied; (b) NF-IL-6/C/EBPβ and NF-κB (p65/RelA) can bind independently to each of their binding sites within the IL-8 promoter; (c) NF-IL-6/C/EBPβ and NF-κB (p65/RelA) binding is cooperative and results in a synergistic ac-

tivation of IL-8 gene transcription, and separation of these two binding motifs by only ten nucleotides completely attenuates the transcriptional response and (d) the NF-κB (p65/RelA) cytosolic inhibitor, IκB, molecule is an important regulator of IL-8 transcriptional activity. These findings were important in delineating the cooperative interaction of the two families of transcriptional factors in the regulation of the IL-8 promoter. While the IL-8 promoter may require both transcriptional binding sites to be occupied for maximal gene expression in response to either IL-1 or TNF, recent studies using deletion mutations of the promoter region of the ENA-78 gene have found that only the NF-κB element is necessary for transcriptional activity.[87] These findings support the notion that not all members of the C-X-C chemokine family require cooperative binding of both NF-IL-6/(C/EBPβ) and NF-κB (p65/RelA), and that NF-κB (p65/RelA) binding alone may be an essential element for transcriptional

Table 1.3. Transcriptional regulatory elements on the IL-8 gene

AP-1
Octamer binding proteins
†NF-κB (p65/RelA)
†NK-IL-6/C/EBPβ

†Denotes binding motifs that are essential to gene activation.

activation of C-X-C chemokine genes.

The C-X-C chemokine family genes encode cDNAs that are characterized by a short 5'-untranslated region (UTR), an open reading frame (ORF) that encodes both the mature polypeptide and the amino terminal signal sequence, and a long 3'-UTR that contains variable numbers of "AUUUA" motifs that are common to a variety of inflammatory cytokines and that have been demonstrated to play a significant role in mRNA stabilization and translational regulation.[25-28,91,92] For example, the identified cDNA for IL-8 is 1.6 kB consisting of a 101-base 5'-UTR, a 297-base coding region that encodes a 99 amino acid polypeptide with a NH_2-terminus having a high degree of hydrophobicity, consistent with a typical signal peptide sequence,[92] and a 1.2 kB 3'-UTR with one region of the TATTTATT motif common to several inflammatory cytokines.[44,93]

PROTEIN STRUCTURE OF THE C-X-C CHEMOKINES

The primary structure of the C-X-C chemokine family is analogous to IL-8. The precursor molecule of IL-8 consists of 99 amino acids with an associated 20 amino acid signal sequence. Several mature forms of IL-8 have been identified that are a result of repeated NH_2-terminal amino acid cleavage.[94,95] One of these NH_2-terminal truncations results in the cleavage of the 20 amino acid residue signal peptide (79 amino acid form), while the remainder of the various NH_2-terminal truncated forms of IL-8 (77-, 72-, 71-, 70- and 69-amino acid

forms) are due to proteolytic cleavage, including the major 72 amino acid mature form.[94] The NH_2-terminus of IL-8, similar to other C-X-C chemokines that bind and activate neutrophils (see below), contain three highly conserved amino acid residues consisting of Glu-Leu-Arg (the ELR motif).[22-28,95] IL-8 is a cationic protein (isoelectric focusing point of pH 8.5) that contains fourteen basic amino acids, such as lysine and arginine. The four cysteine amino acid residues are important for the formation of the disulfide bridges. The COOH-terminus of IL-8 contains the heparin binding domain, consisting of Lys-Phe-Leu-Lys-Arg, that may be important in binding to glycosaminoglycan constituents of the extracellular matrix.[22-28,95,96]

The delineation of the three-dimensional structures of proteins is important to resolve the structure/function relationships that may result in receptor-ligand interaction. Of the C-X-C chemokine family, only the three-dimensional structures of IL-8 and PF4 have been studied by either nuclear magnetic resonance (NMR) or X-ray crystallography.[97-101] The tertiary structure of the IL-8 monomer comprises a COOH-terminus α-helix that lies on top of a three-stranded antiparallel β-sheet arranged in a Greek key.[97-99] The NH_2-terminus containing the ELR motif comprises an irregular strand and a series of turns which enters the first β-sheet strand.[97-99] In solution at high concentrations, IL-8 forms homodimers. The solution structure of the IL-8 quaternary structure (dimer) reveals two symmetrically positioned antiparallel α-helices, lying on top of a six-stranded antiparallel β-sheet platform derived from two three-stranded Greek keys of each of the monomer units. The dimer interface is stabilized by hydrogen bonds between the strands of the β-sheets of each of the monomers.[97-99] The final structure of the IL-8 dimer is globular in shape with the dimensions of 40x42x32 Å.[99] This structural motif is similar to that of the α1/α2 domains of the human class I histocompatibility antigen HLA-A2.[97-99] Furthermore, the comparison of IL-8 quaternary structure by

NMR and X-ray crystallography has demonstrated that the NH_2-terminus of the molecule can undergo conformational transitions in relation to the central loop of the β-strands.[98] This finding suggests that the NH_2-terminus has the potential to change conformations that may have structure/function significance in receptor/ligand interactions.

THE PHYSICOCHEMICAL CHARACTERISTICS OF THE C-X-C CHEMOKINE FAMILY

An ideal neutrophil chemotactic factor is one that demonstrates longevity at the site of inflammation. IL-8, the most studied member of the C-X-C chemokine family, appears to have physicochemical characteristics necessary to allow it to persist in the presence of various proteolytic agents. IL-8 resists proteolysis and denaturation in the presence of either trypsin or chymotrypsin. IL-8 incubated in the presence of either of these proteases for 4 hours has been found to maintain greater than 80% of its bioactivity for the release of neutrophil elastase, whereas IL-8 incubated in the presence of proteinase K for 12 hours loses all of its biological activity.[102] IL-8 is inactivated slowly in response to either cathepsin G, neutrophil elastase or proteinase-3, with half-lives of 2, 4 and 17 hours, respectively. In contrast, NAP-2 and GROα exposed to proteinase-3 have half-lives of 0.2 and 2 hours, respectively.[103] While these studies demonstrated that IL-8 biological activity was relatively resistant to proteolytic degradation, other investigations have shown that physiologically relevant proteases may lead to IL-8 NH_2-terminal truncation and enhanced biological activity for neutrophils.[95,103] Thrombin and plasmin are found to convert IL-8 from the 77 to the 72 amino acid form, whereas urokinase and tissue-type plasminogen activator are unable to induce NH_2-terminus truncation.[95] Moreover, IL-8 incubated in the presence of neutrophil granule lysates and purified proteinase-3 is found to undergo significant conversion from the 77 to 72 amino acid forms of the molecule.[103] The

72 amino acid form of IL-8 binds to neutrophils 2-fold more than the 77 amino acid form, and is 2- to 3-fold more potent in inducing cytochalasin B-treated neutrophil degranulation.[95] Similar studies have been performed examining the NH_2-terminal truncations of ENA-78.[104] ENA-78 incubated with cathepsin G or chymotrypsin for 1-2 hours results in a 3- to 4-fold increase in neutrophil elastase release.[104] The NH_2-terminal truncation of ENA-78 results in a molecule that displays a similar potency to IL-8 for the release of neutrophil elastase.

In the presence of 0.5% SDS, extremes of temperature, pH, 2M lithium chloride, 6M guanidinium chloride and 1% 2-mercaptoethanol, IL-8 is able to maintain 100%, 80%, 75%, 65% and 30% of its neutrophil elastase releasing activity respectively.[102] These conditions suggest that the disulfide bonds of the IL-8 molecule are highly susceptible to reducing agents such as 2-mercaptoethanol, leading to unfolding and inactivation of this chemokine. Moreover, when refolding of the molecule is prevented by alkylation of the exposed cysteine amino acid residues, the molecule is more susceptible to proteolytic degradation, suggesting that the tertiary structure of the molecule is resistant to proteases.[103] In contrast to C5a, that is rapidly inactivated to its des-arg form in the presence of serum/plasma peptidases, IL-8 incubated in the presence of serum can maintain 100% of its activity.[102] Thus the endogenous production of IL-8 and its persistence within an inflammatory milieu may have a significant role in perpetuating neutrophil recruitment and activation necessary to maintain a neutrophil predominant inflammatory response.

PUTATIVE RECEPTOR BINDING DOMAINS OF THE C-X-C CHEMOKINES

The α-helical domain of the IL-8 molecule was originally felt to be important for IL-8 neutrophil binding.[105] However, several studies have now demonstrated that the NH_2-terminus of a majority of the C-X-C chemokine molecules play a significant role in their ability to bind to neutrophils. The evidence, by NMR and X-ray crystallography, that the NH_2-terminus of IL-8 can undergo conformational transitions by pointing away from the core of the protein, and not participate with any intramolecular hydrogen bonds or salt bridges, suggests that this domain may have structure/function significance.[98] In addition, a number of studies either performing scanning mutagenesis or using synthetic analogs of NH_2- or COOH-terminal truncations of the IL-8 molecule have determined that the ELR motif that immediately precedes the first cysteine amino acid residue at the NH_2-terminus is critical for the ability of these chemokines to bind to neutrophils. Hébert and colleagues performed scanning mutagenesis of the IL-8 molecule and systematically replaced charged amino acids with the amino acid alanine.[106] The mutants were compared to wild type IL-8 for their ability to induce a rise in cytosolic free Ca^{2+} in neutrophils.[106] In initial experiments, 11 of the 12 mutants induced a rise in cytosolic free Ca^{2+}, whereas one of the mutants with alanine placed at positions Lys3, Glu4 and Arg6 was inactive. This latter finding lead to further characterization of the NH_2-terminal domain. In a second series of mutations that systematically mutated residues 1-15 with alanine, mutants that replaced Glu4, Leu5 and Arg6 with alanine were all inactive for inducing a rise in cytosolic free Ca^{2+} and in binding assays with neutrophils. The mutation of Glu4, Leu5 or Arg6 to alanine resulted in a 100-, 100- and 1000-fold reduction in neutrophil binding, respectively, suggesting that the highly conserved Arg6 amino acid residue was extremely important in receptor/ligand interaction.

In a similar manner, Clark-Lewis and associates used chemically synthesized analogs of IL-8, as compared to the full-length 72 amino acid synthetic IL-8, to study their ability to stimulate neutrophil elastase release, neutrophil chemotaxis and competitive binding to neutrophils.[107] These investigators found an important dissociation of chemotaxis and exocytosis within the NH_2-terminus. The IL-8 amino acid residue, 5-72 analog, as compared to the full-length IL-8[1-72] molecule, was 80-fold less potent for inducing release of neutrophil elastase, yet equipotent for stimulating neutrophil chemotaxis.[107] IL-8, amino acid residues 6-72, was completely inactive in both assays, but retained detectable receptor binding. In addition, these studies suggested that analogs shortened at the COOH-terminus resulted in reduced potency in neutrophil binding; however, synthetic analogs with the entire COOH-terminal α-helix and β turn missing were still active in neutrophil binding. These studies supported the notion that the Glu4, Leu5 and Arg6 are directly involved in receptor binding, but that the COOH-terminal α helix is important for stabilizing the three-dimensional structure of the molecule. To further support that the ELR motif of the C-X-C chemokines is essential for receptor binding and activation of neutrophils, this same group of investigators replaced the DLQ (Asp-Leu-Gln) of PF4 with the ELR motif at the NH_2-terminus and found that the modified molecule was potent for the stimulation of neutrophil elastase release and chemotaxis.[108] The presence of the ELR motif increased the potency of PF4 by 100- to 1000-fold for neutrophil activation.[108] While these studies suggested that the ELR motif was important for neutrophil binding and activation, studies replacing the TVR (Thr-Val-Arg) of IP-10 or the corresponding positions on monocyte chemoattractant protein-1 (MCP-1) with the ELR motif failed to induce neutrophil binding and activation.[108] However, although IP-10 lacks neutrophil activity and fails to competively inhibit IL-8 binding to neutrophils, when the ELR motif and Gly31 and Pro32 are introduced into IP-10, IP-10 can be converted to a neutrophil activating molecule.[109] These findings suggested that the ELR motif is necessary but not entirely sufficient to dictate neutrophil binding and activation.

Although the above studies support the contention that the ELR motif within the NH_2-terminus of C-X-C chemokines is critical for receptor binding and activation, the role of the heparin-binding domain in the COOH-terminus of these molecules may play an important role in enhancing neutrophil responses to IL-8.[110] The combination of IL-8 and heparan sulfate results in both a significant rise in cytosolic free Ca^{2+} and 4-fold increase in neutrophil chemotaxis, as compared to IL-8 alone.[110] Interestingly, heparin in combination with IL-8 enhances its ability to induce a rise in cytosolic free Ca^{2+}, but not in neutrophil chemotaxis. The affect of these glycosaminoglycans on IL-8 activity is specific, as neither heparan sulfate nor heparin alters the affect of fMLP induced neutrophil activation. These findings together with the importance of the ELR motif in neutrophil binding and activation supports the notion that both the NH_2- and COOH-terminal domains of the C-X-C chemokines interplay in a cooperative fashion to optimize their ability to mediate neutrophil activation and chemotaxis.

C-X-C Chemokine Receptors

The binding of C-X-C chemokines to neutrophils followed by activation is dependent upon its ability to bind to specific cell-surface receptors. While IL-8 activation of neutrophils is similar to the classical neutrophil agonists, fMLP, PAF, C5a or LTB4, it appears that IL-8 must interact with its own specific receptor. This was originally substantiated when IL-8 was found to induce cytosolic free Ca^{2+} that underwent desensitization with repeated IL-8 stimulation.[102] Moreover, IL-8 was able to induce cytosolic free Ca^{2+} in the presence of either fMLP, LTB4, PAF, C5a, PF4 or IP-10,[109,112] suggesting that IL-8 binding results in specific signal coupling and neutrophil activation without evidence for heterologous crossdesensitization with other classical neutrophil agonists or members of the C-X-C chemokine family that do not activate neutrophils.[111,112] Specific binding of radiolabeled IL-8 to neutrophils by Scatchard analysis demonstrated that neutrophils exhibited a single class of high-affinity receptors with Kd between

0.2-4 nM and between 20,000-90,000 binding sites per cell.[113] However, Moser and colleagues demonstrated that increasing concentrations of unlabeled NAP-2 or GROα could competitively inhibit ^{125}I-IL-8 binding to neutrophils.[114] This observation supported the notion of the existence of two classes of IL-8 receptors, 70% of which bind NAP-2 or GROα with high-affinity and a Kd of approximately 0.3 nM, while the remaining 30% bind these two chemokines with low-affinity (Kd = 100-130 nM). However, IL-8 appeared to specifically bind both of the receptors with equivalent affinities.[114] Subsequent desensitization analysis by examination of cytosolic free Ca^{2+}, demonstrated that IL-8 pretreatment resulted in crossdesensitization to a challenge with either NAP-2 or GROα, whereas, pretreatment with either NAP-2 or GROα resulted in only a partial desensitization to a subsequent challenge with IL-8.[114] The regulation of the IL-8 receptor appears to be under its own influence. When neutrophils are exposed to ^{125}I-IL-8, 90% of IL-8 receptor expression is reduced within 10 minutes.[115] The downregulation of the IL-8 receptor is associated with internalization of the ligand with evidence of proteolytic degradation and evidence of trichloroacetic acid-soluble molecules in the supernatants within 60 minutes after challenge with ^{125}I-IL-8. The proteolytic degradation of the IL-8 ligand appears to be due to lysosomal enzymes, as lysosomotropic agents inhibited the ^{125}I-IL-8 degradation.[115] Although receptor expression appears to be under regulation by its own ligand, the removal of excess free IL-8 in the culture media, even in the presence of a protein synthesis inhibitor (cycloheximide), results in a rapid (within 10 minutes) re-expression of cell-surface receptors for IL-8.[115] These findings suggest that the IL-8 receptors can be recycled and dynamically regulated by their ligand.

The functional binding studies predicted two classes of high-affinity IL-8 receptors on neutrophils however, the two IL-8 receptors cloned in 1991; demonstrated that one was of high-affinity and the other was of low-affinity for IL-8. Holmes and colleagues cloned an IL-8 receptor from human neutrophils that structurally and functionally resembled the superfamily of heptahelical, rhodopsin-like, guanine nucleotide binding protein-coupled (G proteins) receptors.[116] This receptor is 29% homologous on the amino acid level with the fMLP and C5a receptors, which are also known to belong to this superfamily and are G protein signal coupled.[116] When the cDNA of this receptor was transfected into mammalian cells, it demonstrated high-affinity binding of IL-8 that corresponded with a rise in cytosolic free Ca^{2+}. This receptor is now known as IL-8RA. In other studies, Murphy and Tiffany cloned a second IL-8 receptor (p2).[117] This receptor is 77% homologous on the amino acid level with IL-8RA, and is also a member of the rhodopsin superfamily of heptahelical, G protein-coupled receptors.[117] However, when this receptor cDNA was expressed in oocytes from *Xenopus laevis*, IL-8 binding is of low-affinity, with an EC_{50} of 20 nM.[117] This receptor is now known as IL-8RB. While these initial findings were confusing, the disparity of the two cloned IL-8 receptors with the original binding studies was clarified with the finding that the two IL-8 receptors were, in fact, two high-affinity receptors for IL-8.[118] Lee and associates subsequently expressed both the IL-8RA and IL-8RB receptors in mammalian cells, and found IL-8 binding to both receptors was of high-affinity, with a Kd of 2 nM.[118] However, GROα binding to IL-8RA was of low-affinity with a Kd of 450 nM, whereas GROα binding to IL-8RB was of high-affinity with a Kd of 2 nM.[118] Functional analysis demonstrated that IL-8 binding to IL-8RA results in a rise of cytosolic free Ca^{2+}, whereas, GROα binding to this receptor fails to induce a Ca^{2+} flux.[118] In contrast, both IL-8 and GROα binding to the IL-8RB receptor resulted in a similar rise in cytosolic free Ca^{2+}.[118] This finding was not unique for GROα, and has been demonstrated using a strategy of crossdesensitization with NAP-2, GROβ,

GROγ and ENA-78, all C-X-C chemokines with the ELR motif.[28,31]

The IL-8RA and IL-8RB receptor genes are found on human chromosome 2 (q34-q35), and may have arisen from duplication of a common ancestral gene.[119] The 5'-UTR of IL-8RA is on 2 exons, whereas 7 distinct mRNAs are found in neutrophils from alternatively spliced 11 exons of the IL-8RB 5'-UTR.[120-123] The ORF of both receptor genes resides on one exon. The mRNA transcripts for IL-8RA and IL-8RB are predominately 2.0 and 2.4 kB and 3.2 and 2.8 kB, respectively in human neutrophils.[120-123] The IL-8RA transcript encodes a 350 amino acid protein with five potential N-linked glycosylation sites, whereas the IL-8RB is 355 amino acids in length, with one potential N-linked glycosylation site. Both of these receptors are characterized by the seven hydrophobic transmembrane spanning stretches characteristic of the rhodopsin superfamily.[120-123] The extracellular NH_2-terminus of both receptors is formed by a number of acidic amino acid residues that are followed by the highly conserved hydrophobic seven transmembrane stretch of the molecule.[120-123] The intracellular COOH-terminus of these receptors is thought to be highly conserved and comprised of a number of serine and threonine amino acid residues that may be important in phosphorylation and signal coupling via G proteins.[120-123]

A number of studies have determined that the NH_2-terminus of these receptors is essential for binding of C-X-C chemokines.[124,125] While the NH_2-terminus, and its predominately acidic amino acid structure, may explain the promiscuous nature of the IL-8RB receptor and interaction with the basic NH_2-terminus (ELR motif) of the C-X-C chemokines, this structure neither accounts for the specificity of the IL-8RA receptor for IL-8 nor other ELR containing C-X-C chemokines. This issue has been resolved with the finding that other domains in the IL-8RA receptor may be essential for IL-8 binding. Recently, Hébert and associates have performed scanning mutagenesis of the IL-8RA receptor by replacing charged amino acids with alanine.[126] They found that the NH_2-terminal amino acid residue (Asp11) and Glu275 and Arg280 of the third extracellular loop of the receptor are critical in ligand binding. These amino acid residues are brought into close proximity by the formation of a disulfide bridge between Cys30 and Cys277. In subsequent studies this group performed complete scanning mutagenesis of the extracellular domain of IL-8RA, and demonstrated, in addition to the importance of the extracellular cysteines, that Arg199, Arg203 and Asp265 were also critical to binding of IL-8.[127] These charged amino acid residues in the IL-8 receptor interact with oppositely charged amino acid counterparts on IL-8, leading to specific and high-affinity binding of IL-8 to IL-8RA. As noted above, this interaction may depend upon the cooperative interaction of both the ELR motif in the NH_2-terminus and amino acid groups in the COOH-terminus of the IL-8 molecule.

The IL-8RA and IL-8RB have been the most studied of the C-X-C chemokine receptors due to their importance in neutrophil activation. However, two other receptors have been identified that bind C-X-C chemokines.[120-123] While viruses often exploit the host's intracellular machinery in order to replicate and survive, recent investigations have identified that viruses may modify the host's immune response by encoding polypeptides that retain both structure and function of various cytokine receptors. For example, the Herpesvirus family encode proteins that resemble the extracellular and binding domains of TNF, IL-1 and IFN-γ. This mimicry may potentially aid the virus in the subversion of the host's immune response.[128,129] Recently another member of the Herpesvirus family has been demonstrated to encode a gene that mimics the C-X-C chemokine IL-8RB receptor.[130] Herpesvirus saimiri's (HVS) natural host is the squirrel monkey; however, in other nonhuman primate hosts this virus has been associated with the cause of fatal lymphomas and leukemias, and can

cause in vitro transformation of human T lymphocytes.[121] Recently Ahuja and Murphy have found that HVS contains a gene, ECRF3, that encodes a putative seven transmembrane domain receptor has significant homology to IL-8RB.[130] This receptor is a functional and specific receptor for the C-X-C chemokines. Moreover, the expression of this receptor, leading to functional binding and signal coupling, may explain a potential role of C-X-C chemokines in mediating the pathogenesis associated with the infection of this virus.

While the IL-8RA and IL-8RB receptors have been demonstrated to have functional activity with ligand binding, another chemokine receptor has been identified that apparently binds chemokines without a subsequent signal coupling event. This receptor was originally found on human erythrocytes and felt to represent a "sink" for interleukin-8.[131] These studies demonstrated that when IL-8 is added to whole blood it rapidly partitions from plasma to the surface of erythrocytes.[131] In addition, they found that ^{125}I-IL-8 binding was specific and of high-affinity on erythrocytes, with a Kd of 5 nM. Two thousand binding sites per red blood cell were found, which represented the potential of one liter of blood to carry 15 nM of IL-8 binding sites.[131] Interestingly, the specific binding of IL-8 to this receptor was inhibited by monocyte chemotactic protein-1 (MCP-1), a member of the C-C chemokine family.[131] This group also determined that other members of both the C-X-C and C-C chemokine family could specifically bind to this receptor.[132] While C-X-C (IL-8, NAP-2 and GROα) and C-C [regulated on activation normal T cell expressed and secreted (RANTES) and MCP-1] appear to bind, macrophage inflammatory protein-1 α and β (MIP-1α and MIP-1β) do not bind to this receptor.[122,123,132] In addition to binding of the chemokine family, this receptor has been found to be shared by the malarial parasites *Plasmodium vivax* and *knowlesi*, and may allow their invasion into erythrocytes.[133] This has been substantiated when IL-8 was found to block the binding and invasion of human erythrocytes by *Plasmodium knowlesi*.[133] This receptor has been cloned and found to be identical to the Duffy blood group antigen, and is now referred to as the Duffy antigen multispecific chemokine receptor, and its structure demonstrates a seven transmembrane spanning receptor motif, similar to IL-8RA and IL-8RB.[122,123,134] However, functional studies of transfected IL-8RA or Duffy antigen cDNAs in human embryonic kidney cells demonstrated that cells expressing the IL-8RA, but not the Duffy antigen receptor, could result in a rise in cytosolic free Ca^{2+}.[134] While these studies suggested that the Duffy antigen multispecific chemokine receptor may only provide a binding site/sink for chemokines without signal coupling, these studies were limited to only the analysis of Ca^{2+} flux, and have not assessed potential Ca^{2+}-independent mechanisms of cellular activation. Furthermore, this receptor has been recently identified on postcapillary venule endothelial cells in kidney.[135] Further studies are required to examine the functional nature of this receptor before assigning it the sole function of a "chemokine sink" it may serve to maintain a chemotactic gradient between the vascular and extravascular compartments (Table 1.4).

While no reported studies have demonstrated a genetic abnormality in the expression of human IL-8Rs, recent studies have demonstrated functional importance of these receptors using an in vivo model of murine homologous deletion of the IL-8 receptor homolog.[136] Although these "knockout" mice appeared healthy, they displayed significant lymphadenopathy unrelated to antigenic challenge. The lymphadenopathy was due to an increase

in B cells and myelopoiesis. In addition, these mice had splenomegaly as a result of an expansion of metamyelocytes, band, and mature forms of neutrophils, and 25% of the animals demonstrated hepatic granulopoiesis in the periportal region. These findings suggested the presence of augmented extramedullary myelopoiesis. The number of circulating neutrophils in these animals was increased 12-fold, and IL-6 was found to be significantly elevated. When the animals with homologous deletion were assessed for neutrophil migration in response to intraperitoneal thioglycollate, neutrophil infiltration was reduced by 80%, as compared to litter mates. However, locomoter function of these neutrophils was not impaired, as in vitro analysis of neutrophil chemotaxis demonstrated that these cells could migrate in response to fMLP, but not to human IL-8 or functional murine homologues of IL-8.[136] Furthermore, the neutrophils from homologous deletion animals were equally efficacious to neutrophils from litter mates for killing of intracellular and extracellular bacteria. These findings suggest that C-X-C chemokine biology may be more complex than mere meditation of leukocyte recruitment.

C-X-C CHEMOKINE BIOLOGICAL ACTIVITIES ON NEUTROPHILS

Binding of IL-8 and other members of the C-X-C chemokine family to their specific receptors on neutrophils results in signal coupling similar to other classical chemotactic/activating agents.[111] This binding is coupled to *B. pertussis* toxin-sensitive G proteins followed by the activation of phosphatidylinositol 4,5-bisphosphate (PIP_2)-specific phospholipase C that leads to the generation of 2 second messenger molecules, 1,4,5-inositoltrisphosphate (IP_3) and diacylglycerol (DAG). IP_3 induces the release of Ca^{2+} from cytosolic stores resulting in the rise of cytosolic free Ca^{2+}, whereas DAG remains membrane-associated and activates protein kinase C (PKC). In addition, phosphatidic acid (PA) released from phosphatidylcholine by phospho-

---

Table 1.4. The C-X-C chemokine receptors

Interleukin-8 Receptor Type A (IL-8RA)
Interleukin-8 Receptor Type B (IL-8RB)
Herpesvirus saimiri protein receptor, ECRF3
Duffy antigen multispecific chemokine receptor

lipase D can form DAG by an alternative pathway via phosphatidic acid phospho-hydrolase, whereas DAG can form additional phosphatidic acid via DAG kinase. Alternatively, phosphatidic acid, released from phosphatidylcholine by phospholipase D, can also generate lysophosphatidic acid and arachidonate via phospholipase A_2.[137] These signal transduction events may be linked, in part, leading to the activation of neutrophils.

For example, neutrophils stimulated with either IL-8 and members of the C-X-C chemokine family that contain the ELR motif or with fMLP all will demonstrate a concentration-dependent rise in cytosolic free Ca^{2+}, change from a spherical to a polarized shape and chemotaxis, enhanced respiratory burst and exocytosis. However, if neutrophils are exposed to either pertussis toxin (an inhibitor of G protein), 17-hydroxywortmannin (an inhibitor of calcium-independent respiratory burst and of exocytosis) or staurosporine (an inhibitor of protein kinase C), they will display a significantly attenuated response to either IL-8 or fMLP.[111] This suggests that neutrophil activation is dependent upon G-binding proteins, PKC and calcium-dependent and -independent signal transduction.[111] Moreover, homologous chemotactic desensitization of neutrophils, that is, a subsequent challenge with the same ligand, is due to a PKC-dependent event. For example, a chemotactic response to IL-8 demonstrates desensitization to a subsequent challenge with IL-8, but not to fMLP. The homologous neutrophil chemotactic desensitization in response to IL-8 can be inhibited by pretreating the cells with the PKC-inhibitor (staurosporine). This effect was not due to alterations in IL-8R expression, affinity for IL-8 binding or rate of IL-8/IL-8R internalization.[138] These findings suggest that specific ligand binding leads to selective desensitization, which is PKC-dependent. However, not all signal coupling events are associated. In other studies, IL-8 or fMLP activation of neutrophils is found to result in a rapid increase in actin polymerization, formation of large cytoplasmic lamellipodia and chemotaxis.[137,139] While the affect of IL-8 and fMLP on neutrophil cytoskeleton and formation of F-actin lamellipodia can be inhibited by pertussis toxin, cells treated with specific inhibitors of PKC and calcium chelators fail to alter the cytoskeletal changes in the presence of either IL-8 or fMLP.[139] These observations support the notion of an important dissociation of G protein signal coupling and PKC and calcium signal transduction leading to neutrophil activation.

While IL-8 and other C-X-C chemokines containing the ELR motif have direct effects in neutrophil activation, it appears that they may have important indirect effects in amplifying this response through the autocrine production of additional neutrophil-derived factors, LTB4 and PAF. IL-8 in a dose-dependent manner stimulates the production and release of LTB4 and 15 HETE from neutrophils as a result of increased 5-lipoxygenase (5-LO) and 15-LO activity, respectively.[140,141] In other studies, IL-8 stimulation of neutrophils can result in the production and release of PAF that can be further augmented in the presence of granulocyte-macrophage colony-stimulating factor (GM-CSF).[142,143] Furthermore, LTB4 activation of neutrophils not only results in the generation of reactive oxygen metabolites, exocytosis and chemotaxis, but also has a direct effect on mediating the further generation of neutrophil-derived IL-8.[49,144] This supports the contention that IL-8 and other C-X-C chemokines may amplify neutrophil function through both autocrine and paracrine mechanisms of LTB4, PAF and additional IL-8 generation, leading to further stimulation and activation of neutrophils.

The ability of neutrophils to migrate to sites of inflammation is dependent not only upon the generation of chemotactic factors, but also on the coordinated expression of specific cell-surface adhesion molecules, such as leukocyte-derived L-selectin and CD11/CD18 complex. IL-8, GROα and NAP-2 can induce the expression of CD11b/CD18, CD11c/CD18 and CR1 by 3- to 10-fold, while causing shedding of L-selectin.[145,146] This expression was associated with functional adhesion and augmented phagocytosis of ligated particles.[146] The rapidity of β_2 integrin expression was correlated with the release of specific granules from neutrophils in response to these chemokines. These findings suggest that C-X-C chemokine stimulation of neutrophils can result in direct activation, direct and indirect amplification, and augmented recruitment at sites of inflammation.

C-X-C CHEMOKINE BIOLOGICAL ACTIVITIES IN OTHER LEUKOCYTE POPULATIONS

Although the majority of C-X-C chemokines have been studied in the characterization of neutrophil activation, a number of studies have clearly demonstrated that IL-8 and members of the C-X-C chemokine family influence the biology of other leukocyte populations. In basophils, IL-8, GROα, GROβ and GROγ in a dose-dependent manner induce both a rise in cytosolic Ca^{2+} and chemotaxis.[147] The order of potency was found to be IL-8 > GROα $\geq$ GROγ > GROβ. Competition binding studies using ^{125}I-IL-8 and ^{125}I-GROα revealed the existence of both IL-8RA and IL-8RB receptors on these cells.[147] While C-X-C chemokines bind and activate basophils leading to a rise in cytosolic Ca^{2+} and chemotaxis, other studies have found that IL-8 either inhibits or stimulates histamine release from basophils.[148,149] High concentrations of IL-8 (100 nM) in the presence of IL-3 induce both histamine release and production of LTB4 from basophils; however, at a 100-fold lower concentration, pretreatment with IL-8 selectively inhibited this response.[148] NAP-2, but not CTAP-III or PF4, partially inhibited either response to IL-8.[148] In similar studies, Kuna and associates using <100 nM concentration of IL-8 failed to find a direct effect of IL-8, and demonstrated that IL-8 pretreatment inhib-

ited histamine release by histamine releasing factor (HRF), which was derived from a mixture of mononuclear cells and platelets.[149] The findings of these two studies were confusing, yet suggested that the effect of IL-8 inhibition may have represented crossdesensitization, since the cells pretreated with IL-8 prior to exposure to HRF may have contained IL-8 or other members of the C-X-C chemokine family. In support of this contention, a subsequent study demonstrated that IL-8 and NAP-2 could both induce significant histamine release by IL-3 pretreated basophils.[150] In studies examining crossdesensitization of either IL-8 or NAP-2 on these cells, each chemokine partially desensitized the rise in cytosolic free Ca^{2+} in response to the other chemokine, suggesting the presence of specific IL-8R on basophils.[150] Basophil migration, similar to that of neutrophils, is also dependent upon the production of chemotactic factors such as C-X-C chemokines, and on the expression of cell-surface adhesion molecules. IL-8 has been found to enhance the binding of basophils to cytokine activated monolayers of endothelial cells, and this adhesion is inhibited by anti-CD18 and anti-CD11c antibodies.[151] These findings suggest that the C-X-C chemokines may play an important role in mediating basophil activation and migration at sites of inflammation.

In eosinophils, IL-8, C5a, PAF and fMLP induce significant rises in cytosolic free Ca^{2+}, shape change and exocytosis of eosinophil peroxidase.[152] In addition, IL-8 has been found to have chemotactic activity for eosinophils both in vitro and in vivo.[153,154] However, the potency of this response is in the following order: C5a > PAF>>>fMLP and IL-8. Pretreatment of eosinophils with pertussis toxin attenuates activation (cytosolic free Ca^{2+}, shape change and exocytosis) in response to the above agonists, suggesting the G proteins are involved in the signal coupling events. Similarly to neutrophils, a dissociation of these events can be found for shape change and exocytosis. Eosinophils exposed to either of the above agonists, in the presence of PKC inhibition (staurosporine) or absence of calcium, results in no shape change, but demonstrates a significant decline in the release of eosinophil peroxidase.[152] This supports the notion that the induction of shape change is through an alternative pathway than classical signal transduction involving phospholipase C.

In monocytes, IL-8 is not a chemotaxin; however, Walz and associates found that IL-8 and GROα, but not NAP-2, stimulation of monocytes results in a dose-dependent activation of monocytes with evidence of a rise in cytosolic free Ca^{2+} and respiratory burst.[155] These findings suggest that C-X-C chemokines may mediate the generation of reactive oxygen species at sites of inflammation by stimulation of both neutrophils and monocytes. In contrast, although IP-10 does not activate neutrophils, this C-X-C chemokine appears to display potent chemotactic activity for both monocytes and T lymphocytes, and induces T cell adhesion to endothelial cells.[156] While IL-8 has been reported to be chemotactic for T cells, its activity appears to be limited, as compared to members of the C-C chemokine family (discussed in chapter 2).[22-28] In addition, IL-8 has been found to induce locomotion in IL-2 activated natural killer cells; however, this activity was found to be related to chemokinesis rather than chemotaxis.[157] Recently, IL-8 has been found to have potential biological effects on B cells. While IL-4 can induce the production of IgE and IgG4, but not IgM, IgG1, IgG2, IgG3 or IgA by tonsillar mononuclear cells, IL-8 can selectively inhibit the IL-4-induced IgE and IgG4 production, but not the generation of the other Igs. This response could not be reversed by IL-5 or IL-6.[158] In other studies, these investigators demonstrated that IL-8 can differentially modulate IL-4- and IL-2-induced human B cell growth. IL-8 in a dose-dependent manner inhibits IL-4-induced growth in response to B cell mitogens, whereas IL-8 does not attenuate the growth of B cells in the presence of IL-2.[159] The above findings suggest that IL-8 and other members of the C-X-C chemokine family may be important factors that modulate the biology of a variety of leukocytes.

C-X-C CHEMOKINE BIOLOGICAL ACTIVITIES IN OTHER CELLS

The role of C-X-C chemokines as mediators of leukocyte activation has been extensively studied. However, it is becoming increasingly clear that C-X-C chemokines may play an important function in regulating parenchymal or stromal cell function. While IL-8 has not been examined in regulating pulmonary epithelial cell chemotaxis or proliferation, IL-8 is an important cytokine for modifying keratinocyte function. Psoriasis has been shown to have accentuated angiogenic activity and keratinocyte hyperplasia.[160] This skin disease is associated with a mononuclear cellular infiltration, and has been demonstrated to contain significant levels of IL-8 expressed within basal keratinocytes.[161-163] In addition, these studies have demonstrated immunoreactivity of IL-8 in normal skin that is predominantly located in the suprabasal keratinocytes.[162,163] Recently, several studies have provided additional insight into the potential function of IL-8 in the epidermis. Michel and associates[164] demonstrated that IL-8 is potent, in a dose-dependent fashion, for the induction of keratinocyte chemotaxis and proliferation. This effect was directly attributable to the presence of specific IL-8 receptors on keratinocytes. The keratinocyte binding studies showed that IL-8 ligand/receptor interaction was specific for the dimeric form of IL-8, and in concentrations compatible with optimal neutrophil chemotactic activity. In addition, this group has recently demonstrated elevated expression of IL-8 receptors in psoriatic lesions, as compared to normal skin.[165] Although IL-8 may have a direct effect on inducing keratinocyte chemotaxis and proliferation, recent work by Valyi-Nagy and colleagues[166] demonstrated that IL-8 stimulation could induce keratinocyte production of TGF-α without changing the expression of TGF-α receptors. These findings suggest that IL-8 directly and indirectly, via the production of TGF-α, may influence the biology of keratinocytes and perhaps other populations of epithelial cells.

IL-8 may play a significant role in regulating vascular biology, and has been identified in the context of atherosclerosis.[167] IL-8 in a dose-dependent manner has been shown to induce vascular smooth muscle cell proliferation and chemotaxis that was inhibited by prostaglandin E_2.[168,169] Recently, IL-8 has been reported to be a potent angiogenic factor.[170-172] Recombinant IL-8 mediates both endothelial cell chemotactic and proliferative activity in vitro and angiogenic activity in vivo.[170-172] In contrast, PF4 has been shown to have angiostatic properties[173] and attenuate growth of tumors in vivo.[174] While the angiostatic activity of PF4 was initially felt to be due to its heparin binding domain (COOH-terminus),[173,174] recent studies have shown that a PF4 mutant lacking both the heparin-binding domain and functional heparin binding, is equipotent to native PF4 for the attenuation of tumor growth.[175] Although it remains unclear whether the COOH-terminus of these chemokines dictates their biological role in angiogenesis, the difference in C-X-C chemokine function can also be explained by other structural domains, the ELR motif.

In further support of this contention, IP-10, a member of the C-X-C chemokine family that lacks the ELR motif, behaves as an angiostatic factor.[176,177] IP-10 in a dose-dependent manner attenuates the in vitro and in vivo angiogenic activity of both IL-8 and bFGF in bioassays of angiogenesis.[176,177] These findings support the contention that the members of the C-X-C chemokine family may exert disparate effects in mediating angiogenesis for primarily four reasons. First, members of the C-X-C chemokine family that display binding and activation of neutrophils share the same NH_2-terminal ELR motif homology that immediately precedes the first cysteine amino acid residue, whereas PF4, IP-10 and MIG lack this motif.[106-108] Second, IL-8

(contains ELR motif) is angiogenic, while PF4 and IP-10 that lack the ELR motif are angiostatic.[173-177] Third, endothelial cells have been recently identified to express IL-8 type A receptors that bind both IL-8 and NAP-2.[178] Finally, the interferons (IFN-α, IFN-β and IFN-γ) are known inhibitors of angiogenesis. While the interferons downregulate the expression of the angiogenic factor, IL-8, from monocytes,[35-37] they induce the expression of IP-10 from a number of cells, including keratinocytes, fibroblasts, endothelial cells and mononuclear phagocytes.[34] The IP-10 produced by these cells may act in an autocrine and paracrine manner as a pivotal angiostatic factor that regulates angiogenesis during wound repair, chronic inflammation and neovascularization associated with tumorigenesis. Thus, the balance in expression of C-X-C chemokines under conditions of neovascularization may be important in regulating net angiogenesis.

CONCLUSION

The discovery of the C-X-C chemokine supergene family has greatly enhanced our understanding of the biology of leukocyte recruitment. These protein mediators of inflammation play an important role during the initiation and maintenance of inflammation. They are responsible for the induction of leukocyte-derived adhesion molecules resulting in enhanced leukocyte-endothelial cell interaction, leukocyte activation and chemotaxis, and subsequent transendothelial extravasation at the site of inflammation. Furthermore, the ability of C-X-C chemokines to exert effects on nonleukocyte cell populations expands their biological role during inflammation and tissue repair.

ACKNOWLEDGMENTS

The work was supported, in part, by NIH grants, CA66180, HL50057, 1P50HL46487 (R.M.S.) and HL31693, HL31936 and HL35276 (S.L.K.). We would like to acknowledge Robin G. Kunkel for her outstanding artwork.

REFERENCES

1. Waller A. Microscopical observations on the perforation of the capillaries by the corpuscles of the blood, and on the origin of mucous and pus-globules. Philos Magazine 1846; 29:397.

2. Massart J, Bordet C. Recherches sur l'irritabilite des leucocytes et sur l'intervention de cette irritabilite dans la nutrition des cellules et dans l'inflammation. J Med Chir Pharm Brux 1890; 90:169.

3. Boyden S. The chemotactic effect of mixtures of antibody and antigens on polymorphonuclear leukocytes. J Exp Med 1962; 115:453.

4. Zigmond SH, Hirsch JG. Leukocyte locomotion and chemotaxis: New methods for evaluation and demonstration of cell-derived chemotactic factor. J Exp Med 1973; 137:387.

5. Ward PA, Newman LJ. A neutrophil chemotactic factor from human C'5. J Immunol 1969; 102:93.

6. Shin HS, Snyderman R, Friedman E et al. Chemotactic and anaphylatoxic fragment cleaved from the fifth component of guinea pig complement. Science 1968; 162:361.

7. Becker EL, Ward PA. Esterases of the polymorphonuclear leukocyte capable of hydrolyzing acetyl DL phenylalanine b-naphthylester. J Exp Med 1969; 129:569.

8. Lee TC, Snyder F. Function, metabolism and regulation of platelet activating factor and related ether lipids. In: Kuo JF, ed. Phospholipids and cellular regulation. Boca Raton: CRC Press Inc, 1985:1-39.

9. Ford-Hutchinson AW, Bray MA, Doig MV et al. Leukotriene B4, a potent chemotactic and aggregating substance released from polymorphonuclear leukocytes. Nature 1980; 286:264-65.

10. Lindley IJ, Westwick J, Kunkel SL. Nomenclature announcement-the chemokines. Immunol Today 1993; 14:24.

11. Issekutag A, Bhimji S. Role for endotoxin in the leukocyte infiltration accompanying E. coli inflammation. Infect Immun 1982; 36:588-96.

12. Remick DG, Strieter RM, Eskandari MK et al. Role of tumor necrosis factor-α in lipopolysaccharide-induced pathologic alter-ations. Am J Pathol 1990; 136:49-60.

13. Cybulsky MI, Chan MKW, Movat HZ. Acute inflammation and microthrombosis induced by endotoxin, interleukin-1, and tumor necrosis factor and their implication in gram-negative infection. Lab Invest 1988; 58:365-78.

14. Cybulsky MI, McComb DJ, Movat HZ. Protein synthesis dependent mechanisms of neutrophil emigration: different mechanisms of inflammation in rabbits induced by interleukin-1, tumor necrosis factor alpha or endotoxin verses leukocyte chemoattractants. Am J Pathol 1989; 135:227-37.

15. Le J, Vilcek J. Tumor necrosis factor and interleukin-1: cytokines with multiple overlapping biological activities. Lab Invest 1987; 56:234-48.

16. Larrick JW, Kunkel SL. The role of tumor necrosis factor and interleukin 1 in the immunoinflammatory response. Pharm Res 1988; 5:129-39.

17. Beutler B, Cerami A. Cachectin and tumor necrosis factor as two sides of the same biological coin. Nature 1986; 320:584-87.

18. Luger TA, Charon JA, Colot M et al. Chemotactic properties of partially purified human epidermal cell-derived thymocyte-activating factor (ETAF) for polymorphonuclear and mononuclear cells. J Immunol 1983; 131:816.

19. Ming WJ, Bersani L, Mantovani A. Tumor necrosis factor is chemotactic for monocytes and polymorphonuclear leukocytes. J Immunol 1987; 138:1469.

20. Sauder DN, Mounessa NL, Katz SI et al. Chemotactic cytokines: The role of leukocyte pyrogen and epidermal cell thymocyte-activating factor in neutrophil chemotaxis. J Immunol 1984; 132:828.

21. Yoshimura TK, Matsushima K, Oppenheim JJ et al. Neutrophil chemotactic factor produced by lipopolysaccharide (LPS)-stimulated human blood mononuclear leukocytes: partial characterization and separation from interleukin 1 (IL-1). J Immunol 1987; 139:788-93.

22. Baggiolini M, Dewald B, Walz A. Interleukin-8 and related chemotactic cytokines. In: Gallin JI, Goldstein IM, Snyderman R, eds. Inflammation: Basic Principles and

Clinical Correlates. New York: Raven Press Ltd, 1992.

23. Baggiolini M, Walz A, Kunkel SL. Neutrophil-activating peptide-1/interleukin 8, a novel cytokine that activates neutrophils. J Clin Invest 1989; 84:1045-49.

24. Matsushima K, Oppenheim JJ. Interleukin 8 and MCAF: Novel inflammatory cytokines inducible by IL-1 and TNF. Cytokine 1989; 1:2-13.

25. Oppenheim JJ, Zachariae OC, Mukaida N et al. Properties of the novel proinflammatory supergene "intercrine" cytokine family. Annu Rev Immunol 1991; 9:617-48.

26. Miller MD, Krangel MS. Biology and biochemistry of the chemokines: a family of chemotactic and inflammatory cytokines. Crit Rev Immunol 1992; 12:17-46.

27. Baggiolini M, Dewald B, Moser B. Interleukin-8 and related chemotactic cytokines-C-X-C and C-C chemokines. Adv Immunol 1994; 55:97-179.

28. Taub DD, Oppenheim JJ. Chemokines, inflammation and immune system. Therapeutic Immunol 1994; 1:229-46.

29. Farber JM. HuMIG: a new member of the chemokine family of cytokines. Biochem Biophys Res Comm 1993; 192:223-30.

30. Proost P, De Wolf-Peeters C, Conings R et al. Identification of a novel granulocyte chemotactic protein (GCP-2) from human tumor cells: in vitro and in vivo comparison with natural forms of GROα, IP-10, and IL-8. J Immunol 1993; 150:1000-10.

31. Walz A, Burgener R, Car B et al. Structure and neutrophil-activating properties of a novel inflammatory peptide (ENA-78) with homology to interleukin-8. J Exp Med 1991; 174:1355-62.

32. Walz A, Baggiolini M. Generation of the neutrophil-activating peptide NAP-2 from platelet basic protein or connective tissue-activating peptide III through monocyte proteases. J Exp Med 1990; 171:449-54.

33. Deutsch E, Kain W. Studies on platelet factor 4. In: Johnson SA, Monto RW, Rebuck JW, Horn RC, eds. Blood Platelets. Boston: Little Brown, 1961:337.

34. Kaplan G, Luster AD, Hancock G et al. The expression of a γ interferon-induced protein (IP-10) in delayed immune responses in human skin. J Exp Med 1987; 166:1098-1108.

35. Gusella GL, Musso T, Bosco MC et al. IL-2 upregulates but IFN-γ suppresses IL-8 expression in human monocytes. J Immunol 1993; 151:2725-32.

36. Schnyder-Candrian S, Strieter RM, Kunkel SL et al. Interferon-α and interferon-γ downregulate the production of interleukin-8 and ENA-78 in human monocytes. J Leuk Biol (in press).

37. Aman MJ, Rudolf G, Goldschmitt J et al. Type-I interferons are potent inhibitors of interleukin-8 production in hematopoietic and bone marrow stromal cells. Blood 1993; 82:2371-81.

38. Oliveira IC, Sciavolino PJ, Lee TH et al. Downregulation of interleukin 8 gene expression in human fibroblasts: unique mechanism of transcriptional inhibition by interferon. Proc Natl Acad Sci USA 1992; 89:9049-53.

39. Oliveira IC, Muaida N, Matsushima K et al. Transcriptional inhibition of the interleukin-8 gene by interferon is mediated by the NF-kappa B site. Mol Cell Biol 1994; 14:5300-08.

40. Ansiowicz A, Zajchowski D, Stenman G et al. Functional diversity of gro gene expression in human fibroblasts and mammary epithelial cells. Proc Natl Acad Sci USA 1988; 85:9645-49.

41. Ansiowicz A, Bardwell L, Sager R. Constitutive overexpression of a growth-regulated gene in transformed Chinese hamster and human cells. Proc Natl Acad Sci USA 1987; 84:7188-92.

42. Richmond A, Thomas HG. Melanoma growth stimulatory activity: isolation from human melanoma tumors and characterization of tissue distribution. J Cell Biochem 1988; 36:185-98.

43. Walz A, Peveri P, Aschauer H et al. Purification and amino acid sequencing of NAF, a novel neutrophil-activating factor produced by monocytes. Biochem Biophys Res Commun 1987; 149:755-61.

44. Matsushima K, Morishita K, Yoshimura T et al. Molecular cloning of a human monocyte-derived neutrophil chemotactic factor (MDNCF) and the induction of MDNCF

mRNA by interleukin-1 and tumor necrosis factor. J Exp Med 1988; 167:1883-93.

45. Strieter RM, Chensue SW, Basha MA et al. Human alveolar macrophage gene expression of interleukin-8 by TNF-α, LPS and IL-1b. Am J Respir Cell Mol Biol 1990; 2:321-26.

46. Rankin JA, Sylvester I, Smith S et al. Macrophages cultured in vitro release leukotriene B4 and neutrophil attractant/activation protein (interleukin 8) sequentially in response to stimulation with lipopolysaccharide and zymosan. J Clin Invest 1900; 86:1556-64.

47. Strieter RM, Kasahara K, Allen R et al. Human neutrophils exhibit disparate chemotactic factor gene expression. Biochem Biophys Res Comm 1990; 173:725-30.

48. Bazzoni F, Cassatella MA, Rossi F et al. Phagocytosing neutrophils produce and release high amounts of the neutrophIL-activating peptide 1/interleukin 8. J Exp Med 1991; 173:771-74.

49. Strieter RM, Kasahara K, Allen RM et al. Cytokine-induced neutrophil-derived interleukin-8. Am J Pathol 1992; 141: 397-407.

50. Kasama T, Strieter RM, Lukacs NW et al. Regulation of neutrophil-derived chemokine expression by IL-10. J Immunol 1994; 152:3559-69.

51. Braun RK, Franchini M, Erard F et al. Human peripheral blood eosinophils produce and release interleukin-8 on stimulation with calcium ionophore. Eur J Immunol 1993; 23:956-60.

52. Takanaski S, Nonaka R, Xing Z et al. Interleukin 10 inhibits lipopolysaccharide-induced survival and cytokine production by human peripheral blood eosinophils. J Exp Med 1994; 180:711-15.

53. Moller A, Lippert U, Lessmann D, Kolde G, Hamann K, Welker P, Schadendorf D, Rosenbach T, Luger T, Czarnetzki BM. Human mast cells produce IL-8. J Immunol 1993; 151:3261-66.

54. Smyth MJ, Zachariae CO, Norihisa Y, Ortaido JR, Hishinuma A, Matsushima K. IL-8 gene expression and production in human peripheral blood lymphocyte subsets. J Immunol 1991; 146:3815-23.

55. Zachariae CO. Chemotactic cytokines and inflammation. Biological properties of the lymphocyte and monocyte chemotactic factors ELCF, MCAF, and IL-8. Acta Derm Venereol Suppl 1993; 181:1-37.

56. Wechsler AS, Gordon MC, Dendorfer U, LeClair KP. Induction of IL-8 expression in T cells uses the CD28 costimulatory pathway. J Immunol 1994; 153:2515-23.

57. Somersalo K, Carpen O, Saksela E. Stimulated natural killer cells secrete factors with chemotactic activity, including NAP-1/IL-8, which supports VLA-4- and VLA-5-mediated migration of T lymphocytes. Eur J Immunol 1994; 24:2957-65.

58. Nickoloff BJ, Karabin GD, Barker JN, Griffiths CE, Sarma V, Mitra RS, Elder JT, Kunkel SL, Dixit VM. Cellular localization of interleukin-8 and its inducer, tumor necrosis factor-alpha in psoriasis. Am J Pathol 1991; 138:129-40.

59. Brown Z, Strieter RM, Chensue SW, Ceska P, Lindley I, Nield GH, Kunkel SL, Westwick J. Cytokine activated human mesangial cells generate the neutrophil chemoattractant - interleukin 8. Kidney International 1991; 40:86-90.

60. Standiford TJ, Kunkel SL, Basha MA, Chensue SW, Lynch JP III, Toews GB, Westwick J, Strieter RM. Interleukin-8 gene expression by a pulmonary epithelial cell line: A model for cytokine networks in the lung. J Clin Invest 1990; 86:1945-53.

61. Elner VM, Strieter RM, Elner SG, Baggiolini M, Lindley I, Kunkel SL. Neutrophil chemotactic factor (IL-8) gene expression by cytokine-treated retinal pigment epithelial cells. Am J Path 1990; 136: 745-50.

62. Nakamura H, Yoshimura K, Jaffe HA, Crystal RG. Interleukin-8 gene expression in human bronchial epithelial cells. J Biol Chem 1991; 266:19611-17.

63. Cromwell O, Hamid Q, Corrigan CJ, Barkans J, Meng Q, Collins PD, Kay AB. Expression and generation of interleukin-8, IL-6, and granulocyte-macrophage colony-stimulating factor by bronchial epithelial cells and enchancement by IL-1 beta and tumor necrosis factor-alpha. Immunology 1992; 77:330-37.

64. Noah TL, Becker S. Respiratory syncytial virus-induced cytokine production by a hu-

man bronchial epithelial cell line. Am J Physiol 1993; 265:L472-78.

65. Levine SJ, Larivee P, Logun C, Angus CW, Shelhamer JH. Corticosteroids differentially regulate secretion of IL-6, IL-8, and G-CSF by human bronchial epithelial cell line. Am J Physiol 1993; 265:L360-68.

66. Becker S, Quay J, Koren HS, Haskill JS. Constitutive and stimulated MCP-1, GRO alpha, beta, and gamma expression in human airway epithelium and bronchoalveolar macrophages. Am J Physiol 1994; 266: L278-86.

67. Kwon OJ, Au BT, Collins PD, Baraniuk JN, Adcock IM, Chung KF, Barnes PJ. Inhibition of interleukin-8 expression by dexamethasone in human cultured airway epithelial cells. Immunology 1994; 81: 389-94.

68. Thornton AJ, Strieter RM, Lindley I, Baggiolini M, Kunkel SL. Cytokine-induced gene expression of a neutrophil chemotactic factor/interleukin-8 by human hepatocytes. J Immunol 1990; 144:2609-13.

69. Strieter RM, Phan SH, Showell HJ, Remick DG, Lynch JP, Genord M, Raiford C, Eskandari M, Marks RM, Kunkel SL. Monokine-induced neutrophil chemotactic factor gene expression in human fibroblasts. J Biol Chem 1989; 264:10621-26.

70. Rolfe MW, Kunkel SL, Standiford TJ, Chensue SW, Allen RM, Evanoff HL, Phan SH, Strieter RM. Pulmonary fibroblast expression of interleukin-8: a model for alveolar macrophage-derived cytokine networking. Am J Respir Cell Mol Biol 1991; 5:493-501.

71. Wang JM, Sica A, Peri G, Walter S, Padura IM, Libby P, Ceska M, Lindley I, Colotta F, Mantovani A. Expression of monocyte chemotactic protein and interleukin-8 by cytokine-activated human vascular smooth cells. Arterioscler Thromb 1991; 11: 1166-74.

72. Lukacs NW, Kunkel SL, Allen R, Evanoff H, Shaklee C, Sherman J, Burdick MD, Strieter RM. Stimulus and cell-specific expression of C-X-C and C-C chemokines by pulmonary stromal cell populations. Am J Physiol: Lung Cell Mol Physiol (in press).

73. Goodman RB, Wood RG, Martin TR, Hanson-Painton O, Kinasewitz GT. Cytokine-stimulated human mesothelial cells produce chemotactic activity for neutrophils including NAP-1/IL-8. J Immunol 1992; 148:457-65.

74. Antony VB, Hott JW, Kunkel SL, Godbey SW, Burdick MD, Strieter RM. Pleural mesothelial cell expression of C-C (monocyte chemotactic peptide [MCP-1]) and C-X-C (interleukin-8 [IL-8]) chemokines. Am J Respir Cell Mol Biol (in press).

75. Griffith DE, Miller EJ, Gray LD, Idell S, Johnson AR. Interleukin-1-mediated release of interleukin-8 by asbestos-stimulated human pleural mesothelial cells Am J Respir Cell Mol Biol 1994; 10:245-52.

76. Strieter RM, Kunkel SL, Showell HJ, Marks RM. Monokine-induced gene expression of human endothelial cell derived neutrophil chemotactic factor. Biochem Biophys Res Commun 1998; 156:1340-45.

77. Strieter RM, Kunkel SL, Showell H, Remick DG, Phan SH, Ward PA, Marks RM. Endothelial cell gene expression of a neutrophil chemotactic factor by TNF-α, LPS, and IL-1b. Science 1989; 243:1467-69.

78. Brown Z, Gerritsen ME, Carley WW, Strieter RM, Kunkel SL, Westwick J. Chemokine expression and secretion by cytokine-activated human microvascular endothelial cells. Differential regulation of monocyte chemoattractant protein-1 and interleukin-8 in response to interferon-gamma. Am J Pathol 1994; 145:913-21.

79. Griffin CA, Emanuel BS, LaRocco P, Schwartz E, Poncz M. Human platelet factor 4 gene is mapped to 4q12-21. Cytogent Cell Genet 1987; 45:67-69.

80. Majundar S, Gonder D, Koutsis B, Poncz M. Characterization of the human β-thromboglobulin gene. Comparison with the gene for platelet factor 4. J Biol Chem 1991; 266:5785-89.

81. Mukaida N, Shiroo M, and Matsushima K. Genomic structure of the human monocyte-derived neutrophil chemotactic factor IL-8. J Immunol 1989; 143:1366-71.

82. Modi WS, Dean M, Seuanez HN, Mukaida N, Matsushima K, O'Brien SJ. Monocyte-derived neutrophil chemotactic factor (MDNCF/IL-8) resides in a gene cluster

along with several other members of the platelet factor 4 gene superfamily. Hum Genet 1990; 84:185-87.

83. Richmond A, Balentien E, Thomas HG, Flaggs G, Barton DE, Spiess J, Bordoni R, Francke U, Derynck R. Molecular characterization and chromosomal mapping of melanoma growth stimulatory activity, a growth factor structurally related to β-thromboglobulin. EMBO J 1988; 7: 2025-33.

84. Haskill S, Peace A, Morris J, Sporn SA, Anisowicz A, Lee SW, Smith T, Martin G, Ralph P, Sager R. Identification of three related human GRO genes encoding cytokine functions. Proc Natl Acad Sci USA 1990; 87:7732-36.

85. Luster AD, Jhanwar SC, Chaganti RS, Kersey JH, Ravetch JV. Interferon-inducible gene maps to a chromosomal band associated with a (4;11) translocation in acute leukemia cells. Proc Natl Acad Sci USA 1987; 84:2868-71.

86. Luster AD, Ravetch JV. Genomic characterization of a gamma-interferon-inducible gene (IP-10) and identification of an interferon-inducible hypersensitive site. Mol Cell Biol 1987; 7:3723-31.

87. Chang MS, McNinch J, Basu R, Simonet S. Cloning and characterization of the human neutrophil-activating peptide (ENA-78) gene. J Biol Chem 1994; 269:25277-82.

88. Corbett MS, Schmitt I, Riess O, Walz A. Characterization of the gene for human neutrophil-activating peptide 78 (ENA-78). Biochem Biophys Res Comm 1994; 205: 612-17.

89. Mukaida N, Shiroo M, Matsushima K. Molecular mechanism of interleukin-8 gene expression. J Leuk Biol 1994; 56:554-58.

90. Kunsch C, Lang RK, Rosen CA, Shannon MF. Synergistic transcriptional activation of the IL-8 gene by NF-κB p65 (RelA) and NF-IL-6. J Immunol 1994; 153:153-64.

91. Caput D, Beutler B, Hartog K, Thayer R, Brown-Shimer S, Cerami A. Identification of a common nucleotide sequence in the 3'-untranslated region of mRNA molecules specifying inflammatory mediators. Proc Natl Acad Sci USA 1986; 83:1670.

92. von Heijne G. Patterns of amino acids near signal-sequence cleavage sites. Eur J Biochem 1983; 133:17.

93. Schmid J, Weissmann C. Induction of mRNA for a serine protease and a beta-thromboglobulin-like protein in mitogen-stimulated human leukocytes. J Immunol 1987; 139:250-56.

94. Yoshimura T, Robinson EA, Appella E, Matsushima K, Showalter SD, Skeel A, Leonard EJ. Three forms of monocyte-derived neutrophil chemotactic factor (MDNCF) distinguished by different lengths of the amino-terminal sequence. Mol Immunol 1989; 26:87-93.

95. Hébert CA, Baker JB. Interleukin-1: a review. Cancer Invest 1993; 11:743-50.

96. Witt DP, Lander AD. Differential binding of chemokines to glycosaminoglycan subpopulations. Curr Biol 1994; 4:394-400.

97. Clore GM, Appella E, Yamada M, Matsushima K, Gronenborn AM. Determination of the secondary structure of interleukin-8 by nuclear magnetic resonance spectroscopy. J Biol Chem 1989; 264: 18907-11.

98. Clore GM, Gronenborn AM. Comparison of the solution nuclear magnetic resonance and crystal structures of interleukin-8. Possible implications for the mechanism of receptor binding. J Mol Biol 1991; 217:611-20.

99. Clore GM, Gronenborn AM. Three-dimensional structures of α and β chemokines. FASEB J 1995; 9:57-62.

100. Lodi PJ, Garrett DS, Kuszewski J, Tsnag MLS, Weatherbee JA, Leonard WJ, Gronenborn AM, Clore GM. High-resolution solution structure of the β chemokine hMIP-1b by multidimensional NMR. Science 1994; 263:1762-67.

101. St Charles R, Walz DA, Edwards BFP. The three dimensional structure of bovine platelet factor x at 3.0-A resolution. J Biol Chem 1989; 264:2092-99.

102. Peveri P, Walz A, Dewald B, Baggiolini M. A novel neutrophil-activating factor produced by human mononuclear phagocytes. J Exp Med 1988; 167:1547-59.

103. Padrines M, Wolf M, Walz A, Baggiolini M. Interleukin-8 processing by neutrophil elastase, cathepsin G, and proteinase-3.

FEBS Lett 1994; 352:231-35.

104. Walz A, Strieter RM, Schnyder S. Neutrophil-activating peptide ENA-78. Adv Exp Med Biol 1993; 351:129-37.

105. Clore GM, Appella E, Yamada M, Matsushima K, Gronenborn AM. Three-dimensional structure of interleukin 8 in solution. Biochemistry 1990; 29:1689-96.

106. Hébert CA, Vitangcol RV, Baker JB. Scanning mutagenesis of interleukin-8 identifies a cluster of residues required for receptor binding. J Biol Chem 1991; 266: 18989-94.

107. Clark-Lewis I, Schumacher C, Baggiolini M, Moser B. Structure-activity relationships of interleukin-8 determined using chemically synthesized analogs. Critical role of NH2-terminal residues and evidence for uncoupling of neutrophil chemotaxis, exocytosis, and receptor binding. J Biol Chem 1991; 266:23128-34.

108. Clark-Lewis I, Dewald B, Geiser T, Moser B, Baggiolini M. Platelet factor 4 binds to interleukin 8 receptors and activates neutrophils when its N terminus is modified with Glu-Leu-Arg. Proc Natl Acad Sci USA 1993; 90:3574-77.

109. Clark-Lewis I, Dewald B, Loetscher M, Moser B, Baggiolini M. Structural requirements for interleukin-8 function identified by design of analogs and C-X-C chemokine hybrids. J Biol Chem 1994; 269:16075-81.

110. Webb LMC, Ehrengruber MU, Clark-Lewis I, Baggiolini M, Rot A. Binding to heparan sulfate or heparin enhances neutrophil responses to interleukin 8. Proc Natl Acad Sci USA 1993; 90:7158-62.

111. Thelen M, Peveri P, Kernen P, Von Tscharner V, Walz A, Baggiolini M. Mechanisms of neutrophil activation by NAF, a novel monocyte-derived peptide agonist. FASEB J 1988; 2:2702-19.

112. Dewald B, Moser B, Barella L, Schumacher C, Baggiolini M, Clark-Lewis I. IP-10, a gamma-interferon-inducible protein related to interleukin-8, lacks neutrophil activating properties. Immunol Lett 1992; 32:81-84.

113. Samanta AK, Oppenheim JJ, Matsushima K. Identification and characterization of specific receptors for monocyte-derived neutrophil chemotactic factor (MDNCF) on human neutrophils. J Exp Med 1989; 169:1185-89.

114. Moser B, Schumacher C, von Tschamer V, Clark-Lewis I, Baggiolini M. Neutrophil-activating peptide 2 and gro/melanoma growth-stimulatory activity interact with neutrophil-activating peptide 1/interleukin 8 receptors on human neutrophils. J Biol Chem 1991; 266:10666-71.

115. Samanta AK, Oppenheim JJ, Matsushima K. Interleukin 8 (monocyte-derived neutrophil chemotactic factor) dynamically regulates its own receptor expression on human neutrophils. J Biol Chem 1990; 265:183-89.

116. Holmes WE, Lee J, Kuang WJ, Rice GC, Wood WI. Structure and functional expression of a human interleukin-8 receptor. Science 1991; 253:1278-80.

117. Murphy PM, Tiffany HL. Cloning of complementary DNA encoding a functional human interleukin-8 receptor. Science 1991; 253:1280-83.

118. Lee J, Horuk R, Rice GC, Bennett GL, Camerato T, Wood WI. Characterization of two high affinity human interleukin-8 receptors. J Biol Chem 1992; 267:16283-87.

119. Lloyd A, Modi W, Sprenger H, Cevario S, Oppenheim JJ, Kelvin D. Assignment of the genes for interleukin-8 receptors (IL-8R) A and B to human chromosome band 2q35. Cytogenet Cell Genet 1993; 63:238-40.

120. Ahuja SK, Gao JL, Murphy PM. Chemokine receptors and molecular mimicry. Immunol Today 1994; 15:281-87.

121. Murphy PM. The molecular biology of leukocyte chemoattractant receptors. Annu Rev Immunol 1994; 12:593-633.

122. Horuk R. The interleukin-8-receptor family from chemokines to malaria. Immunol Today 1994; 15:169-74.

123. Horuk R. Molecular properties of the chemokine receptor family. Trends Pharmacol Sci 1994; 15:159-65.

124. LaRosa GJ, Thomas KM, Kaufmann ME, Mark R, White M, Taylor L, Gray G, Witt D, Navarro J. Amino terminus of the interleukin-8 receptor is a major determinant of receptor subtype specificity. J Biol Chem 1992; 267:25402-06.

125. Gayle RB, Sleath PR, Srinivason S,

Birks CW, Weerawarna KS, Cerretti DP, Kozlosky CJ, Nelson N, Vanden Bos T, Beckman MP. Importance of the amino terminus of the interleukin-8 receptor in ligand interaction. J Biol Chem 1993; 268:7283-89.

126. Hébert CA, Chuntharapal A, Smith M, Colby T, Kim J, Horuk R. Partial functional mapping of the human interleukin-8 type A receptor. Identification of a major ligand domain. J Biol Chem 1993; 268: 18549-53.

127. Leong SR, Kabakoff RC, Hébert CA. Complete mutagenesis of the extracellular domain of the interleukin-8 (IL-8) type A receptor identifies charged residues mediating IL-8 binding and signal transduction. J Biol Chem 1994; 269:19343-48.

128. Smith CA, Davis T, Wignall JM, Din WS, Farrah T, Upton C, McFadden G, Goodwin RG. T2 open reading frame from the shope fibroma virus encodes a soluble form of the TNF receptor. Biochem Biophys Res Comm 1991; 176:335-40.

129. Spriggs CA, Hruby DE, Maliszewski CR, Pickup DJ, Sims JE, Buller RML, Van Slyke J. Vaccina and cowpox viruses encode a novel secreted IL-1 binding protein. Cell 1992; 71:145-53.

130. Ahuja SK, Murphy PM. Molecular piracy of mammalian interleukin-8 receptor type B by herpesvirus saimiri. J Biol Chem 1993; 268:20691-94.

131. Darbonne WC, Rice GC, Mohler MA, Apple T, Hebert CA, Valente AJ, Baker JB. Red blood cells are a sink for interleukin-8, a leukocyte chemotaxin. J Clin Invest 1991; 88:1362-69.

132. Neote K, Darbonne W, Ogez J, Horuk R, Schall T. Identification of a promiscuous inflammatory peptide receptor on the surface of red blood cells. J Biol Chem 1993; 268:12247-49.

133. Horuk R, Chitnis CE, Darbonne WC, Colby TJ, Rybicki A, Hadley TJ, Miller LH. A receptor for the malarial Plasmodium vivax: the erythrocyte chemokine receptor. Science 1993; 261:1182-84.

134. Neote K, Mak JY, Kolakowski LF, Schall TJ. Functional and biochemical analysis of the clone Duffy antigen: identity with the red blood cell chemokine receptor. Blood 1994; 84:44-52.

135. Hadley TJ, Lu ZH, Wasniowska K, Martin AW, Pieper SC, Hesselgesser J, Horuk R. Postcapillary venule endothelial cells in kidney express a multispecific chemokine receptor that is structurally and functionally identical to the erythroid isoform, which is the Duffy blood group antigen. J Clin Invest 1994; 94:985-91.

136. Cacalano G, Lee J, Kikly K, Ryan AM, Pitts-Meek S, Hultgren B, Wood WI, Moore MW. Neutrophil and B cell expansion in mice that lack the murine IL-8 receptor homolog. Science 1994; 265:682-84.

137. Baggiolini M, Boulay F, Badwey JA, Curnutte JT. Activation of neutrophil leukocytes: chemottractant receptors and respiratory burst. FASEB J 1993; 7:1004-10.

138. Johnston JA, Ferris DK, Wang JM, Longo DL, Oppenheim JJ, Kelvin DJ. Staurosporine restores signaling and inhibits interleukin-8-induced chemotactic desensitization. Eur J Immunol 1994; 24: 2556-62.

139. Sham RL, Phatak PD, Ihne TP, Abboud CN, Packman CH. Signal pathway regulation of interleukin-8-induced actin polymerization in neutrophils. Blood 1993; 82: 2546-51.

140. Schroder JM. The monocyte-derived neutrophil activating peptide (NAP/interleukin 8) stimulates human neutrophil arachidonate-5-lipoxygenase, but not the release of cellular arachidonate. J Exp Med 1989; 170:847-63.

141. Fogh K, Larsen CG, Iversen L, Kragballe K. Interleukin-8 stimulates the formation of 15-hydroxy-eicosatetraenoic acid from human neutrophils in vitro. Agents Actions 1992; 35:227-31.

142. Bussolino F, Sironi M, Bocchietto E, Mantovani A. Synthesis of platelet-activating factor by polymorphonuclear neutrophils stimulated with interleukin-8. J Biol Chem 1992; 267:14598-14603.

143. McDonald PP, Pouliot M, Borgeat P, McColl SR. Induction by chemokines of lipid mediator synthesis in granulocyte-macrophage colony-stimulating factor-treated human neutrophils. J Immunol 1993; 151:6399-6409.

144. McCain RW, Holden EP, Blackwell TR, Christman JW. Leukotriene B4 stimulates human polymorphonuclear leukocytes to synthesize and release interleukin-8 in vitro. Am J Respir Cell Mol Biol 1994; 10: 651-57.

145. Detmers PA, Lo SK, Olsen-Egbert E, Walz A, Baggiolini M, Cohn ZA. Neutrophil-activating protein 1/interleukin 8 stimulates the binding activity of the leukocyte adhesion receptor CD11b/CD18 on human neutrophils. J Exp Med 1990; 171:1155-62.

146. Detmers PA, Powell DE, Walz A, Clark-Lewis I, Baggiolini M, Cohn ZA. Differential effects of neutrophil-activating peptide 1/IL-8 and its homologues on leukocyte adhesion and phagocytosis. J Immunol 1991; 147:4211-17.

147. Geiser T, Dewald B, Ehrengruber MU, Clark-Lewis I, Baggiolini M. The interleukin-8-related chemotactic cytokines GRO alpha, beta, and GRO gamma activate human neutrophil and basophil leukocytes. J Biol Chem 1993; 268:15419-24,.

148. Bischoff SC, Baggiolini M, deWeck AL, Dahinden CA. Interleukin 8-inhibitor and inducer of histamine and leukotriene release in human basophils. Biochem Biophys Res Comm 1991; 179:628-33.

149. Kuna P, Reddigari SR, Kornfeld D, Kaplan AP. IL-8 inhibits histamine release from human basophils induced by histamine-releasing factors, connective tissue activating peptide III, and IL-3. J Immunol 1991; 147:1920-24.

150. Krieger M, Brunner T, Bischoff SC, von Tschamer V, Walz A, Moser B, Baggiolini M, Dahinden CA. Activation of human basophils through the IL-8 receptor. J Immunol 1992; 149:2662-67.

151. Bacon KB, Flores-Romo L, Aubry JP, Wells TN, Power CA. Interleukin-8 and RANTES induce the adhesion of the human basophilic cell line KU-812 to human endothelial cell monolayers. Immunology 1994; 82:473-81.

152. Kernen P, Wymann MP, von Tsharner V, Deranieau DA, Tai PC, Spry CJ, Dahinden CA, Baggiolini M. Shape changes, exocytosis, and cytosolic free calcium changes in stimulated human eosinophils. J Clin Invest 1991; 87:2012-17.

153. Schweizer RC, Welmers BA, Raaijmakers JA, Zanen P, Lammers JW, Koenderman L. RANTES- and interleukin-8-induced responses in normal human eosinophils: effects of priming with interleukin-5. Blood 1994; 83:3697-3704.

154. Collins PD, Weg VB, Faccioli LH, Warson ML, Moqbel R, Williams TJ. Eosinophil accumulation induced by human interleukin-8 in the guinea-pig in vivo. Immunology 1993; 79:312-18.

155. Walz A, Meloni F, Clark-Lewis I, von Tscharner V, Baggiolini M. {Ca+2}i changes and respiratory burst in human neutrophils and monocytes induced by NAP-1/interleukin-8, NAP-2, and GRO/MGSA. J Leuk Biol 1991; 50:279-86.

156. Taub DD, Lloyd AR, Conlon K, Oppenheim JJ. Recombinant human interferon-inducible protein 10 is a chemoattractant for human monocytes and T lymphocytes and promotes T cell adhesion to endothelial cells. J Exp Med 1993; 177:1809.

157. Sebok K, Woodside D, al-Aoukaty A, Ho AD, Gluck S, Maghazachi AA. IL-8 induces the locomotion of human IL-2-activated natural killer cells. Involvement of a guanine nucleotide binding (Go) protein. J Immunol 1993; 150:1524-34.

158. Kimata H, Yoshida A, Ishioka C, Lindley I, Mikawa H. Interleukin 8 (IL-8) selectively inhibits immunoglobulin E production induced by IL-4 in human B cells. J Exp Med 1993; 176:1227-31.

159. Kimata H, Lindley I. Interleukin-8 differentially modulates interleukin-4- and interleukin-2-induced human B cell growth. Eur J Immunol 1994; 24:3237-40.

160. Nickoloff BJ. The cytokine network in psoriasis. Arch Dermatol 1991; 127:871-84.

161. Nickoloff BJ, Karabin GD, Barker JNWN, Giffiths CEM, Sarma V, Mitra RS, Elder JT, Kunkel SL, Dixit VM. Cellular localization of interleukin-8 and its inducer, tumor necrosis factor-alpha in psoriasis. Am J Pathol 1991; 138:129-40.

162. Sticherling M, Bornscheuer E, Schroder JM, Christophers E. Localization of neutrophil-activating peptide-1/interleukin-8-immunoreactivity in normal and psoriatic skin. J Invest Dermatol 1991; 96:26-30.

163. Anttila HSI, Reitamo S, Erkko P, Ceska M, Moser B, Baggiolini M. Interleukin-8 immunoreactivity in the skin of healthy subjects and patients with palmoplantar pustulosis and psoriasis. J Invest Dermatol 1992; 98:96-101.

164. Michel G, Kemeny L, Peter RU, Beetz A, Ried C, Arenberger P, Ruzicka T. Interleukin-8 receptor-mediated chemotaxis of normal human epidermal cells. FEBS 1992; 305:241-43.

165. Schulz BS, Michel G, Wagner S, Suss R, Beetz A, Peter RU, Kemeny L, Ruzicka T. Increased expression of epidermal IL-8 receptor in psoriasis. J Immunol 1993; 151:4399-4406.

166. Valyi-Nagy I, Jensen PJ, Albelda SM, Rodeck U. Cytokine-induced expression of transforming growth factor-α and the epidermal growth factor receptor in neonatal skin explants. J Invest Dermatol 1992; 99:350-56.

167. Koch AE, Kunkel SL, Pearce WH, Shaw M, Parikh D, Evanoff HL, Haines GK, Burdick MD, Strieter RM. Enhanced production of the chemotactic cytokines interleukin-8 (IL-8) and monocyte chemoattractant protein-1 (MCP-1) in human abdominal aortic aneurysms. Am J Pathol 1993; 142:1423-31.

168. Yue TL, McKenna PJ, Gu JL, Feuerstein GZ. Interleukin-8 is chemotactic for vascular smooth muscle cells. Eur J Pharmacol 1993; 240:81-84.

169. Yue TL, Wang X, Sung CP, Olson B, McKenna PJ, Gu JL, Feuerstein GZ. Interleukin-8. A mitogen and chemoattractant for vascular smooth muscle cells. Circ Res 1994; 75:1-7.

170. Koch AE, Polverini PJ, Kunkel SL, Harlow LA, DiPietro LA, Elner VM, Elner SG, Strieter RM. Interleukin-8 (IL-8) as a macrophage-derived mediator of angiogenesis.

Science 1992; 258:1798-1801.

171. Strieter RM, Kunkel SL, Elner VM, Martonyl CL, Koch AE, Polverini PJ, Elner SG. Interleukin-8: A corneal factor that induces neovascularization. Am J Pathol 1992; 141:1279-84.

172. Hu DE, Hori Y, Fan TPD. Interleukin-8 stimulates angiogenesis in rats. Inflammation 1993; 17:135-43.

173. Maione TE, Gray GS, Petro J, Hunt AJ, Donner AL, Bauer SI, Carson HF, Sharpe RJ. Inhibition of angiogenesis by recombinant human platelet factor-4. Science 1990; 247:77-79.

174. Sharpe RJ, Byers HR, Scott CF, Bauer SI, Maione TE. Growth inhibition of murine melanoma and human colon carcinoma by recombinant human platelet factor 4. J Natl Cancer Inst 1990; 82:848-53.

175. Maione TE, Gray GS, Hunt AJ, Sharpe RJ. Inhibition of tumor growth in mice by an analogue of platelet factor 4 that lacks affinity for heparin and retains potent angiostatic activity. Cancer Res 1991; 51:2077-83.

176. Strieter RM, Kunkel SL, Arenberg DA, Burdick MD, Polverini PJ. Interferon γ-inducible protein 10 (IP-10) a member of the C-X-C chemokine family is an inhibitor of angiogenesis. Biochem Biophys Res Comm 1995; 210:51-57.

177. Strieter RM, Polverini PJ, Kunkel SL, Arenberg DA, Burdick MD, Kasper J, Dzuiba J, VanDamme J, Walz A, Marriott D, Chan S-Y, Roczniak S, Shanafelt AB. The functional role of the ELR motif in C-X-C chemokine-mediated angiogenesis. J Biol Chem 1995; 270:27348-57.

178. Schonbeck U, Brandt E, Peterson F, Hans-Dieter F, Loppnow H. IL-8 specifically binds to endothelial but not to smooth muscle cells. J Immunol 1995; 154:2374-83.

CHAPTER 2

C-C CHEMOKINES: AN OVERVIEW

Dennis D. Taub*

The recruitment of leukocytes into a site of tissue damage is dependent upon a dynamic and complex series of events. The steps which lead to leukocyte recruitment include: endothelial cell activation and expression of endothelial cell-derived adhesion molecules, leukocyte activation and expression of leukocyte-derived adhesion molecules, leukocyte-endothelial cell adhesion, leukocyte diapedesis and leukocyte migration beyond the vascular barrier via established chemotactic gradients.[1-6] While adhesive interactions between leukocytes (L-selectin, β1 and β2 integrins) and endothelial cells (P- and E-selectin, ICAM-1 and VCAM-1) are prerequisite events for successful leukocyte extravasation at sites of inflammation, the subsequent steps leading to diapedesis and migration beyond the vascular compartment are dependent upon both the continued expression of β1 and β2 integrins and the movement along a leukocyte-specific chemotactic gradient.[1-6] Recent studies have dramatically increased our knowledge concerning these various steps of leukocyte extravasation. This is especially true for research leading to the identification of cytokines mediating leukocyte chemotaxis. Information gained from studying chemotactic cytokines and other immunomodulators have generated exciting new concepts regarding the genesis of inflammatory responses.

Early studies of chemoattractants have identified a number of agents as inducers of leukocyte migration, including activated serum components, platelet activating factor (PAF), casein, eicosanoids, bacterial-derived peptides (i.e., fMLP), mast cell-, neutrophil- and lymphocyte-derived chemoattractant factors, β-thromboglobulin, cytokines (i.e., IL-2, IL-4, IL-10, IL-12) and opioids.[7-10] Recent studies have defined a novel family of structurally related *chemo*tactic cyto*kines* termed "chemokines" which

* The contents of this publication do not necessarily reflect the views and policies of the Department of Health and Human Services, nor does mention of trade names, commercial products, or organizations imply endorsement by the U.S. Government.

Chemokines in Disease, edited by Alisa E. Koch and Robert M. Strieter.
© 1996 R.G. Landes Company.

are secreted by many different cell types and have been shown to elicit the selective accumulation of inflammatory leukocytes in vivo.[11-12] Since the cloning and characterization of interleukin-8 (IL-8) in 1988,[13] over 30 unique human and mouse cytokines have been identified as members of the chemokine superfamily of peptides that have between 20-70% homology in their amino acid sequences and are related, for the most part, by a conserved motif containing four cysteine residues (Figs. 2.1 and 2.2).[14-18] The family has been divided into three subfamilies, the C-X-C, C-C, and C subfamilies, based on differences in their genetic and biochemical structures and biological activities.[14-18] Each of these chemokines has been shown to induce the directional migration of a number of inflammatory cell types including neutrophils, monocyte/macrophages, lymphocytes, eosinophils, basophils and mast cells. All of these proteins are basic heparin-binding peptides that are active over a wide concentration range (0.001-10 nM) and are produced by a wide variety of cell types in response to exogenous irritants such as LPS, phorbol esters, and silicon and endogenous inflammatory mediators such as IL-1, TNF-α, PDGF and IFN-γ[14-18] (Table 2.1). Chemokines have also been shown to be produced at inflammatory sites and in many pathologic conditions, including rheumatoid arthritis, osteoarthritis, sepsis, inflammatory bowel disease, atherosclerosis, asthma, leprosy, granulomatous disease, psoriasis, ischemia/reperfusion injury, autoimmune responses and a variety of pulmonary disease states.[14-18]

THE CHEMOKINE SUPERFAMILY

The chemokine superfamily can be separated into the C-X-C and C-C subfamilies based on the presence (the α subfamily) or absence (the β subfamily) of an intervening amino acid residue located between the first two of the four conserved cysteines[14-18] (Figs. 2.1 and 2.2). Chemokine

family members show considerable similarity in their amino acid sequence, exhibiting between 20-50% sequence homology (Fig. 2.2).[14-18] The cDNA codes for a precursor protein which contains a leader sequence which presumably enables the chemokines to be produced, cleaved and secreted to yield a mature form at the cell membrane by a wide variety of cell types.[14-18] Many chemokines form dimers, trimers and tetramers upon secretion. Several laboratories have recently proposed that chemokine dimer formation is necessary for optimal ligand interaction with its chemokine-specific receptor. However, the biological role of chemokine dimers is still controversial, since monomers have been shown to be active.

Other features of the individual subfamilies include their apparent leukocyte specificity.[14-18] Many of the C-X-C chemokines including IL-8/neutrophil activating peptide-1 (NAP-1), *gro*wth related peptide (GROα)/melanoma growth and stimulating activity (MGSA), macrophage inflammatory protein-2 (MIP-2)/GROβ, GROγ, NAP-2, ENA-78 and GCP-2 induce both neutrophil migration and activation but have no effect on monocytes. However, members of this family are not restricted to interactions with neutrophils as several C-X-C chemokines act on other cell types (e.g., basophils, T cells, endothelial cells, melanocytes, muscle cells, keratinocytes, etc.). In addition, the C-X-C chemokine IP-10 has been shown to chemoattract monocytes and T lymphocytes rather than neutrophils[19] while PF-4 and β-TG attract fibroblasts, but not neutrophils.[20] In contrast, C-C chemokines including MIP-1α, MIP-1β, <u>r</u>egulated upon <u>a</u>ctivation, <u>n</u>ormal <u>T</u> cell <u>e</u>xpressed and <u>s</u>ecreted (RANTES), macrophage chemotactic protein-1 (MCP-1)/macrophage chemotactic activating factor (MCAF), MCP-2, MCP-3, I-309/TCA-3, fic and C10 predominantly chemoattract and activate monocytes/macrophages and T lymphocytes and have very little to no effects on neutrophils.Although eosinophils,

Subfamily:	C-X-C Chemokines		C-C Chemokines	
Structure:	$NH_2\text{-}X_{6\text{-}12}\text{-}C\text{-}X\text{-}C\text{-}X_{23\text{-}24}\text{-}C\text{-}X_{15\text{-}16}\text{-}C\text{-}X_n\text{-}COOH$		$NH_2\text{-}X_{10\text{-}11}\text{-}C\text{-}C\text{-}X_{22\text{-}23}\text{-}C\text{-}X_{15}\text{-}C\text{-}X_{18\text{-}24}\text{-}COOH$	
Species:	<u>Human</u>	<u>Mouse</u>	<u>Human</u>	<u>Mouse</u>
Chromosome:	4q12-21	–	17q11-q21	11
Members:	IL-8/NAP-1 GCP-1	–	MCP-1/MCAF hJE/LDCF/HC11 GDCF/MCP-1α MCP-1β	JE
	GROα/MGSA	KC	MCP-2	HC14
	GROβ/MIP-2α	MIP-2	MCP-3	fic/MARC
	GROγ/MIP-2β	–	RANTES/hSISδ	RANTES
	ENA-78	ENA-78	MIP-1α/LD78 pLD78/PAT464 GOS19/hSISα/hSISβ	MIP-1α
	NAP-2	–	MIP-1β/ACT2 pAT744/G-26/HC21 HIMAP/MAD-5 hH400/hSISα/SISγ	MIP-1β
	NAP-4	–	I-309/hSISε SISε	TCA-3/p500
	GCP-2	–	–	C10/MRP-1
	PF-4	–	–	MRP-2
	IP-10	IP-10/C7/CRG-2		
	–	mig		

Fig. 2.1. Members of the C-X-C and C-C chemokine superfamily.

Fig. 2.2. Amino acid sequence analysis of the C-C chemokine subfamily.

```
                  1         10        20        30        40        50        60        70
                  .          .         .         .         .         .         .         .

hMCP-1    QPDAINAPVTC-CYNFTNRKISVQRLASYRRITSS-KCPKE-AVIFKTIVAK-EICADPKQKWVQDSMDHLDKQYQTPKT
JE        QPDAVNAPLTC-CYSFTSKMIPMSRLESYKRITSS-RCPKE-AVVFVTKLKREVCADPKKEWVQTYIKNLDRNQMRSEP
hMCP-2   AQPDSVSIPITC-CFNVINRKIPIQRLESYTRI-TNIQCPKE-AVIFKTKRGKEVCADPKERWVRDSMKHLDQIFQNLKP
hMCP-3            KSTTC-CYRFINKKIPKQRLESYRRTTSSHCPRE-AVIFK————DKEICADPTQKWVQDFMKHLDKKTQTPKL
hMIP-1α   ASLAADTPTAC-CFSYTSRQIPQNFIADYFE——TSSQCSKP-GVIFLTKR-SRQVCADPSEEWVQKYVSDLELSA
mMIP-1α   APYGADTPTAC-CFSY-SRKIPRQFIVDYFE——TSSLCSQP-GVIFLTKR-NRQICADSKETWVQETITDLELNA
hACT2     APMGSDPPTAC-CFSYTARKLPRNFVVDYYE-TSSLCSQP-AVVFQTKRSKQVCADPSESWVQEYVYDLEIN
hMIP-1β   APMGSDPPTAC-CFSYT-REASSNFVVDYYE-TSSLCSQP-AVVFQTKRS-KQVCADPSESWVQEYVYDLEIN
mMIP-1β   APMGSDPPTSC-CFSYTSRQLHRSFVMDYYETSSLCSKP-AVVFLTKR-GRQICANPSEPWTEYMSDLEIN
hRANTES   SPYSSDTTPC-CFAYIARPLPRAHIKEYFY-TSGKCSNP-AVVFVTRK-NRQVCANPEKKWVREYINSLEMS
mRANTES   SPYGSDTTPC-CFAYLSLALPRAHVKEYFYTSSKCSNL-AVVFVTRR-NRQVCANPEKKWVQEYINYLEMS
hI-309    KSMQVPFSRC-CFSFAEQEIPLRAILCYRN-TSSICSNE-GLIFKLKRG-KEA-CALDTVGWVQRHRKMLRHCPSKRK
mTCA3     KSMLTVSNSC-CLNTLKKELPLKFIQCYRKMGSSCPDPPAVVFRLNKGRESCASTNKTWVQNHLKKVNPC
mfic      QPDGPNASTC-CYVKKQKIPKRNLKSYRRI-TSSRCPWE-AVIFKTKK-MEV-CREAHQKWVEEAIAYLDMKTPTPKP
mC10      GLIQEMEKEDRRYNPPIIHQGFQDT-
            SSDC-CFSY-ATQIPCKRFIYFP——TSGGCIKPGIIFISRRGTQV——CADPSDRRVQRCLSTLKQGPR-
                                                               -SGNKVIA
```

Table 2.1. Stimulants and cellular sources of C-C chemokines

Chemokine	Stimulants	Cell Source(s)
MCP-1,MCP-2, MCP-3	IL-1, TNF, PDGF, EGF, IFN-γ PHA, LPS, hydroxyurea, silica, poly (rI):poly (rC), viruses, *Listeria* anti-CD3, Ag activation	Monocytes/macrophages, endothelial cells, fibroblasts, keratinocytes, T cells
MIP-1α	IL-2, TNF, IL-7 PHA, PMA, anti-CD3, ConA, LPS, Ag activation IgE/Fcε crosslinking	T cells, monocytes, mast cell
MIP-1β/ACT2	IL-2, TNF PHA, PMA, anti-CD3, Con A, LPS, Ag activation	T cells, monocytes
RANTES	PHA, PMA, anti-CD3,LPS Ag activation	T cells, platelets
I-309	PHA, Anti-CD3, Ag activation IgE/Fcε crosslinking	T cells, mast cells

basophils and mast cells are developmentally linked to neutrophils, they are primarily chemoattracted and activated by the C-C chemokines.[14-18] The remainder of this chapter will focus on C-C chemokines and their role in leukocyte infiltration and cellular activation.

C-C CHEMOKINE SUBFAMILY: ISOLATION AND CLONING

The best described C-C chemokine family member MCP-1, also known as MCAF, was initially purified independently by two groups from the conditioned media of various cell types, including LPS- and PHA-activated human peripheral blood mononuclear cells, a glioblastoma cell line and the human myelomonocytic cell line, THP-1.[21-25] The protein was purified based on its monocytic chemotactic activity. After the cloning and sequencing of human MCP-1, it became clear that human MCP-1 was highly homologous to the mouse early activation gene product, JE. The JE gene, which was originally described in platelet-derived growth factor (PDGF)-stimulated fibroblasts,[26] is now considered the murine MCP-1 homolog. A

number of tumor cell lines have been shown to constitutively express MCP-1.[14-18] However, several normal cell types including monocytes, macrophages, B cells, T cells, endothelial cells, astrocytes and smooth muscle cells also produce MCP-1 upon stimulation with various exogenous and endogenous stimuli.[14-18,21] MCP-1 homologs have been purified and cloned from baboon, bovine, rabbit, guinea pig, mouse and rat.[27-30] In addition to MCP-1, two highly related human monocyte chemotactic proteins (MCP-2/HC14 and MCP-3) have been biochemically isolated from cultures of osteosarcoma cells.[31] The genes of both of these proteins have been cloned and sequenced.[32] The gene for the murine MCP-2 homolog, HC14, was identified in activated T cells by differential screening.[33] The gene has been subsequently cloned and sequenced.[34] The murine homolog of MCP-3, fic, was isolated by differential screening of a cDNA library of mRNA from a serum-stimulated NIH 3T3 fibroblasts.[35]

The cDNA of RANTES was initially discovered by subtractive hybridization as a T cell specific sequence.[36] More recently, a product of thrombin-stimulated platelets with eosinophil-chemotactic activity has been found to be identical to RANTES.[37] Using probes based on the human RANTES, a murine cDNA highly homologous to the human RANTES cDNA has been isolated and cloned.[38] Murine RANTES is highly homologous to human RANTES (>90%) at both the nucleotide and deduced amino acid level. A number of cell types have been shown to express RANTES including the organs kidney, liver and spleen as well as epithelial cells, T cells, B cells and NK cells (see refs. 14-18, 39; unpublished observations).

Macrophage inflammatory protein-1 (MIP-1) was a term originally applied to a protein preparations derived from the medium of LPS-stimulated murine macrophages that contains two distinct molecules.[40] The two murine proteins called MIP-1α and MIP-1β were originally characterized by their neutrophil chemokinetic activity and by footpad inflammation and were subsequently cloned and sequenced.[41-42] The human counterparts of mMIP-1α as well as mMIP-1β were independently discovered by several groups. Human MIP-1α has also been independently cloned and sequenced as LD78, pAT464 and GOS19.[14-18,43-44] Human MIP-1β has also been independently cloned and sequenced as several different proteins, Act-2, pAT744, hH400, G-26, HI-MAP, HC21 and MAD-5.[14-18,45-47] All of these proteins are highly homologous and exhibit between 94-98% identity.

The T cell activation gene-3 (TCA-3) like RANTES was also identified by subtractive hybridization.[48] A cDNA clone called P500 has also been cloned and found to be homologous to TCA-3.[49] The human homolog to TCA-3, I-309, was subsequently identified in 1989 and was shown to only be 42% homologous to murine TCA-3.[50] I-309 is expressed specifically in activated T cells upon secondary stimulation and is also expressed in a human mast cell line.[51] TCA-3 has also been shown to be expressed in T cell lines and mast cells.[51]

Two additional murine C-C chemokines, C10[52-53] and MRP-2,[54] have subsequently been cloned and sequenced. C10, a C-C chemokine with a unique N-terminal region, was cloned by differential screening of a cDNA library from GM-CSF stimulated mouse bone marrow cells.[53] Expression is limited to hematopoietic cells and is stimulated by exposure to GM-CSF and IL-4.

C-C CHEMOKINES: SEQUENCES

The C-C chemokine family members from mouse and man exhibit a great deal of homology in their amino acid sequences.[14-18] The intraspecies homology in amino acid sequence of the chemokine C-C subfamily ranges from 28-45%, while the interspecies homology ranges from 25-55% (Fig. 2.2).[14-18] There is about 20-40% homology between members of the C-X-C and C-C subfamilies (Fig. 2.2).[14-18] All C-C chemokines share a typical primary structure: a cleaved signal sequence of about 20-24 amino acids and a mature secreted protein of 68 to 76 amino acids. This signal sequence presumably enables the chemokines to be secreted and enzymatically cleaved to yield a mature form. Each of the four cysteine residues are conserved in the primary sequence of these molecules, as are a number of other amino acids. Similarly to the C-X-C chemokines, the conserved four cysteine residues form disulfide bridges folding the molecule into several looped domains. The disulfide bridge links the first cysteine to the third cysteine and the second cysteine to the fourth cysteine. The C-C chemokines have a short N-terminal sequence preceding the first cysteine (6-10 amino acids) and a longer C-terminal domain following the fourth cysteine (18-24 amino acids). The primary sequences of many of the C-C chemokine family predict secreted molecules with molecular masses of 7800-8700 daltons.[14-18,51] While all the C-C chemokines act on monocytes and T cells, they lack a common N-terminal sequence, in analogy to the ELR motif in C-X-C chemokines. In contrast to C-X-C chemokines, several of the C-C chemokines contain N- and/or O-linked glycosylation sites, which may also account for electrophoretically distinct forms of these chemokines.

The most biochemically studied of the C-C chemokines is MCP-1. The open reading frame of human MCP-1 cDNA encodes a 99 amino acid residue precursor protein with a 23 residue hydrophobic signal peptide that is cleaved to generate a 76 residue mature protein.[14-18, 23] The amino acid sequence similarities between human MCP-1 and bovine, rabbit, guinea pig, mouse and rat MCP-1s are 71, 74, 56, 55 and 52%, respectively.[27-30] Rabbit, guinea pig, mouse and rat MCP-1s have an extra amino acid at the C-terminus.[27-30] There are two major forms of human MCP-1: MCP-1α (15 kDa) and MCP-1β (13 kDa).[30] The 8700 core protein is modified to higher molecular mass forms by O-linked carbohydrates and addition of terminal sialic acid residues, which probably accounts for the different migrating positions of MCP-1s on acrylamide gels.[55] Heterogeneity of MCP-1 appears to be due to variations in O-linked carbohydrate processing. Glycosylation is not required for biological activity.[30] Truncated forms of MCP-1 with up to five fewer amino acids at the N-terminus has been reported.[30] MCP-1 like all C-C chemokines has two disulfide bridges, Cys11-Cys36 and Cys12-Cys52. Reductive cleavage of MCP-1 and other C-C chemokines causes a loss of biological activity (see refs. 30, 55; also unpublished observations).

Recently, MCP-2 and MCP-3 show approximately 62% and 72% homology with MCP-1.[31] MCP-3 appears to be more closely related to human MCP-1 (73% similarity) as well as rabbit and bovine MCP-1 and to a lesser extent mouse JE and rat MCP-1. MCP-2 is only 60% homologous to human MCP-1. The number of conserved and identical residues for all the MCP-1s is 17 out of 76 residues. All MCP proteins appear to contain a blocked glutamate residue at the N-terminus. The fic (also called MARC) cDNA, which is the mouse homolog of human MCP-3, contains an open reading frame of 291 nucleotides, encoding a 97 amino acid protein with a predicted molecular weight of 11 kDa.[35] The predicted protein contains a highly hydrophobic N-terminus and an N-linked glycosylation site.[35]

The human RANTES cDNA encodes a highly basic, 91 amino acid residue precursor polypeptide with a 23 amino acid residue hydrophobic signal peptide that is cleaved to generate the 68 amino acid residue mature protein.[36] Human RANTES contains no potential N-linked glycosylation sites and does not appear to be glycosylated. Naturally-derived RANTES isolated from human platelets are composed of two isoforms that differ in molecular size due to the presence of O-glycosylation.[37]

The cDNAs for both human and mouse MIP-1α and MIP-1β encode precursor proteins with signal peptides (with a predicted translation product of 92 amino acids) that are cleaved to generate mature proteins of 69 amino acids.[14-18,49,56] The products of murine MIP-1α and MIP-1β genes are both secreted, nonglycosylated proteins of about 8 kDa.[14-18,49,56] Although the mouse MIP-1β sequence has a potential site for N-linked glycosylation, the presence of a proline residue within the site makes this site inactive. Several distinct cDNA clones have been identified for human MIP-1α and MIP-1β.[14-18,49] Subsequently, two groups have identified multiple nonallelic genes for both MIP-1α and MIP-1β present in the human genome; the number varies among individuals.[51] It is believed that the multiple cDNA forms of the MIP-1s isolated were derived from distinct genes.[14-18,51] The mature forms of human MIP-1α and MIP-1β, similarly to murine MIP-1α and MIP-1β, share approximately 70% homology with one another. Both the murine and human proteins show cross-species activity.[14-18]

The TCA-3 cDNA clone encodes a protein of 92 amino acid protein that displays the amino terminal sequence and a single site for N-linked glycan attachment. The P500 cDNA clone is identical to TCA-3 through about 260 nucleotides but diverges thereafter.[15,51] Similar to TCA-3, the human I-309 cDNA also encodes a 92 amino acid protein and contains a N-linked glycan attachment site.[50-51] Both TCA-3 and I-309 contain an extra pair of cysteine residues that are not found in most C-X-C or C-C chemokines. TCA-3 and I-309 are approximately 42% homologous (Fig. 2.2).[51] The product of the TCA-3 and I-309 genes are secreted as a 15-16 kDa glycoprotein. As with the MIP-1s, these two chemokines demonstrate cross-species activity (unpublished observations).

The amino acid sequence of the murine C10 cDNA revealed the primary translation product to be 116 amino acids long including a putative amino terminal signal peptide.[14-18,52-53,58-59] There are no N- or O-linked glycosylation sites within the sequence. The C10 molecule contains an extra pair of cysteine residues not found in the other C-X-C or C-C family members and distinct from the extra cysteine residues found in TCA-3 and I-309. C10 also possess a significant amino terminal extension relative to the other C-C chemokine family members. While other C-C chemokines have an amino terminal region length of 9 to 10 amino acids, the N-terminal region of C10 is 28 amino acids in length. No human homolog of this protein has been described.

Utilizing a combination of HPLC purification and the in vivo detection of eosinophil chemoattractant activity similar to previously described techniques,[60-61] Williams and colleagues[62] initially set forth to identify an eosinophil chemoattractant present in BAL fluids from allergen challenged guinea pigs. The chemokine, eotaxin, was isolated and biochemically purified yielding a single protein band on SDS-PAGE of 8-9 kDa.[62] The amino terminal 37 residues of eotaxin shows the closest homology to MCP-1 (53%), MCP-2 (54%) and MCP-3 (51%). Eotaxin is 37% homologous to MIP-1β, 31% homologous to MIP-1α and 26% homologous to RANTES. This is quite interesting, as adhesion factors and RANTES exhibit the most potent effects on eosinophils. The various molecular masses (8.4, 8.8, 8.2 and 9 kDa) observed for purified adhesion factors may reflect differential glycosylation. The sequence contains no N-linked glycosylation sites but does contain a potential O-linked glycosylation attachment site.

The 3-D structure of MCP-1 has been modeled based on the NMR derived structure of IL-8.[63] While the degree of homology between MCP-1 and IL-8 is quite low, the computer modeling exhibits a high degree of analogous folding and secondary structure.[55,64] These results strongly suggest that C-C chemokines have a similar structure and behavior to C-X-C chemokines in solution. As IL-8 and MCP-1 are predicted to have a similar backbone structure but bind to different receptors, it is believed that specific side chains in the structure control receptor binding and cell specificity. Substitution of amino acid residues 28 and 30 of MCP-1 with the corresponding residues of IL-8 converted the new molecule into a neutrophil, but not monocyte, chemotactic protein.[65] Computer graphic analysis predicts that this substitution would convert the binding groove of MCP-1 to one topographically similar to IL-8. More recent studies have elucidated that part of the 3-D structure of human MIP-1β using solution multidimensional heteronuclear magnetic resonance spectroscopy.[66] As is predicted for MCP-1, the structure of monomeric MIP-1β is similar to that of IL-8. However, the quaternary structures of IL-8 and MIP-1β are entirely distinct and the dimer interface is formed by a completely different set of residues. While the IL-8 molecule is globular, the human MIP-1β molecule is elongated and cylindrical. This may account for the lack of crossbinding and reactivity between C-X-C and C-C chemokines.

C-C CHEMOKINES: GENOMIC STRUCTURE

Many of the human C-C chemokine genes, including MCP-1, MCP-3, RANTES, MIP-1α, MIP-1β and I-309 have been localized and assigned to human chromosome 17q11-q21.[14-18,67-70] In mice, these C-C chemokines have been mapped to chromosome 11 between *Evi-2* and *Hox-2* loci forming a tightly linked cluster with the other members of the family including MIP-1α, MIP-1β and TCA-3.[14-18,51] This region of the mouse chromosome is evolutionarily conserved and corresponds to the q11.2 to q21.1 region of human chromosome 17. While the precise distance between each of these genes has not yet been determined, it seems likely that this family, like the C-X-C chemokines, arose through gene duplication and subsequent divergence. The MCP-1, RANTES, MIP-1α, MIP-1β and I-309 genes consists of three exons and two introns. The first and second introns appear to be conserved within this family and the first intron separates the leader sequence from the mature protein. The first exon contains a 5' untranslated sequence and coding nucleotides for the leader peptide. The second exon encodes the N-terminal half of the mature protein while the third exon encodes the carboxyl region as well as the 3' untranslated region of the protein. The structure of these genes are highly conserved, revealing a similarity in the placement of the second exon, number of exons and intron junctions.[14-18] Studies of the genomic structures of many of the C-C chemokines have not yet been fully investigated. The MCP-1 gene typically generates a single mRNA transcript of 0.8 kb as do many of the C-C chemokines. Recent studies have described that RANTES gene and shown it to span approximately 7.1 kb, being composed of three exons of 133, 112, 1075 bases and two introns of approximately 1.4 and 4.4 kb with the position of the intron/exon boundaries conserved relative to the other C-C chemokine family members.[71]

C-C chemokine cDNAs have been recognized by their characteristic conserved single open reading frames, typical signal sequences in the 5' region, and AT rich sequences in their 3' untranslated regions.[14-18] Expression of mRNA for C-C chemokines in both macrophages and T cells increases rapidly after stimulation, reaches a maximum in 3-4 hours, then in many cases declines. Interestingly, the expression and production of RANTES is quite different from that of the other C-C chemokines. RANTES has been shown to be constitutively expressed by unstimulated T lymphocytes.[14-18,36,72] However, upon pharmacological stimulation with anti-CD3 antibody and lectins, RANTES mRNA and protein expression are dramatically decreased.[36,72] Expression of the other C-X-C and C-C chemokine mRNAs is only observed after cellular activation.[14-18,49,72]

The human genomic MCP-1 DNA has been cloned.[67] The gene comprises three 45, 118 and 478 base pair exons, and two introns of 800 and 385 base pairs in length. There are two putative consensus phorbol ester response sequences (at position -156 and -128) and an NFκB-binding motif (at position -48) in the 5'-flanking region of the MCP-1 gene.[73] The 5'-flanking region of the MCP-1 gene shows no overall sequence similarity with that of the C-X-C genes. However, like IL-8, the mouse and human MCP-1 gene contains several potential binding elements for known nuclear factors including AP-1, AP-2, NF-IL-6 and NFκB.[14-18,51,55] In the rat MCP-1 gene, the AP-1 binding site is involved in the basal expression of the MCP-1 gene but not phorbol-induced gene expression.[55] NF-IL-6 (C/EPB), NF-κB and c-Ets sites have been identified in the promoter for MIP-1α.[15,51,74] More recently, studies examining the human MIP-1α (GOS19) gene transcription revealed that a set of widely-expressed transcription factors of the ICK-1 family affects the MIP-1α promoter.[75] ICK-1A, which normally behaves as a negative regulator of transcription, did not function in this manner in U937 cells.[75] In addition, another binding site, termed the MIP-1α nuclear protein (MNP) site, which overlaps the

ICK-1 site, appears to be an important regulator of MIP-1α transcription.[75] Much less is known about the factors regulating C-C chemokine gene expression than for IL-8. Octamer transcription factor binding site, inteferon consensus sequence, lymphokine decanucleotide core sequence, EIA enhancer core, PU-1 transcription factor binding site, Ig octamer, HIV-1 enhancer, CK-2 transcription factor binding site, SRE core sequence, GASNE negative regulatory element motif, and the HTLV-1 tax response site are but a few possible regulatory elements found within C-C chemokine genes. Approximately 1 kb of DNA from the immediate 5' upstream region of RANTES was sequenced and found to contain a large number of these potential DNA binding elements for tissue specific expression.[71] Much remains to be discovered about the activation elements regulating C-C chemokine expression.

Many different cell types have been shown to produce chemokines in response to a variety of stimuli (Table 2.1). In addition to leukocytes, endothelial cells, fibroblasts, synovial cells, keratinocytes, melanocytes, chondrocytes, astrocytes, hepatocytes and muscle cells can produce C-C chemokines. Chemokine production occurs in response to either exogenous or endogenous stimuli including lectins, LPS, urate crystals, silicon, phorbol esters, antigenic stimulation, anti-CD3 mAb, injurious stimuli, infectious agents and various inflammatory cytokines.[14-18] The role of chemokine production by these various cell populations in biological responses remains to be determined.

C-C CHEMOKINES: BIOLOGICAL ACTIVITIES

The biological properties of many of the C-C chemokines have been identified.[14-18] In contrast to many of the C-X-C chemokines, all of the C-C chemokines have been shown to be potent monocyte/macrophage, but not neutrophil, chemoattractants.[14-18] In addition, MCP-1 can stimulate the monocytes/macrophages to generate and release superoxide anion, ni-

tric oxide, mobilize intracellular calcium, release enzymes and inhibit tumor cell growth (Table 2.2).[14-18] Many of the C-C chemokines tested also appear to induce the migration of peripheral blood T lymphocytes.[76-82] Recent studies within our laboratory show that MCP-1, MCP-2 and MCP-3 are all chemotactic for T cells.[80-82] This is also true for RANTES, MIP-1α, MIP-1β, C10 and fic (see refs. 18, 76-79; unpublished observations). In addition, recent studies from this laboratory have shown that MIP-1α as well as the other C-C chemokines is a potent chemoattractant for natural killer cells.[83] Schall and coworker have reported MIP-1α to be a B cell chemoattractant.[79] Several of the C-C chemokines, namely MCP-1 and RANTES as well as MIP-1α, have potent chemoattraction for basophils and mast cells.[84-89] RANTES, MIP-1α and adhesion factor are also potent chemoattractants for eosinophils.[61-62,90-91] MCP-1 and RANTES as well as MIP-1α have been shown to induce mast cell migration in vitro.[89] In addition, MIP-1α has also been shown to induce histamine release from peritoneal exudate cells, believed to be derived from mast cells.[87]

Chemokine activities are not restricted to chemotaxis; multiple other pro-inflammatory effects have been described. They have been shown to induce granulocyte, mast cell and lymphocyte degranulation; to increase expression of cell adhesion molecules and enhance adhesion to endothelial cells and extracellular matrix proteins; to enhance the cytostatic effects of neutrophils and monocytes on pathogens such as *Candida albicans*; to enhance the cytolytic activity against CTL and NK cell target cells; and to costimulate T cell and antigen presenting cell functions (see refs. 14-18; unpublished observations). In addition, many chemokines selectively recruit leukocytes to sites of injection, supporting an in vivo role for these peptides (Table 2.3).[14-18] We have recently determined that C-C chemokines can modulate the level and isotype of immunoglobulin release by human B cells in combination with anti-μ mAb in the presence or absence of IL-4 (unpublished observations).

Recent studies have proposed that chemokines, rather than remaining in solution, are preferentially immobilized through binding to heparin-containing proteoglycans on cell surfaces or to extracellular matrix proteins at inflammatory sites.[6,92-93] Chemokines are basic proteins, glycosaminoglycan (GAG) binding sites, and their carboxyl termini bind heparin.[92-93] Recent studies have proposed that chemokines, rather than remaining in solution, are preferentially immobilized by binding to proteoglycans on cell surfaces at inflammatory sites or to extracellular matrix proteins.[92-94] The bound chemokines promote "haptotaxis" of leukocytes by triggering adhesion of leukocyte subsets to vascular cell adhesion molecules on endothelial cells; thus facilitating the extravasation of leukocytes from the blood stream.[6]

Several C-C chemokines have been implicated as negative regulators of hematopoiesis.[18] A number of hematopoietic growth factors and cytokines regulate the proliferation and differentiation of hematopoietic stem and progenitor cells in vitro and in vivo. Initial studies using the murine C-C chemokines MIP-1α and MIP-1β demonstrated that MIP-1α, but not MIP-1β, is a specific inhibitor of hematopoietic stem cell proliferation.[95] The addition of 10- to 100-fold excess MIP-1β to the stem cell cultures can specifically block the suppressive effects of MIP-1α.[96-99] Similarly, MCP-1 also are reported to suppress in a dose-dependent fashion colony formation of immature subsets of myeloid progenitor cells stimulated by GM-CSF plus stem cell factor.[98] MIP-1β and RANTES were not suppressive nor were they synergistically suppressive with the other chemokines. Other studies have shown that MIP-1α and MIP-1β each can synergize with GM-CSF and M-CSF to enhance the formation of granulocyte-macrophage colonies by granulocyte/macrophage progenitor cells (CFU-GM), but this needs to be confirmed.[18,99] None of the chemokines directly stimulated colony formation in the absence of CSF, or influenced colony formation by growth factors such as GM-CSF or erythropoietin.

Several studies have demonstrated the expression of C-C chemokines in neoplastic cells.[14-18,100-102] Immune cells must confront a variety of physical and biochemical barriers upon entering a site of tumor development. The mechanisms by which these cells are attracted to tumor tissues remains to be defined. Glioblastoma and melanoma cancer cells were also reported to express MCP-1 mRNA and increased numbers of infiltrating macrophages were observed within tumor sections.[101] Recent studies from this laboratory have shown that a wide variety of tumor cells including breast, kidney, lung and prostate cancers as well as melanomas, sarcomas, lymphomas, myelomas, astrocytomas, glioma, neuroblastoma and neuroglioma produce C-C chemokines either constitutively or upon stimulation with inflammatory cytokines (unpublished observations). A number of these chemokines appear to be cell cycle-dependent tumor growth factors.[103] Transfection with cytokine genes has also been used to define the influence of local production of cytokines on tumors. In particular, transfection of tumor cells to overproduce MCP-1 has been shown to partially or completely inhibit tumor cell growth, without the subsequent development of tumor immunity.[104] RANTES-transfected tumor cells have also been shown to inhibit tumor cell growth (B. Averbrook, personal communication).

C-C CHEMOKINE RECEPTORS

While the following chapter of this book deals with the chemokine receptors, a brief description is required to give a full overview of C-C chemokines. The chemokine receptors belong to the serpentine superfamily of G-protein coupled receptors.[105] Many similarities exist between chemokine receptors and other members of the G-protein coupled receptor family, yet

Table 2.2. *In vitro effects of C-C chemokine family members*

Chemokine	Target	Effect
MCP-1/JE	Monocytes	Chemotaxis; increased superoxide anion release; increased cytosolic Ca^{2+}; increased adhesion to endothelial cells and extracellular matrix proteins; increased N-acetyl β-glucuronaminidase; increased cytostatic augmenting activity; increased intracellular calcium; induced arachidonic acid release, actin polymerization
	T cells	Chemotaxis; enhanced T cell proliferation, actin polymerization
	B cells	Enhanced anti-mu induced proliferation; isotype switching; inhibits IL-4 induced IgE production
	Mast cells	Chemotaxis; histamine release
	Basophils	Chemotaxis; increased histamine release; increased intracellular calcium; increased leukotriene release
	Stem cells	Suppresses colony formation of immature myeloid progenitor
MCP-2	Monocytes	Chemotaxis
	T cells	Chemotaxis
	Mast cells	Chemotaxis; histamine release
MCP-3	Monocytes	Chemotaxis; increased intracellular calcium; induced arachidonic acid release
	T cells	Chemotaxis
	Mast cells	Chemotaxis
MIP-1α	Monocytes	Chemotaxis; increased respiratory burst; increased intracellular calcium
	T cells	Chemotaxis; increased adhesion to extracellular matrix proteins and cytokine-activated endothelial cell monolayers; increased collagenase release; increased CTL killing of tumor cell targets; degranulation; inhibits anti-CD3-mediated proliferation; enhanced antigen-specific T cell proliferation
	B cells	Chemotaxis; enhanced anti-mu induced B cell proliferation; B cell isotype switching; inhibits IL-4induced IgE production
	NK cells	Chemotaxis; increased killing of tumor targets; increased adhesion to extracellular matrix proteins
	Mast cells	Chemotaxis; histamine release
	Eosinophils	Chemotaxis; induces cationic protein release; increased intracellular calcium
	Basophils	Chemotaxis; histamine release
	Stem cells	Suppresses colony formation of immature myeloid progenitor
	Neutrophils	Weak increases in intracellular calcium; increased shape change
MIP-1β	Monocytes	Chemotaxis; degranulation
	T cells	Chemotaxis; increased adhesion to extracellular matrix proteins and cytokine-activated endothelial cell monolayers; actin polymerization
	B cells	Enhanced anti-mu induced B cell proliferation; B cell isotype switching; inhibits IL-4 induced IgE production
	NK cells	Chemotaxis
	Stem cells	Antagonizes anti-proliferative effects of MIP-1α
RANTES	Monocytes	Chemotaxis
	T cells	Chemotaxis; increased adhesion to extracellular matrix proteins and cytokine-activated endothlial cell monolayers; enhanced CD3-mediated T cell proliferation; enhanced antigen-specific T cell proliferation

Table 2.2. (continued)

Chemokine	Target	Effect
	B cells	Enhanced anti-mu induced B cell proliferation; B cell isotype switching; inhibits IL-4 induced IgE production
	Eosinophils	Chemotaxis; increased cell surface CD11b/CD18 expression; increased cationic protein release; increased intracellular calcium
	Basophils	Chemotaxis; increased histamine release
	NK cells	Chemotaxis
TCA-3	Monocytes	Chemotaxis; increased intracellular calcium, nitric oxide production; degranulation; enzyme release; respiratory burst; increased cell adhesion to fibrinogen
	Neutrophils	Chemotaxis; increased intracellular calcium, nitric oxide production; degranulation; enzyme release; respiratory burst; increased cell adhesion to fibrinogen
	Tumor cells	Lymphocyte-independent anti-tumor effect
I-309	Monocytes	Chemotaxis; increased intracellular calcium
	T cells	Chemotaxis
Eotaxin	Eosinophils	Chemotaxis
fic	Monocytes	Chemotaxis
C10	Monocytes	Chemotaxis; increased intracellular calcium
	T cells	Chemotaxis

Table 2.3. In vivo effects of C-C chemokine family members

Chemokine	Biological Effects
MCP-1	Induction of monocyte infiltration in mice, rabbits and rats Induction of human T cell infiltration in SCID mice
MCP-2	Induction of monocyte infiltration in rabbits
MCP-3	Induction of monocyte infiltration in rabbits
MIP-1α/β	Induction of neutrophil infiltration in mice and rabbits Non-prostaglandin mediated fever induction
MIP-1α	Induction of monocyte infiltration in rabbits and rats Non-prostaglandin mediated fever induction Induction of human T cell infiltration in SCID mice
MIP-1β	Induction of monocyte infiltration in rabbits and rats Non-prostaglandin mediated fever induction Induction of human T cell infiltration in SCID mice
RANTES	Induction of eosinophil and monocyte infiltration in mice and dogs Induction of human T cell infiltration in SCID mice
Eotaxin	Induction of eosinophil migration in guinea pigs
fic	Induction of monocyte infiltration in mice
C10	Induction of monocytic infiltration in mice

chemokine receptors initiate unique and specific cellular activities. A number of receptor cDNAs (for chemoattractants from various species) have been cloned and functionally expressed, including IL-8, MIP-1α/RANTES, MCP-1, C5a, PAF, fMLP and an ubiquitous chemokine receptor on red blood cells, known as the Duffy (Fy) antigen.[105-108] Recent studies by Schall, Horuk and co-workers at Genentech[109-111] have demonstrated that a unique chemokine receptor exists on the surface of human red blood cells. This receptor appears even more promiscuous than the IL-8RB and the described β chemokine receptors as it binds both α and β chemokines. Further analysis of this red blood cell receptor has revealed that chemokines fail to bind to erythrocytes that have a Duffy blood group negative phenotype,[112] suggesting that the Duffy antigen may actually be the red cell chemokine receptor. While it is believed that red blood cells are not directly affected by chemokine binding, it is believed that this receptor acts as a sink for excess chemokine leaking into the peripheral circulation. Further characterization of this receptor may provide insight into the role of this receptor in the systemic regulation of cell migration into inflammatory sites.

These receptors are members of the rhodopsin or serpentine receptor superfamily, and have the characteristic seven hydrophobic spanning transmembrane regions. These receptors have been difficult to purify biochemically, but molecular cloning has led to the identification of several chemokine receptors with varying degrees of homology. Several laboratories have initially attempted to define the presence of specific and promiscuous C-C chemokine receptors on various leukocyte populations by evaluating both Ca²⁺ mobilization and radiolabeled ligand binding. Studies by Wang and colleagues[113] have demonstrated that the chemokines MCP-1 and MIP-1α crosscompete for RANTES binding and Ca²⁺ mobilization on human monocytes and monocytic tumor cell lines. However, this competition was unidirectional and RANTES failed to block either MCP-1 or MIP-1α binding or Ca²⁺ mobilization, suggesting that distinct MCP-1 and MIP-1α receptors as well as a shared MCP-1/RANTES and/or MIP-1α/RANTES receptor are present on the surface of monocytes. Similar cross utilization studies were performed on basophils demonstrating that a distinct RANTES receptor and a shared MIP-1α/RANTES receptor are present on the surface of these populations.[11,114] Additional studies using radiolabeled MIP-1α and MIP-1β revealed that they utilize a common MIP receptor on human monocytes and monocytic cell lines.[115] However, the dissociation of activities of MIP-1α and MIP-1β on other cell types such as T lymphocytes and hematopoietic stem cells suggests the existence of unique receptors as well.

To date, two human β chemokine receptors have been identified. Schall and Neote[107] as well as Murphy[108] identified a cDNA from a neutrophil library (CKR1) that could bind MIP-1α with high affinity (approximately 6.5 nM). Ligation of this receptor by MIP-1α and RANTES induces Ca²⁺ mobilization in transfected fibroblasts. This receptor has also been shown to bind MCP-3. Further characterization of the binding specificity of this transfected receptor may elucidate the specificity of this receptor. The relationship of this cloned receptor to the shared receptors detected by Wang and colleagues[113] remains unclear. More recently, Charo and co-workers[116-117] have cloned two alternatively spliced 7-transmembrane domain receptors (MCP-1RA/MCP-1RB) that differ only in their carboxyl-terminal tails and that confer calcium mobilization when expressed in *Xenopus* oocytes.[116] Both receptors have been shown to bind MCP-1, while more recently MCP-1RB has been shown to bind MCP-3.[117] The genomic localization and organization of some of the genes for these receptors as well as of inactive isoforms and psuedogenes have also been established.[105]

Human cytomegalovirus has also been shown to encode several proteins with high similarity to seven transmembrane domain receptors.[118] The product of the US28 gene has been shown to bind C-C chemokines with high affinity. Binding specificity of this receptor is highly promiscuous with many of the C-C chemokines cross competing for receptor binding. Recent studies have also shown that CMV-infected fibroblasts acquire the ability to migrate in response to C-C chemokines while non-infected cells remain inactive (A. Lloyd, personal communication). The role of this receptor in CMV pathogenesis remains to be defined.

A critical and contentious issue about chemokine-receptor interaction is whether the ligands bind to their receptors as monomers or dimers. Published estimates for the affinity of chemokine dimerization place the Kd for dimer dissociation several logs above the 50% effective concentration for biological activity and receptor binding.[119-120] Recent studies using variants of IL-8 have shown that, while these proteins are unable to dimerize in solution, they possess full biological activity. Although these results suggest that dimerization may not be a prerequisite for biological activity, there is contradictory evidence that IL-8 binds to its receptors as dimers even at low concentrations.[121] More recently, studies using N-terminal deletion variants of MCP-1 that prevents dimerization have been shown to antagonize wild type MCP-1 activity and receptor binding.[122] These studies strongly suggest that MCP-1 activates its receptor as a dimer while the monomeric form may act as a dominant negative inhibitor.

Signal transduction through these receptors is believed to operate through G proteins, phosphoinositol hydrolysis, arachidonic acid metabolism and the rapid elevation of diacylglycerol and cytosolic Ca^{2+} levels [as reviewed by Lefkowitz[123]]. Chemokine-receptor interactions initiates a characteristic pattern of responses including shape change, chemotaxis, degranulation and respiratory burst. The only receptor whose signaling mechanism seems to deviate from the general scheme is MCP-1R. MCP-1 stimulation of human monocytes does not result in phosphati-

dylinositol 4,5-biphosphate (PIP_2) turnover and production of inositol 1,4,5-triphosphate (IP_3).[117] Unlike many other ligands, the MCP-1- and MCP-3-induced rise in $[Ca^{2+}]i$ depends on external Ca^{2+}.[122] MCP-2 is also an exception since it does not induce increase in $[Ca^{2+}]i$ when assayed at chemotactic concentrations.[124] The activation of protein kinase C and a number of additional serine/threonine kinases was demonstrated in response to MCP-1, MCP-2 and MCP-3.[124] Studies by Sozzani and colleagues demonstrated that the monocyte chemotactic response induced by MCP-1, RANTES and MIP-1α could be inhibited by C-I, a serine/threonine kinase inhibitor, as well as erbstatin and genistein, tyrosine kinase inhibitors.[124] This suggests that protein phosphorylation is also crucial to the signal transduction of these ligands. More recent studies have shown that RANTES induces the activation of phosphoinositol 3-kinase.[125] However, the physiological role of each of these signaling pathways remains to be determined.

C-C CHEMOKINES: IN VIVO EFFECTS

The most common in vivo study performed to assess chemokine activity is the ability of a given chemokine to recruit leukocytic subpopulations to sites of challenge. In vivo injection of both C-X-C and C-C chemokines into rodent and rabbit models have been shown to induce a number of pro-inflammatory effects (Table 2.3).[14-18] Injections of some of the C-C chemokines such as MIP-1α, MIP-1β, RANTES, MCP-1 and I-309/TCA-3 have been reported to cause edema and a mild early neutrophil accumulation followed by a more prominent monocytic infiltration.[14,16,18,22,40,50,126] In contrast, subcutaneous injection of human MCP-1 into the ears of rats induces a monocytic but not neutrophilic infiltrate beginning as early as 3 hours and peaking by 18-24 hours.[55,126] Purified preparations of mixtures of MIP-1α/β have also been reported to induce local acute neutrophil accumulation at injection sites, whereas intracisternal injection of such mixtures of MIP-1α/β cause an influx of neutrophils into the cerebrospinal fluid by 4-6 hours, followed by a later monocytic infiltrate.[40,56] Intradermal injection of MCP-2 and MCP-3 in rabbits resulted in selective monocyte recruitment in vivo.[126] Guinea pig adhesion has been shown to induce eosinophil accumulation in the skin of intradermally injected guinea pigs while the C-C chemokines RANTES, MIP-1α and MCP-1 were found to be ineffective.[61] More recent studies in mice with severe combined immunodeficiency (SCID) engrafted with human peripheral blood lymphocytes (huPBL-SCID) have demonstrated that human CD3+ T cells migrate by 72 hours into injection sites in response to recombinant preparations of human MIP-1α, MIP-1β, RANTES and MCP-1 (see refs. 81, 127; unpublished observations). The injection of human MCP-1, MIP-1α, MIP-1β and RANTES as well as murine C10 and fic into this chimeric SCID mice also led to an early (4 hours) infiltration by murine macrophages and in some cases neutrophils at 4 hours (see refs. 81, 127; unpublished observations). Additional studies of C-C chemokines in the huPBL-SCID mouse model has revealed that MIP-1β and RANTES promote human T cell trafficking to the thymus and various peripheral lymphoid tissues upon injection into these mice (unpublished observations). Together, the in vivo effects of chemokine injection suggest that chemokines contribute to the development of both acute and chronic inflammatory responses as well as the trafficking of cells to peripheral lymphoid tissues.

C-C CHEMOKINES: INFLAMMATORY DISEASE STATES

In a number of inflammatory, noninflammatory and respiratory disease states, C-C chemokines play a key role in the accumulation of leukocytes at the site of the lesion.[14-18] A number of respiratory disease states exhibit increased C-C chemokine expression at both the protein and RNA levels and both are detected in histological sections and interstitial lung fluids as well as associated with increased neutrophils and monocytes present within the lung compared to normal lavage controls.[11,14,16,18,55] These disease states include idiopathic pulmonary fibrosis, active sarcoidosis and bronchial carcinoma.[11,128] Studies examining *Pseudomonas*-induced airway inflammation in cystic fibrosis patients revealed the presence of significant levels of MCP-1 in both bronchoalveolar lavage (BAL) fluid and sputum specimens.[128-130] The levels of MCP-1 in lung tissue correlated with the severity of pulmonary disease. MCP-1 mRNA and protein levels are increased in a number of respiratory disease states.[128] Elevated levels of these chemokines have also been detected in histological sections and interstitial lung fluids, and were associated with neutrophilic and monocytic infiltrates within the lungs of respiratory disease patients.[128-134] IPF is an immunologically-mediated lung disorder characterized by the sequestration of activated neutrophils and macrophages in the distal airspace. An increase in the number of macrophages and neutrophils in the BAL fluids and lung tissues have been demonstrated in IPF patients.[128,133-134] Cells isolated from the lungs of active IPF patients were found to express increased levels of MCP-1 mRNA as well as cell-associated protein while healthy nonsmoking volunteers failed to express any steady-state levels of MCP-1 mRNA.[128,134] Additionally, immunohistochemical analysis of lung tissues and cells isolated from BAL fluids demonstrated a strong correlation between MCP-1 antigen expression, monocyte accumulation and disease activity. The levels of these chemokines dropped significantly with disease resolution. Additionally, patients undergoing rejection of a lung transplant showed an increase in MCP-1 expression by day 3 and peaking by day 6.[11,128] MCP-1 and other C-C chemokines have also been observed in patients with pneumonia, respiratory distress syndrome, lung injury, immune complex-induced alveolitis and pulmonary granulomatosis.[135-137]

The release of LPS during a bacterial infection results in the sequential release of IL-1 and TNF by the host leading to the accumulation of leukocytes in several organ systems.[138-139] Chemokines have been associated with the neutrophilic influx into organs during endotoxemia.[140-141] In experimentally induced inflammation, MCP-1 and RANTES as well as C-X-C chemokines can be detected in the plasma at concentrations up to 5-10 ng/ml.[146-148] In addition, the presence of chemokines in plasma and BAL fluids correlated to influx of leukocytes in the lung as well as lung capillary leakage. Furthermore, the presence of these chemokines also correlated with early mortality due to endotoxemia. Perhaps the most characterized murine sepsis model involves the bolus i.p. injection of LPS resulting in a systemic sepsis response including cachexia, granulocytosis, multiple organ failure and eventually death as well as the accumulation of neutrophils in several organ systems.[139,141] C-C chemokines were found to be upregulated in the lungs of mice after LPS injection.[141-142,144-145] The presence of MIP-1α and RANTES correlated with the accumulation of mononuclear phagocytes within the lungs of LPS challenged mice. Pretreatment of mice with antibodies to these chemokines significantly inhibited the influx of lung macrophages but not neutrophils or lymphocytes at 24 hours post-LPS challenge.[144-145] In addition, administration of a mixture of murine MIP-1α and MIP-1β had a pyrogenic effect in rabbits, suggesting a role for chemokines in fever induction.[146] In contrast to IL-1- and TNF-induced fevers, the pyrogenic effects of MIP-1α/β were found to be prostaglandin-independent. These results suggest that C-C chemokines play a role in septic responses leading to monocytic accumulation as well as a possible role in mediating fever development.

Rheumatoid arthritis is characterized by persistent synovial inflammation, destruction of bone and cartilage and numerous systemic manifestations.[147] Chemokines are produced within the inflamed synovial tissues that are believed to account for a number of the pathological and clinical manifestations of rheumatoid arthritis.[128] The mechanism by which monocytes, lymphocytes and neutrophils are recruited into inflamed synovial tissue has not been fully elucidated. Several laboratories have shown that high levels of MCP-1, MIP-1α and RANTES are present in the synovial fluids of inflamed joints of patients with rheumatic diseases, including rheumatoid arthritis, osteoarthritis and gout.[128,141,148-150] The monocyte chemotactic activity of these synovial fluids did not correlate with the levels of each of these chemokines, suggesting that all of these chemokines participate in the chemotactic activity of these rheumatoid samples. Synovial fluids and sera from rheumatoid arthritis, but not osteoarthritis, have subsequently been shown to possess increased levels of MCP-1, MIP-1α and RANTES, which presumably accounts for the increased numbers of neutrophils and monocytes in collected fluids.[148-150] A recent study by Koch et al has described the preferential production of MIP-1β in the synovial fluids of osteo- but not rheumatoid-arthritic patients (Robert Strieter, personal communication). While the precise role of this C-C chemokine in these arthritic lesions remains to be defined, these findings suggest that chemokine production may play an important role in the recruitment of neutrophils and macrophages to RA synovial tissues and that synovial macrophages may be the primary source of these chemokines. Similarly, analysis of type II collagen-induced arthritis in mice has demonstrated a correlation between the expression of MIP-1α and MCP-1 with the onset and severity of clinical disease.[151] Depletion of these chemokines by administration of antichemokine antisera decreased the influx of monocytes to the joint and delayed the onset of joint inflammation. The above studies indicate that disruption of monocyte accumulation could significantly alter the onset and severity of joint inflammation.

Granulomatous lesions are typically characterized by the infiltration of various mononuclear cells, depending on the stage of the disease, resulting in prolonged inflammation, tissue destruction and fibrosis.[152] The selective infiltration of mononuclear cells into these lesions suggests a role for C-C chemokines in granuloma development. Studies by Lukacs and colleagues have demonstrated that significant levels of MIP-1α mRNA and protein are expressed in the primary (acute) and secondary (chronic) lesions of *Schistosoma mansoni* egg-induced granulomatous inflammation.[153-154] Treatment of *S. mansoni*-infected mice with polyclonal antimouse MIP-1α abrogated the development of granuloma formation in acutely, but not chronically, infected mice. Mononuclear phagocytes were found to be the primary source of MIP-1α in these lesions as determined by immunohistological analysis.[153] These results suggest that MIP-1α plays a greater role in leukocyte recruitment during primary rather than secondary granuloma formation. In contrast, additional studies examining JE in primary and secondary granulomas revealed that JE mRNA and protein were strongly expressed in lungs of secondary but less so in primary granulomas.[154-155] In contrast to MIP-1α, neutralization of JE in vivo with specific antisera decreased the formation of secondary, but not primary lesions.[155] Smooth muscle cells were shown to be the primary source of JE in these secondary granulomas. In a β-glucan-induced model of granuloma formation, rat MCP-1 has also been shown to mediate mononuclear cell recruitment as well as granuloma formation in vivo.[156] The differential expression of chemokines during the various stages of inflammation may indicate a differential role of chemokines during disease development.

Recent support has been given to the hypothesis that arteriosclerosis may be an inflammatory disease initiated injury of the blood vessel wall and mediated by the production of chemokines and other cytokines in areas of arterial damage. Chemokines attract and activate monocytes to associate with the arterial plaque.[157] In situ analysis of intact rat aortas subjected to balloon dilation demonstrated rapid expression of high levels of the mRNA of JE.[158-159] Interestingly, this same report demonstrates that JE appears to be a chemoattractant for vascular smooth muscle cells. Additional reports have demonstrated, using in situ analysis, that in human carotid endarterectomy specimens, MCP-1 is detected only in diseased but not normal arteries.[160-161] MCP-1 was detected primarily in macrophage-rich regions underlying the necrotic core of the plaque and in organizing thrombi. Expression appeared to be detected only in localized smooth muscle cells and not in endothelium. Similarly, MCP-1 has also been detected in the proliferative neointimal lesions of heart transplant developing arteriosclerosis.[162-163] A role for MCP-1 in the initiation of atherosclerotic lesions was further supported by a recent study looking at hypercholesterolemic primates.[164] Using in situ hybridization techniques, primates fed high levels of cholesterol were demonstrated to express increased levels of MCP-1 in vascular smooth muscle cells and on the inner surfaces of lesions within the arteries. A report by Schall[15] has described the presence of high levels of mRNA specific for MIP-1α, MIP-1β and RANTES in normal carotid plaques, atherosclerotic lesions and in atherosclerosing allogeneic heart transplant.

C-C chemokines have been identified in a number of inflammatory disease states. Elevated levels of MCP-1 can also be detected in skin cells and biopsies and are believed to be present in scales of psoriatic lesions.[11,165] MCP-1 has also been detected in adult periodontal disease, inflammatory gingivitis, inflammatory bowel disease, gastritis and in the circulation of patients with post major surgery, nephritis, septic shock, endometritis and in various peritonitis models.[14-18,166-173] Human fat storing cells have also been shown to express MCP-1 upon stimulation with IL-1, IFN-γ and TNF.[174] It is believed that MCP-1 release from fat storing cells in the liver may participate in the recruitment and activation of monocytes at sites of liver injury. MCP-1 has also been recently shown to be expressed in dermal wound repair.[171] It is likely that more C-C chemokines will be detected at many inflammatory sites when probes and antibodies become available. It should be noted that the presence of chemokines in various inflammatory states does not indicate that they play a role in disease progression or resolution. Additional studies are required using chemokine-specific antagonists and antibodies to better characterize their role in these various disease states.

SUMMARY

The C-C chemokines comprise a subfamily of small secreted chemotactic proteins that with the exception of RANTES are not expressed in resting cells but are rapidly induced in response to various inflammatory and mitogenic stimuli. These proteins are believed to function primarily as chemoattractants and activating agents for inflammatory cells. At present, it appears that each of the C-C chemokines have both unique and overlapping activities. C-C chemokines are implicated as major participants in acute as well as chronic inflammatory reactions and inhibition of hematopoiesis. C-C chemokines that act on monocytes and T lymphocytes presumably influence the recruitment of immunocompetent cells to inflammatory sites. There is recent evidence from this laboratory demonstrating that C-C chemokines play a role in the induction of immune reactions and promote the effector limb of immunity. The likely possibility that C-C chemokines may also contribute to the normal homing and distribution of leukocytes also needs to be evaluated. These chemokines obviously have major differentiative effects on the functions of target cells and appear to act as costimulants of leukocyte and tumor cell growth. Finally, C-C chemokines are attractive targets for the development of new anti-inflammatory agents. Inhibition of their activities may be an effective anti-inflammatory strategy

while promoting their activity might enhance wound healing and tissue repair.

REFERENCES

1. Colditz IG. Margination and emigration of leukocytes. Surv Synth Pathol Res 1985; 4:44.
2. Ward P. Leukotaxis and leukotactic disorders. Am J Pathol 1974; 77:520.
3. Butcher EC. Leukocyte-endothelial cell recognition: Three (or more) steps to specificity and diversity. Cell 1991; 67:1033.
4. Springer TA. Traffic signals for lymphocyte recirculation and leukocyte emigration: the multistep paradigm. Cell 1994; 76:301.
5. Carlos TM. Leukocyte-endothelial adhesion molecules. Blood 1994; 84:2068.
6. Shimizu Y, Newman W, Tanaka Y, Shaw S. Lymphocyte interactions with endothelial cells. Immunol Today 1992; 13:106.
7. El-Naggar AK, Van Epps DE, Williams RC Jr. Effect of culturing on the human lymphocyte locomotion response to casein, C5a, and fMet-Leu-Phe. Cell Immunol 1981; 60:43.
8. Schiffmann E, Corcoran BA, Wahl SM. Formylmethionyl peptides as chemoattractants for leukocytes. Proc Natl Acad Sci USA 1975; 72:1059-1066.
9. Lewis RA, Austen KF. The biologically active leukotrienes. J Clin Invest 1984; 73:889.
10. Heagy W, Laurance M, Cohen E, Finberg R. Neurohormones regulate T cell function. J Exp Med 1990; 171:1625.
11. Taub DD, Oppenheim JJ. Review of the chemokine meeting: The third international symposium of chemotactic cytokines. Cytokine 1993; 5(3):175.
12. Baggiolini M. Chemotactic and inflammatory cytokines—C-X-C and C-C proteins. In: Westwick J, Kunkel S, Lindley IJD, eds. Chemotactic Cytokines: Biology of the Inflammatory Peptide Gene Superfamily. London: Plenum Press, 1991:1-11.
13. Matsushima K, Morishita K, Yoshimura T, Lavu S, Kobayashi Y, Lew W, Appella E, Kung HF, Leonard EJ, Oppenheim JJ. Molecular cloning of cDNA for a human monocyte derived neutrophil chemotactic factor (MDNCF) and the induction of

MDNCF mRNA by interleukin-1 and tumor necrosis factor. J Exp Med 1988; 167:1883.

14. Oppenheim JJ, Zachariae COC, Mukaida N, Matsushima K. Properties of the novel proinflammatory supergene "intercrine" cytokine family. Ann Rev Immunol 1991; 9:617.

15. Schall TJ. Biology of the rantes/sis cytokine family. Cytokine 1991; 3:165.

16. Baggiolini M, Dewald B, Moser B. Interleukin-8 and related chemotactic cytokines—C-X-C and C-C Chemokines. Adv Immunol 1994; 55:97.

17. Matsushima K, Baldwin ET, Mukaida N. Interleukin-8 and MCAF: Novel leukocyte recruitment and activating cytokines. Chem Immunol 1992; 51:236.

18. Taub DD, Oppenheim JJ. Chemokines, inflammation and the immune system. Ther Immunol 1994; 1:229.

19. Taub DD, Lloyd AR, Conlon K, Wang JM, Ortaldo JR, Harada A, Matsushima K, Kelvin DJ, Oppenheim JJ. Recombinant human interferon-inducible protein 10 is a chemoattractant for human monocytes and T lymphocytes and promotes T cell adhesion to endothelial cells. J Exp Med 1993; 177:1809.

20. Senior RM, Griffin GL, Huang JS, Walz DA, Deuel TF. Chemotactic activity of platelet alpha granule proteins for fibroblasts. J Cell Biol 1983; 96:283.

21. Yoshimura T, Robinson EA, Tanaka S, Appella E, Kuratsu J-I, Leonard EJ. Purification and amino acid analysis of two human glioma-derived monocyte chemoattractants. J Exp Med 1989; 169:1449.

22. Robinson EA, Yoshimura T, Leonard EJ, Tanaka S, Griffin PR, Shabanowitz J, Hunt DF, Appella E. Complete sequence of a human monocyte chemoattractant, a putative mediator of cellular immune reactions. Proc Natl Acad Sci USA 1989; 86:1850.

23. Yoshimura T, Yuhki N, Moore SK, Appella E, Lerman MI, Leonard EJ. Human monocyte chemoattractant protein-1 (MCP-1): Full-length cDNA cloning, expression in mitogen-stimulated blood mononuclear leukocytes, and sequence similarity to mouse competence gene JE. FEBS Lett 1989;

244:487.

25. Matsushima K, Larsen CG, DuBois GC, Oppenheim JJ. Purification and characterization of a novel monocyte chemotactic and activating factor produced by a human myelomonocytic cell line. J Exp Med 1989; 169:1485.

24. Furutani Y, Nomura H, Notake M, Oyamada Y, Fukue T, Yamada M, Larsen CG, Oppenheim JJ, Matsushima K. Cloning and sequencing of the cDNA for human monocyte chemotactic and activating factor (MCAF). Biochem Biophys Res Comm 1989; 159:249.

25. Matsushima K, Larsen CG, DuBois GC, Oppenheim JJ. Purification and characterization of a novel monocyte chemotactic and activating factor produced by a human myelomonocytic cell line. J Exp Med 1989; 169:1485.

26. Rollins BJ, Morrison ED, Stiles CD. Cloning and expression of JE, a gene inducible by platelet-derived growth factor and whose product has cytokine-like properties. Proc Natl Acad Sci USA 1988; 85:3738.

27. Yoshimura T. cDNA cloning of guinea pig monocyte chemoattractant protein-1 and expression of the recombinant protein. J Immunol 1993; 150:5025.

28. Yoshimura T, Leonard EJ. Interleukin 8 (NAP-1) and related chemotactic cytokines. In: Baggiolini M, Sorg C, ed. Cytokine. Vol. 4. Basel: Karger, 131-152.

29. Yoshimura T, Yuhki N. Neutrophil attractant/activating protein-1and monocyte chemoattractant protein-1 in rabbit: cDNA cloning and their expression in spleen cells. J Immunol 1991; 146:3483.

30. Yoshimura T, Takeya M, Takahashi K. Molecular cloning of rat monocyte chemoattractant protein-1 (MCP-1) and its expression in rat spleen cells and tumour cell lines. Biochem Biophys Res Commun 1991; 174:504.

31. Van Damme J, Proost P, Lenaerts J-P, Opdenakker G. Structural and functional identification of two human, tumor-derived monocyte chemotactic proteins (MCP-2 and MCP-3) belonging to the chemokine family. J Exp Med 1992; 176:59.

32. Opdenakker G, Froyen G, Fiten P, Proost

P, Van Damme J. Human monocyte chemotactic protein-3 (MCP-3): molecular cloning of the cDNA and comparison with other chemokines. Biochem Biophys Res Commun 1993; 191:535.

33. Chang HC, Hsu F, Freeman GJ, Griffin JD, Reinherz EL. Cloning andexpression of a γ-interferon-inducible gene in monocytes: a new member of a cytokine gene family. Int Immunol 1989; 1:388.

34. Thirrion S, Nys G, Fiten P, Masure S, Van Damme J, Opendaker G. Mouse macrophage derived chemotactic protein-3: cDNA cloning and identification as MARC/FIC. Biochem Biophys Res Commun 1994; 201:493.

35. Heinrich JN, Ryseck RP, MacDonald-Bravo H, Bravo R. The product of a novel growth factor-activated gene, fic, is a biologically active "C-C"-type cytokine. Mol Cell Biol 1993; 13:2020.

36. Schall TJ, Jongstra J, Dyer BJ, Jorgenson J, Clayberger C, Davis MM, Krensky AM. A human T cell-specific molecule is a member of a new gene family. J Immunol 1988; 141:1018.

37. Kameyoshi Y, Dorschner A, Mallet AI, Christophers E, Schroder JM. Cytokine RANTES released by thrombin-stimulated platelets is a potent attractant for human eosinophils. J Exp Med 1992; 176:587.

38. Schall TJ, Simpson NJ, Mak JY. Molecular cloning and expression of the murine RANTES cytokine: structural and functional conservation between mouse and man. Eur J Immunol 1992; 22:1477.

39. Rovin BH, Yoshimura T, Tan L. Cytokine-induced production of monocyte chemoattractant protein-1 by cultured human mesangial cells. J Immunol 1992; 148:2148.

40. Wolpe SD, Davatelis G, Sherry B, Beutler B, Hesse DG, Nguyen HT, Moldawer LL, Nathan CF, Lowry SF, Cerami A. Macrophages secrete a novel heparin-binding protein with inflammatory and neutrophil chemokinetic properties. J Exp Med 1988; 167:570.

41. Sherry B, Tekamp-Olson P, Gallegos C, Bauer D, Davatelis G, Wolpe SD, Masiarz F, Cort D, Cerami A. Resolution of the two components of macrophage inflammatory protein 1, and cloning and characterization of one of those components, macrophage inflammatory protein 1β. J Exp Med 1988; 168:2251.

42. Davatelis G, Tekamp-Olson P, Wolpe SD, Hermsen K, Luedke C, Gallegos C, Coit D, Merryweather J, Cerami A. Cloning and characterization of a cDNA for murine macrophage inflammatory protein (MIP), a novel monokine with inflammatory and chemokine properties. J Exp Med 1988; 167:1939.

43. Nakao M, Nomiyama H, Shimada K. Structures of human genes coding for cytokine LD78 and their expression. Mol Cell Biol 1990; 10:3646.

44. Widmer U, Yang Z, Van Deventer S, Manogue KR, Sherry B, Cerami A. Genomic structure of murine macrophage inflammatory protein-1-alpha and conservation of potential regulatory sequences with a human homolog, LD78. J Immunol 1991; 146:4031.

45. Napolitano M, Modi WS, Cevario SJ, Gnarra JR, Seuanez HN, Leonard WJ. The gene encoding the Act-2 cytokine. J Biol Chem 1991; 266:17531.

46. Chang HC, Reinherz EL. Isolation and characterization of a cDNA encoding a putative cytokine which is induced by stimulation via the CD2 structure on human T lymphocytes. Eur J Immunol 1989; 19:1045.

47. Sporn SA, Eierman DF, Johnson CE, Morris J, Martin G, Ladner M, Haskill S. Monocyte adherence results in the selective induction of novel genes sharing homology with mediators of inflammation and tissue repair. J Immunol 1990; 144:4434.

48. Burd PR, Freeman GJ, Wilson SD, Berman M, DeKruyff R, Billings PR, Dorf ME. Cloning and charcaterization of a novel T cell activation gene. J Immunol 1987; 139:3126.

49. Brown KD, Zurawski SM, Mossmann TR, Zurawaski G. A family of small inducible proteins secreted by leukocytes are members of a new superfamily that includes leukocyte and fibroblast inflammatory agents, growth factors, and indicators of various activation processes. J Immunol 1989; 142:679.

50. Miller MD, Hata S, Maleyft RDW, Krangel MS. A novel polypeptide secreted by activated T lymphocytes. J Immunol 1989; 143:2907.

51. Miller MD, Krangel MS. Biology and biochemistry of the chemokines: A family of chemotactic and inflammatory cytokines. Crit Rev Immunol 1992; 12:17.

52. Orlofsky A, Berger MS, Prystowsky MB. Novel expression pattern of a new member of the MIP-1 family of cytokine-like genes. Cell Regulation 1991; 2:403.

53. Berger MS, Orlofsky A, Kleyman TR, Coupaye-Gerard B, Eisner D, Cohen SA. The chemokine C10: Immunological analysis of the sequence encoded by the novel second exon. (submitted for publication)

54. Youn B-S, Jang I-K, Broxmeyer HE, Cooper S, Jenkins N, Gilbert D, Copeland NG, Elick TA, Fraser MJ Jr, Kwon BS. A novel chemokine, macrophage inflammatory protein-related protein-2, inhibits colony formation of bone marrow myeloid progenitors. J Immunol 1995; 155:2661.

55. Matsushima K, Baldwin ET, Mukaida N. In: Kishimoto T, ed. Interleukins: Molecular Biology and Immunology. Vol. 51. Basel: Karger, 1992:236-265.

56. Wolpe SD, Cerami A. Macrophage inflammatory proteins 1 and 2: members of a novel superfamily of cytokines. FASEB J 1989: 3:2565.

57. Irving SG, Zipfel PF, Balke J, McBride OW, Morton CC, Burd PR, Siebenlist U, Kelly K. Two inflammatory mediator cytokine genes are closely linked and variably amplified on chromosome 17q. Nucleic Acid Res 1989; 18:3261.

58. Berger MS, Kozak CA, Prystowsky MB. The gene for C10, a member of the beta chemokine family, is located on mouse chromosome 11 and contains a novel second exon not found in other chemokines. DNA Cell Biol 1993; 12:839.

59. Orlofsky A, Lin EY, Prystowsky MB. Selective induction of the beta chemokine C10 by IL-4 in mouse macrophages. J Immunol 1994; 152:5084.

60. Collins PD, Jose PJ, Williams TJ. The sequential generation of neutrophil chemoattractant proteins in acute infalmmation

in the rabbit in vivo: relationship between C5a and a protein with the charcateristics of IL-8. J Immunol 1991; 146:677.

61. Jose PJ, Collins PD, Perkins JA, Beaubein NF, Totty NF, Waterfield MD, Hsuan J, Williams TJ. Identification of a second neutrophil chemoattractant cytokine generated during an inflammatory reaction in the rabbit peritoneal cavity in vivo: purification, partial amino acid sequence and structural relationship to melanoma growth stimulating activity. Biochem J 1991; 278:493.

62. Jose PJ, Griffiths-Johnson DA, Collins PD, Walsh DT, Moqbel R, Totty NF, Truong O, Hsuan JJ, Williams TJ. Eotaxin: A potent eosinophil chemoattractant cytokine detected in a guinea pig model of allergic airways inflammation. J Exp Med 1994; 179:881.

63. Clore GM, Gronenborn AM. NMR and X-ray analysis of the three dimentional structure of interleukin-8 In: Baggiolini M, Sorg C, eds. Cytokine. Vol. 4. Basel:Karger, 18-40.

64. Gronenborn AM, Clore GM. Modeling the three dimentional structure of the monocyte chemoattractant and activating factor MCAF/MCP-1 on the basis of the solution structure of interleukin-8. Protein Eng 1991; 4:263.

65. Beall CJ, Sangeeta M, Kolattukudy E. 1992. Conversion of monocyte chemoattractant protein-1 into a neutrophil attractant by substitution of two amino acids. J Biol Chem 267:3455.

66. Lodi PJ, Garrett DS, Kuszewski J, Tsang ML-S, Weatherbee JA, Leonard WJ, Gronenborn AM, Clore GM. High resolution solution structure of the β chemokine MIP-1β by multidimensional NMR. Science 1994; 263:1762.

67. Mehrabian M, Sparkes RS, Mohandas T, Fogelman AM, Lusis A. Localization of monocyte chemotactic protein-1 gene (SCYA2) to human chromosome 17q11.2-q21.1. Genomics 1991; 9:200.

68. Irving SG, Zipfel PF, Balke J, McBride OW, Morton CC, Burd PR, Siebenlist U, Kelly K. Two inflammatory mediator cytokine genes are closely linked and variably ampli-

fied on chromosome 17q. Nucleic Acid Res 1990; 18:3261.

69. Donlon TA, Krensky AM, Wallace MR, Collins FS, Lovett M, Clayberger C. Localization of a human T cell-specific gene, RANTES (D17S136E), to chromosome 17q11.2-q12. Genomics 1990; 6:548.

70. Miller MD, Wilson SD, Dorf ME, Seuanez HN, O'Brien SJ, Krangel MS. Sequence and chromosomal localization of the I309 gene: Relationship to genes encoding a family of inflammatory cytokines. J Immunol 1990; 145:2737-2744.

71. Nelson PJ, Kim HT, Manning WC, Goralski TJ, Krensky AM. Genomic organization and transcriptional regulation of the RANTES chemokine gene. J Immunol 1993; 151:2601.

72. Conlon K, Lloyd A, Chattopadhyay U, Lukacs N, Kunkel S, Schall T, Taub D, Morimoto C, Osborne J, Oppenheim J, Young H, Kelvin D, Ortaldo J. CD8+ and CD45RA+ human peripheral blood lymphocytes are potent sources of macrophage inflammatory protein-1α, interleukin-8 and RANTES. Eur J Immunol 1995; 25:751.

73. Li Y-S, Kolattukudy E. Functional role of the cis-acting elements in human monocyte chemotactic protein-1 gene in the regulation of its expression by phorbol ester in human glioblastoma cells. Mol Cell Biochem 1994; 141:121.

74. Grove M, Plumb M. C/EBP, NF-κB, and c-Ets family members and transcriptional regulation of the cell-specific and inducible macrophage inflammatory protein 1α immediate-early gene. Mol Cell Biol 1993; 13:5276.

75. Ritter LM, Bryans M, Abdo O, Sharma V, Wilkie NM. MIP-1α nuclear protein (MNP), a novel transcription factor expressed in hematopoetic cells that is crucial for transcription of the human MIP-1α gene. Mol Cell Biol 15:3110.

76. Schall TJ, Bacon K, Toy KI, Goedell DV. Selective attraction of monocytes and T lymphocytes of the memory phenotype by the cytokine RANTES. Nature 1990; 347:669.

77. Taub DD, Conlon K, Lloyd AR, Oppenheim JJ, Kelvin DJ. Preferential migration of activated CD4+ and CD4+ T cells in re-

sponse to MIP-1α and MIP-1β. Science 1993; 260:355.

78. Tanaka Y, Adams DH, Hubscher S, Hirano H, Siebenlist U, Shaw S. T cell adhesion induced by proteoglycan-immobilized cytokine MIP-1β. Nature 1993; 361:81.

79. Schall TJ, Bacon K, Camp RDR, Kaspari JW, Goeddel DV. Human macrophage inflammatory protein-1α (MIP-1α) and MIP-1β chemokines attract distinct populations of lymphocytes. J Exp Med 1993; 177:1821.

80. Carr MW, Roth SJ, Luther E, Rose SS, Springer TA. Monocyte chemoattractant protein 1 acts as a T lymphocyte chemoattractant. Proc Natl Acad SCi USA 1994; 91:3652.

81. Taub DD, Proost P, Murphy WJ, Anver M, Longo DL, Van Damme J, Oppenheim JJ. Monocyte chemotactic protein-1 (MCP-1), -2, and -3 are chemotactic for human T lymphocytes. J Clin Invest 1995; 95:1370.

82. Loetscher P, Seitz M, Clark-Lewis I, Baggiolini M, Moser B. Monocyte chemotactic proteins MCP-1, MCP-2, and MCP-3 are major attractants for human CD4+ and CD8+ T lymphocytes. FASEB J 1994; 8:1055.

83. Taub DD, Sayers T, Carter C, Ortaldo J. α and β Chemokines induce NK cell migration and enhance NK cell cytolytic activity via cellular degranulation. J Immunol 1995; in press.

84. Kuna P, Reddigari SR, Rucinski D, Oppenheim JJ, Kaplan AP. Monocyte chemotactic and activating factor is a potent histamine-releasing factor for basophils. J Exp Med 1992; 175:489.

85. Kuna P, Reddigari SR, Schall TJ, Rucinski D, Viksman MY, Kaplan AP. RANTES, a monocyte and T lymphocyte chemotactic cytokine releases histamine from human basophils. J Immunol 1992; 149:636.

86. Bischoff SC, Krieger M, Brunner T, Rot A, Tscharner Vv, Baggiolini M, Dahinden CA. RANTES and related chemokines activate human basophil granulocytes through different G protein-coupled receptors. Eur J Immunol 1993; 23:761.

87. Alam R, Forsythe PA, Stafford S, Lett-

Brown MA, Grant JA. Macrophage inflammatory protein-1α activates basophils and mast cells. J Exp Med 1992; 176:781.

88. Kuna P, Reddigari SR, Schall TJ, Rucinski D, Sadick M, Kaplan AP. Characterization of the human basophil response to cytokines, growth factors, and histamine releasing factors of the intercrine/chemokine family. J Immunol 1993; 150:1932.

89. Taub DD, Dastych J, Inamura N, Upton J, Kelvin D, Metcalfe D, Oppenheim JJ. Bone marrow-derived murine mast cells migrate, but do not degranulate, in response to chemokines. J Immunol 1995; 154:2393.

90. Rot A, Krieger M, Brunner T, Bischoff SC, Schall TJ, Dahinden CA. RANTES and macrophage inflammatory protein 1α induce the migration and activation of normal human eosinophil granulocytes. J Exp Med 1992; 176:1489.

91. Kameyoshi Y, Dorschner A, Mallet AI, Christophers E, Schroder JM. Cytokine RANTES released by thrombin-stimulated platelets is a potent attractant for human eosinophils. J Exp Med 1992; 176:587.

92. Rot A. Endothelial binding of NAP-1/IL-8: role in neutrophil emigration. Immunol Today 1992; 13:291.

93. Rot A. Chemokines link the two steps of leukocyte adhesion to endothelium. Immunologist 1993; 1(5):145.

94. Webb LMC, Ehrengruber MU, Clark-Lewis I, Baggiolini M, Rot A. Binding of heparin sulfate or heparin enhances neutrophil responses to interleukin-8. Proc Natl Acad Sci USA 1993; 90:7158.

95. Graham GJ, Pragnell IB. SCI/MIP-1α: A potent stem cell inhibitor with potential roles in development. Development Biology 1992; 151:377.

96. Maze R, Sherry B, Kwon S, Cerami A, Broxmeyer HE. Myelosuppressive effects in vivo of purified recombinant murine macrophage inflammatory protein-1α. J Immunol 1992; 149:1004.

97. Broxmeyer HE, Sherry B, Cooper S, Ruscetti FW, Williams DE, Arosio P, Kwon BS, Cerami A. Macrophage inflammatory protein (MIP)-1β abrogates the capacity of MIP-1α to suppress myeloid progenitor cell growth. J Immunol 1991; 147:2586.

98. Broxmeyer HE, Sherry B, Cooper S, Lu L, Maze R, Beckmann MP, Cerami A, Ralph P. Comparative analysis of the human macrophage inflammatory protein family of cytokines (chemokines) on proliferation of human myeloid progenitor cells: Interacting effects involving suppression, synergistic suppression, and blocking suppression. J Immunol 1993; 150:3448.

99. Broxmeyer HE, Sherry B, Lu L, Cooper S, Carow C, Wolpe SD, Cerami A. Myelopoietic enhancing effects of murine macrophage inflammatory proteins 1 and 2 in vitro on colony formation by murine and human bone marrow granulocyte-macrophage progenitor cells. J Exp Med 1989; 170:1583.

100. Graves DT, Jiang YL, Williamson MJ, Valente AJ. Identification of monocyte chemotactic activity produced by malignant cells. Science 1989; 245:1490.

101. Kuratsu J, Yoshizato K, Leonard EJ, Takeshima H, Ushio Y. Quantitative study of monocyte chemoattractant protein-1 (MCP-1) in cerebrospinal fluid and cyst fluid from patients with malignant glioma. JNCI 1993; 85(22):1836.

102. Negus RPM, Stamp GW, Relf MG, Burke F, Malik STA, Bernasconi S, Allavena P, Sozzani S, Mantovani A, Balkwill FR. The detection and localization of monocyte chemoattractant protein-1 (MCP-1) in human ovarian cancer. J Clin Invest 1995; 95:2391.

103. Richmond A, Lawson DH, Nixon DW, Chawla RK. Characterization of autostimulatory and transforming growth factors from human melanoma cells. Cancer Res 1986; 45:6390.

104. Bottazzi B, Walter S, Govoni D, Colotta F, Mantovani A. Monocyte chemotactic cytokine gene transfer modulates macrophage infiltration, growth, and susceptibility to IL-2 therapy of a murine melanoma. J Immunol 1992; 148:1280.

105. Kelvin DJ, Michiel D, Johnston JA, Lloyd AR, Sprenger H, Oppenheim JJ, Wang JM. Chemokines and Serpentines: The molecular biology of chemokine receptors. J Leuk Biol 1993; 54:604.

106. Murphy PM, Tiffany HL. Cloning of

complementary DNA encoding a functional interleukin-8 receptor. Science 1991; 253:1280.

107. Neote K, DiGregorio D, Mak JY, Horuk R, Schall TJ. Molecular cloning, functional expression, and signaling characteristics of a C-C chemokine receptor. Cell 1993; 72:415.

108. Gao J-L, Kuhns DB, Tiffany HL, McDermott, Li X, Francke U, Murphy PM. Structure and functional expression of the human macrophage inflammatory protein 1α/RANTES receptor. J Exp Med 1993; 177:1421.

109. Darbonne WC, Rice GC, Mohler MA, Apple T, Herbert CA, Valente AJ, Baker JB. Red blood cells are a sink for interleukin 8, a leukocyte chemotaxin. J Clin Invest 1991; 88(4):1362.

110. Neote K, Darbonne W, Ogez J, Horuk R, Schall TJ. Identification of a promiscuous inflammatory peptide receptor on the surface of red blood cells. J Biol Chem 1993; 268(17):12247.

111. Horuk R, Colby TJ, Darbonne WC, Schall TJ, Neote K. The human erythrocyte inflammatory peptide (chemokine) receptor. Biochemical characterization, solubilization, and development of a binding assay for the soluble receptor. Biochemistry 1993; 32(22):5733.

112. Horuk Chitnis C, Darbonne W, Colby T, Rybicki A, Hadley T, Miller L. The erythrocyte chemokine receptor is a receptor for the malarial parasite Plasmodium vivax. Science 1993; 261:1182.

113. Wang JM, McVicar DW, Oppenheim JJ, Kelvin DJ. Identification of RANTES receptors on human monocytic cells: Competition for binding and desensitization by homologous chemotactic cytokines. J Exp Med 1993; 177:699-705.

114. Van Riper G, Sicilano S, Fischer PA, Meurer R, Springer MS, Rosen H. Characterization and species distribution of high affinity GTP-coupled receptors for human RANTES and monocyte chemoattractant protein-1. J Exp Med 1993; 177:851.

115. Wang JM, Sherry B, Fivash M, Kelvin DJ, Oppenheim JJ. Human recombinant macrophage inflammatory protein-1α (MIP-1α)

and β (MIP-1β) and monocyte chemotactic and activating factor (MCAF) utilize common and unique receptors on human monocytes. J Immunol 1993; 150:3022.

116. Charo IF, Myers SJ, Herman A, Franci C, Connolly AJ, Coughlin SR. Molecular cloning and functional expression of two monocyte-chemoattractant protein 1 receptors reveals alternative splicing of the carboxyl-terminal tails. Proc Natl Acad Sci USA 1994; 91:2752.

117. Franci C, Wong LM, Damme JV, Proost P, Charo IF. Monocyte chemoattractant protein-3, but not monocyte chemoattractant protein-2, is a functional ligand of the human monocyte chemoattractant protein-1 receptor. J Immunol 1995; 154:6511.

118. Kuhn DE, Beall CJ, Kolattukudy PE. The cytomegalovirus US28 protein binds multiple C-C chemokines with high affinity. Biochm Biophys Res Commun 1995; 211:325.

119. Paolini JF, Willard D, Consler T, Luther M, Krangel MS. The chemokines Il-8, monocyte chemoattractant protein-1 and I-309 are monomers at physiologically relevant concentrations. J Immunol 1994; 153:2704.

120. Rajarathnam K, Sykes BD, Kay CM, Dewald B, Geiser T, Baggiolini M, Clark-Lewis I. Neutrophil activation by monomeric interleukin-8. Science 1994; 264:90.

121. Schnitzel W, Monschein U, Besemer J. Monomer-dimer equilibria of interleukin-8 and neutrophil activating peptide 2. Evidence for IL-8 binding as a dimer and oligmer to IL-8 receptor. J Leuk Biol 1994; 55:763.

122. Zhang Y, Rollins BJ. A dominant negative inhibitor indicates that monocyte chemoattractant protein 1 functions as a dimer. Mol Cell Biol 1995; 15:4851.

123. Lefkowitz RJ. G protein-coupled receptor kinases. Cell 1993; 74:409.

124. Sozzani S, Luini W, Molino M, JiLek P, Bottazzi B, Cerletti C, Matsushima K, Montovani A. The signal transduction pathway involved in the migration induced by a monocyte chemotactic cytokine. J Immunol 1991; 147:2215.

125. Turner L, Ward SG, Westwick J. RANTES-

activated human T lymphocytes: A role for phosphoinositol 3-kinase. J Immunol 1995; 155:2437-2444.

126. Yoshimura T, Matsushima K, Tanaka S, Robinson EA, Appella E, Oppenheim JJ, Leonard EJ. Purification of a human monocyte-derived neutrophil chemotactic factor that has peptide sequence similarity to other host defense cytokines. J Exp Med 1987; 169:1449.

127. Murphy WJ, Taub DD, Anver M, Conlon K, Oppenheim JJ, Kelvin DJ, Longo DL. Human RANTES induces the migration of human T lymphocytes into the peripheral tissues of mice with severe combined immune deficiency. Eur J Immunol 1994; 24(8):1823.

128. Streiter RM, Kunkel SL. The immunopathology of chemotactic cytokines. In: Westwick J, Lindley J, Kunkel S, eds. The Chemokines. New York: Plenum Press, 1993:19-28.

129. Massion PP, Inoue H, Richman-Eisenstat J, Grunberger D, Jorens PG, Housset B, Pittet J-F, Wiener-Kronish JP, Nabel JA. Novel *Pseudomonas* product stimulates interleukin-8 production in airway epithelial cells in vitro. J Clin Invest 1994; 93:26.

130. McElvaney NG, Nakamura H, Birrer P, Hebert CA, Wong WL, Alphonso M, Baker JB, Catalano MA, Crystal RG. Modulation of airway inflammation in cystic fibrosis. In vivo suppression of interleukin-8 levels on the respiratory epithelial surface by aerosolization of recombinant secretory leukoprotease inhibitor. J Clin Invest 1992; 90:1296.

131. Merrill WW, Naegel GP, Matthay RA, Reynolds HY. Alveolar macrophage-derived chemotactic factor: Kinetics of in vitro production and partial characterization. J Clin Invest 1980; 65:268.

132. Lynch JP III, Standiford TJ, Rolfe MW, Kunkel SL, Strieter RM. Neutrophilic alveolitis in idiopathic pulmonary fibrosis: The role of interleukin-8. Am Rev Respir Dis 1992; 145:1433.

133. Car BD, Meloni F, Luisetti M, Semenzato G, Gialdroni-Grassi G, Walz A. Elevated IL-8 and MCP-1 in the broncoalveolar lavage fluids of patients with idiopathic pulmo-nary fibrosis and pulmonary sarcoidosis. Am J Respir Crit Care Med 1994; 149:655.

134. Zhang K, Gharaee-Kermani M, Jones ML, Warren JS, Phan SH. Lung monocyte chemoattractant protein-1 gene expression in bleomycin-induced pulmonary fibrosis. J Immunol 1994; 153:4733.

135. Brieland JK, Jones ML, Clarke SJ, Baker JB, Warren JS, Fantone JC. Effect of acute inflammatory lung injury on the expression of monocyte chemoattractant protein-1 (MCP-1) in rat pulmonary alveolar macrophages. Am J Respir Cell Mol Biol 1992; 7:134.

136. Jones ML, Mulligan MS, Flory CM, Ward PA, Warren JS. Potential role of monocyte chemoattractant protein 1/JE in monocyte/macrophage-dependent IgA immune complex alveolitis in the rat. J Immunol 1992; 149:2147.

137. Jones ML, Warren JS. Monocyte chemoattractant protein 1 in a rat model of pulmonary granulomatosis. Lab Invest 1992; 66:498.

138. Ghosh S, Latimer RD, Gray BM, Harwood RJ, Oduro A. Endotoxin-induced organ injury. Crit Care Med 1993; 21:S19.

139. Evans GF, Snyder YM, Butler LD, Zuckerman SH. Differential expression of interleukin-1 and tumor necrosis factor in murine septic shock models. Cir Shock 1989; 29:279.

140. Rampart M, Herman AG, Grillet B, Opdenakker G, Van Damme J. Different proinflammatory profiles of the macrophage-derived cytokines IL-1, IL-8, and TNF. Lab Invest 1992; 66:512.

141. Lukacs NW, Streiter RM, Standiford TJ, Kunkel SL. Characterization of chemokine function in animal models of diseases. Immunomethods on Chemokines: Characterization and Activity 1995:(in press).

142. Xing Z, Jordana M, Kirpalani H, Driscoll KE, Schall TJ, Gauldie J. Cytokine expression by neutrophils and macrophages in vivo: endotoxin induces tumor necrosis factor-α, macrophage inflammatory protein-2, interleukin-1β, and interleukin-6 but not RANTES or transforming growth factor-β1 mRNA expression in acute lung inflammation. Am J Resp Cell Mol Biol 1994;

10:148.

143. Standiford TJ, Kunkel SL, Lukacs NW, Greenberger MJ, Danforth JM, Kunkel RG, Strieter RM. Macrophage inflammatory protein-1α mediates lung leukocyte recruitment, lung capillary leak, and early mortality in murine endotoxemia. J Immunol 1995; 155:1515.

144. Van Otteren GM, Strieter RM, Kunkel SL, Paine R, Greenberger MJ, Danforth JM, Burdick MD, Standiford TJ. Compartmentalized expression of RANTES in a murine model of endotoxemia. J Immunol 1995; 154:1900.

145. Standiford TJ, Kunkel SL, Lukacs NW, Greenberger MJ, Danforth JM, Kunkel RG, Strieter RM. Macrophage inflammatory protein-1α mediates lung leukocyte recruitment, lung capillary leak, and early mortality in murine endotoxemia. J Immunol 1995; (in press).

146. Davatelis G, Wolpe SD, Sherry B, Dayer JM, Chicheportiche R, Cerami A. Macrophage inflammatory protein-1: a prostaglandin-independent endogenous pyrogen. Science 1989; 243:1066.

147. Harris ED. Rheumatoid arthritis: pathophysiology and implications for therapy. N Eng J Med 1990; 322:1277.

148. Rathanaswami P, Hachicha M, Sadick M, Schall TJ, McColl SR. Expression of the cytokine RANTES in human rheumatoid synovial fibroblasts. Differential regulation of RANTES and interleukin-8 genes by inflammatory cytokines. J Biol Chem 1993; 268:5834.

149. Koch AE, Kunkel SL, Harlow LA, Johnson B, Evanoff HL, Haines GK, Burdick MD, Pope RM, Strieter RM. Enhanced production of monocyte chemoattractant protein-1 in rheumatoid arthritis. J Clin Invest 1992; 90:772.

150. Koch AE, Kunkel SL, Harlow LA, Mazarakis DD, Haines GK, Burdick MD, Pope RM, Strieter RM. Macrophage inflammatory protein-1 alpha. A novel chemotactic cytokine for macrophages in rheumatoid arthritis. J Clin Invest 1994; 93:921.

151. Kasama T, Strieter RM, Lukacs NW, Lincoln PM, Burdick MD, Kunkel SL. Interleukin-10 expression and chemokine regulation during the evolution of murine type II collagen-induced arthritis. J Clin Invest 1995; (in press).

152. Boros DL. Immunopathology of Schistosoma mansoni infection. Clin Microbiol Rev 1989; 2:250.

153. Lukacs NW, Kunkel SL, Strieter RM, Warmington K, Chensue SW. The role of macrophage inflammatory protein 1α in Schistosoma mansoni egg-induced granulomatous inflammation. J Exp Med 1993; 177:1551.

154. Lukacs NW, Chensue SW, Smith RE, Strieter RM, Warmington K, Wilke C, Kunkel SL. Production of monocyte chemoattractant protein-1 and macrophage inflammatory protein-1 alpha by inflammatory granuloma fibroblasts. Am J Pathol 1993; 144:711.

155. Chensue SW, Warmington KS, Lukacs NW, Lincoln PM, Burdick MD, Strieter RM, Kunkel SL. Monocyte chemotactic protein expression during schistosome egg granuloma formation: Sequence of production, localization, contribution, and regulation. Am J Pathol 1995; 146:130.

156. Flory CM, Jones ML, Warren JS. Pulmonary granuloma formation in the rat is partially dependent on monocyte chemoattractant protein-1. Lab Invest 1993; 69:396.

157. Edgington SM. Chemokines in cardiovascular disease. Biotechnology 1993; 11:676.

158. Marmur JD, Friedrich VL, Rossikhina M, Rollins BJ, Taubman M. The JE gene encodes a smooth muscle chemotactic factor that is induced by vascular injury. Circulation 1990; 82:698.

159. Taubman M, Rollins B, Poon M, Marmur J, Green R, Berk B, Nadal-Ginard B. JE mRNA accumulated rapidly in aortic injury and in platelet-derived growth factor-stimulated vascular smooth muscle cells. Circ Res 1992; 70:314.

160. Yla-Herttuala S, Lipton BA, Rosenfeld ME, Sarkioja T, Yoshimura T, Leonard EJ, Witztum JL, Steinberg D. Expression of monocyte chemoattractant protein 1 in macrophage-rich areas of human and rabbit atherosclerotic lesions. Proc Natl Acad Sci USA 1991; 88:5252.

161. Nelken NA, Coughlin SR, Gordon D, Wilcox JN. Monocyte chemoattractant protein-1 in human atheromatous plaques. J Clin Invest 1991; 88:1121.

162. Cushing S, Berliner J, Valente A, Territo M, Navab M, Parhami F, Gerrity R, Schwart C, Fogelman A. Minimally modified low-density lipoprotein induces monocyte chemotactic protein 1 in human endothelial cells and smooth muscle cells. Proc Natl Acad Sci USA 1990; 87:5134.

163. Navab M, Imes S, Hama S, Hough G, Ross L, Bork R, Valente A, Berliner J, Drinkwater D, Laks H, Fogleman A. Monocyte transmigration induced by modification of low-density lipoprotein in cocultures of human aortic wall cells is due to induction of monocyte chemotactic protein 1 synthesis and is abolished by high density lipoprotein. J Clin Invest 1991; 88:2039.

164. Yu Xiaohui, Dluz S, Graves DT, Zhang L, Antoniades HN, Hollander W, Prusty S, Valente AJ, Schwartz CJ, Sonenshein GE. Elevated expression of monocyte chemoattractant protein 1 by vascular smooth muscle cells in hypercholesterolemic primates. Proc Natl Acad Sci USA 1992; 89:6953.

165. Deleuran MS. Regulation of the chemotactic cytokines IL-8 and MCAF and their induction in different cell types related to the skin. Act Derm Venereal Suppl 1994; 189:1.

166. Russell ME, Adams DH, Wyner LR, Yamashita Y, Halnon NJ, Karnovsky MJ. Early and persistent induction of monocyte chemoattractant protein 1 in rat cardiac allografts. Proc Natl Acad Sci USA 1993; 90:6086.

167. Koch AE, Kunkel SL, Pearce WH, Shah MR, Parikh D, Evanoff HL, Haines GK, Burdick MD, Strieter RM. Enhanced production of the chemotactic cytokines interleukin-8 and monocyte chemoattractant protein-1 in human abdominal aortic aneurysms. Am J Path 1993; 142:1423.

168. Yu X, Antoniades HN, Graves DT. Expression of monocyte chemoattractant protein 1 in human inflamed gingival tissues. Infect Immun 1993; 61(11):4622.

169. Marra F, Valente AJ, Pinzani M, Abboud HE. Cultured human liver fat-storing cells produce monocyte chemotactic protein-1: Regulation by proinflammatory cytokines. J Clin Invest 1993; 92:1674.

170. Jansen PM, Van Damme J, Put W, de Jong IW, Taylor FB, Hack CE. Monocyte chemotactic protein 1 (MCP-1) is released during lethal and sublethal bacteremia in baboons. J infect Dis 1995; (in press).

171. DiPietro LA, Polverini PJ, Rahbe SM, Kovacs EJ. Modulation of JE/MCP-1 expression in dermal wound repair. Amer J Pathol 1995; 146:868.

172. Hanazawa S, Kawata Y, Takeshita A, Kumada H, Okithu M, Tanaka S, Yamamoto Y, Masuda T, Umemoto T, Kitano S. Expression of monocyte chemoattractant protein 1 (MCP-1) in adult peridontal disease: Increased monocyte chemotactic activity in crevicular fluids and induction of MCP-1 expression in gingival tissues. Infect Immun 1993; 61:5219.

173. Yu X, Antoniades HN, Graves DT. Expression of monocyte chemoattractant protein 1 in human inflamed gingival tissues. Infect Immun 1993; 61(11):4622.

174. Marrs F, Valente AJ, Pinzani M, Abboud HE. Cultured human liver fat-storing cells produce monocyte chemotactic protein-1: Regulation by prinflammatory cytokines. J Clin Invest 1995; 92:1674.

CHAPTER 3

CHEMOKINE RECEPTORS

Philip M. Murphy, Sunil K. Ahuja,
Christophe Combadiere and Ji-Liang Gao

INTRODUCTION

Chemokines activate leukocytes by binding to specific plasma membrane receptors.[1] The hypothesis that chemokines are involved in the pathogenesis of inflammatory diseases, which comprises the major focus of this volume, originated before specific information was available about chemokine receptors. Nevertheless, testing the hypothesis and developing specific chemokine antagonists may be greatly facilitated by detailed knowledge of the receptors. In addition, new leads linking chemokines to malaria and herpesvirus infections have come directly from the study of chemokine receptors.[2,3] The nature of the receptors and the way they work has become clearer in the past four years in large part due to molecular studies, which will be the primary focus of this chapter. From this beginning, new studies are being carried out in animal models that may clarify further the physiologic and pathologic roles played by chemokine receptors and their agonists.

Like chemokines themselves, chemokine receptors constitute a structurally and functionally related family of proteins, currently amounting to eight known human members. Unlike chemokines, the receptors form part of a much larger protein superfamily, the rhodopsin-like, seven-transmembrane-domain (7TMD), G protein-coupled receptors.[2-4] 7TMD receptors have diverse functions, such as light and odor perception, hormone action, neurotransmission and leukocyte chemotaxis, yet they probably all originated by replication and divergence of a common ancestral gene. The 7TMD structural motif is perhaps nature's most functionally adaptable protein foundation.

Knowing the DNA sequence of one 7TMD receptor has often made it possible to clone DNA for another owing to the presence of certain especially well-conserved sequence motifs located principally in the TMDs that can be used to make crosshybridizing probes.[5,6] This strategy has been used to clone most of the known chemokine receptor genes and

Chemokines in Disease, edited by Alisa E. Koch and Robert M. Strieter.
© 1996 R.G. Landes Company.

cDNAs.[6] *Xenopus* oocytes and human embryonic kidney 293 cells have been most widely used for expression and functional characterization of cloned chemokine receptors.

CLASSIFICATION OF CHEMOKINE RECEPTORS

Chemokine receptor cDNAs and genes have been cloned primarily from human, mouse and rabbit. Surprisingly, functional chemokine receptor genes have also been found in two mammalian viruses, human cytomegalovirus and Herpesvirus saimiri.[3,7-11] Chemokine receptors currently can be classified into four groups based on their ligand and/or agonist selectivity (Table 3.1): (1) receptors restricted to C-X-C chemokines (e.g., human IL-8 receptors A and B, and open reading frame ECRF3 of Herpesvirus saimiri);[11-13] (2) receptors restricted to C-C chemokines (e.g., human C-C chemokine receptors 1, 2A, 2B and 4, and open reading frame US28 of human cytomegalovirus);[8,9,14-18] (3) a promiscuous C-C and C-X-C chemokine binding protein also known as the Duffy antigen of red blood cells[19-22] and (4) "orphan" chemokine receptors whose sequences are strongly related to known chemokine receptors, but whose ligands have not yet been identified (human examples include CMKBRL1, GPR5, HUMSTSR, EBI1 and BLR1).[23-28]

Whereas most mammalian cells produce one or more chemokines when appropriately stimulated (see ref. 29 for an exhaustive review of chemokine sources), expression of their receptors appears to be much more restricted.[17,24,30,31] Exhaustive surveys have not been reported, however it is already clear that all cloned chemokine receptors are expressed in at least one type of leukocyte in peripheral blood, and that in general the expression patterns are distinct and relatively selective for different chemokine receptors. For example, IL-8 receptors are neutrophil selective, and C-C chemokine receptor (C-C CKR) 2 is monocyte selective. It is reasonable therefore to speculate that chemokine receptors may be

host factors that regulate the types of leukocytes appearing in inflammatory infiltrates in disease states.

If so, chemokine receptors may be good targets for the development of new cell type-selective anti-inflammatory agents. However, all chemokine receptors, with the possible exception of interleukin-8 receptor A, bind multiple chemokines, and most chemokines activate more than one chemokine receptor even on the same cell type, greatly complicating the issue of signaling specificity. The biologic responses in a given cell type elicited by each set of agonists for a given receptor are at least broadly overlapping, but differences have also been observed suggesting that even closely related chemokines may not be completely redundant in function.[32] Although the biologic relevance of chemokines to leukocyte trafficking and activation is supported by an abundance of strong data, work connecting chemokines and their receptors to other cell types such as erythrocytes, endothelial cells, brain, skin, placenta, skeletal muscle and other cell types and tissues [2,24,25,33-37] is in its embryonic phase of development and merits close attention in the future.

RELATIONSHIP OF CHEMOKINE RECEPTORS TO RHODOPSIN

Ten amino acid residues are invariant for all members of the rhodopsin superfamily, and many others are highly conserved (Fig. 3.1).[4] Based on analogy with the transmembrane topology established by structural studies for rhodopsin, and earlier for the prototype bacteriorhodopsin, a general model for plasma membrane insertion for 7TMD proteins has been proposed.[38,39] In this model, the receptor polypeptide is stitched into the membrane with the N-terminus lodged in the extracellular space, the C-terminus in the intracellular space, and each of seven hydrophobic domains passing as α helices through the plane of the membrane. This arrangement defines four potential extracellular and four potential intracellular domains: a total of

Table 3.1. Properties of cloned human, mouse and viral chemokine receptors

Receptor	Length	RNA[a]	Antigen[b]	Radioligands	Ca²⁺ Flux	Ref.
CXC						
hIL8RA	350	N>>M[c]	N, M, NK	IL-8	IL-8>>GROα	12, 30, 31
hIL8RB	360	N>>M	N, M, NK	IL-8, GROα, NAP-2	IL-8=GROα=NAP-2	13, 30, 31
mIL8RB	360	ND	ND	KC	ND	76-78
HVS-ECRF3	321	–	ND	GROα	GROα>NAP-2>IL-8	11
CC						
hCC CKR1	355	M, L_B, N, L_T, Eo, Br, Ht, Sp, SM Pa, Pl, Li Ki, Lu	ND	MIP-1α, RANTES, MCP-3	MIP-1α>RANTES>> MIP-1β~MCP-1	8, 14, 15, 24, 103
hCC CKR 2A	374	M Lu, Li, Sp	ND	ND	MCP-1	16
hCC CKR 2B	360	M Lu, Li, Sp	ND	MCP-1, MCP-3	MCP-1~MCP-3	16, 24, 103, 104
hCC CKR3[d]	355	Eo	ND	ND	eotaxin	17, 103a
hCC CKR4	360	L	ND	ND	MIP-1α, RANTES, MCP-1	18
mMIP-1αR	355	L, Ht, Lu, Sp	ND	MIP-1α, RANTES	MIP-1α>RANTES	37
HCMV-US28	354	Fb	ND	MIP-1α	RANTES>>MIP-1α =MIP-1β=MCP-1	8, 9, 131
CC/CXC						
DARC	339	BM, Br, Lu, Ki, Ht, Sp, SM, Pa, Li	E, EC RANTES	GROα,	–	19-22, 121-124
Human, Mouse and Viral Orphans						
hHUMSTSR	352	N, M, L	ND	ND	ND	26
hBLR1	372	L_B	L_B	ND	ND	28
hEBI1	378	L_B	ND	ND	ND	23
hCMKBRL1	355	N, M, Br, Li, SM, Lu	ND	ND	ND	24
hGPR1	355	ND	ND	ND	ND	136
hGPR2	>354	ND	ND	ND	ND	136
hGPR5	333	ND	ND	ND	ND	25
mMIP-1αRL1	356	L, Sk	ND	ND	ND	37
mMIP-1αRL2	359	L, Sp, Lu, Li	ND	ND	ND	37
SPV-K2R	370	ND	ND	ND	ND	128
EHV-2 ORF 74	330	ND	ND	ND	ND	129
EHV-2 ORF E1	383	ND	ND	ND	ND	129

[a] Only the RNA distributions determined by Northern blot hybridization for normal human tissues and cell types are listed.

[b] Cell types staining with receptor-specific antibodies

[c] Abbreviations: h, human; m, mouse; ND, not determined; E, erythrocyte; N, neutrophil; NK, natural killer cells; M, monocyte; Eo, eosinophil; EC, endothelial cell; L, leukocyte; L_B, B lymphocyte; L_T, T lymphocyte; Fb, fibroblast; Lu, lung; Br, brain; Sp, spleen; Li, liver; Ki, kidney; SM, skeletal muscle; Pl, placenta; Pa, pancreas; Ht, heart; HCMV, human cytomegalovirus; HVS, Herpesvirus saii•iri; HUMSTSR, human seven-transmembrane-segment-receptor; BLR1, Burkitt's lymphoma receptor-1; EBI1, Epstein-Barr virus-induced receptor; CMKBRL1, chemokine β receptor-like I; GPR, G protein-coupled receptor; SPV, swinepox virus; EHV, equine herpesvirus; MIP-1αRL, MIP-1α receptor-like

[d] CC CKR3 was originally reported to be a MIP-1α, RANTES and MIP-1β receptor. This agonist profile actually belongs to another CC CKR, named CCCKR5, owing to a mislabeled sample (C Combadiere, SK Ahuja, and PM Murphy, manuscript submitted).

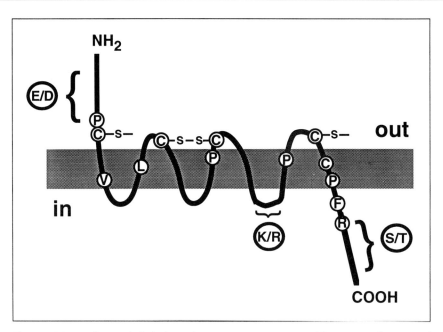

Fig. 3.1. Mammalian and viral chemokine receptors: conserved features and proposed transmembrane topography. Shaded rectangle, plasma membrane spanned seven times by the receptor protein; NH₂, amino terminus; COOH, carboxy terminus; solid line, core peptide; -S-S-, disulfide bond; circled K/R, lysine and arginine-rich domain 16 amino acids in length; circled E/D, aspartate/glutamate-rich domain; circled S/T, sites of multiple serine and threonine residues for potential phosphorylation; circled single letters, invariant residues. Orphan sequences that have these features are good chemokine receptor candidates.

six loops (i1-3 and e1-3) connecting the seven TMDs, and the free N- and C-terminal extensions. Antibody studies have verified that the N-terminal segments of the IL-8 receptors and the Duffy antigen are indeed extracellular.[21,30] 7TMD receptor proteins lack a signal sequence but can correctly self-orient in lipid bilayers in vitro without accessory factors.[40]

Chemokine receptors are relatively small members of the rhodopsin superfamily, ranging in size from 339 to 373 amino acids. As a group they stand out from other rhodopsin superfamily members by virtue of the following sequence features (Fig. 3.1): (1) a short i3 loop 16 amino acids long; (2) 25-80% amino acid identity to each other; (3) numerous aspartate and glutamate residues in the N-terminal segment prior to TMD1, making this domain acidic (C-C CKR2 is an exception) and (4) a conserved cysteine residue in the N-terminal segment and the e3 loop. By

analogy with other rhodopsin-like receptors, the e1 and e2 loop cysteines of chemokine receptors probably form a disulfide bond. The N-terminal and e3 loop cysteines could also form a disulfide bond, further constraining the arrangement of the α helical TMDs which are envisioned, again by analogy to rhodopsin, to be arranged as seven staves in a barrel oriented counterclockwise to the plane of the membrane, from the intracellular perspective.[38] Treatment of neutrophils with reducing agents abrogates IL-8 binding, suggesting that these linkages actually occur in the IL-8 receptors.[41]

Chemokines exist as monomers at physiologic concentrations, although all chemokines tested have been shown to dimerize at high concentrations.[42,43] They probably bind to the receptor ectodomain as monomers, although this remains controversial.[44] There is no evidence at present for receptor dimerization after activation.

Chemokine signal transduction pathways involving pertussis toxin sensitive heterotrimeric G proteins, phospholipases and tyrosine kinases have been reviewed previously.

MAMMALIAN CHEMOKINE RECEPTORS

C-X-C CHEMOKINE RECEPTORS

Human IL-8 Receptors

IL-8 was the first chemokine shown to be a leukocyte chemoattractant and activating factor.[45,46] Based on: (1) the ability of pertussis toxin to abolish IL-8's actions on neutrophils and (2) the discovery of high affinity ^{125}I-IL-8 binding sites on neutrophils, it was expected that IL-8 action was mediated by 7TMD G protein-coupled receptors.[47,48] It was later shown that the related C-X-C chemokines GROα and NAP-2 mimicked IL-8's actions on neutrophils and could compete partially for ^{125}I-IL-8 binding sites, suggesting the presence of at least two distinct receptors.[49,50] cDNAs encoding two related human neutrophil IL-8 receptors, one of which was also a receptor for GROα and NAP-2, were then isolated by expression and homology hybridization cloning strategies.[12,13,51,52] The names of these receptors have not been standardized, but they are most commonly referred to as IL8RA (IL-8 selective) and IL8RB (IL-8, GROα and NAP-2 selective). No other human C-X-C chemokine-restricted receptor cDNAs have been cloned.

The longest open reading frames for IL8RA and IL8RB encode 350 and 360 amino acids respectively; the sequences can be aligned easily since they possess 78% amino acid identity (Fig. 3.2A). IL8RB could be 355 instead of 360 amino acids in length since codon six encodes methionine and is flanked by sequences that fit the consensus criteria established by Kozak for the start of translation.[53] Chemokine selectivity has been established for the cloned receptors by receptor binding assays as well as by calcium mobilization and chemotaxis assays of receptor function.[12,13,51,52,54-57] IL-8

is the only potent agonist and high affinity ligand identified for IL8RA. In contrast, IL8RB is selective for all members so far tested of the subset of C-X-C chemokines that, like IL-8, possess the amino acid sequence motif glutamic acid-leucine-arginine (ELR) in the unordered domain N-terminal to the first cysteine. In addition to GROα and NAP-2, this group includes GROβ, GROγ and ENA-78 (SK Ahuja and PM Murphy, manuscript submitted). The ELR motif has been shown by alanine substitutions and N-terminal truncations to be critical for receptor binding and activation by IL-8, and data confirming its importance for GROα have recently been reported.[58-60] Three other human C-X-C chemokines, platelet factor 4, Mig and γIP-10, lack the ELR motif, and do not bind to IL8RB or IL8RA.

IL-8 Receptor Expression

The genes for IL8RA and IL8RB appear to be coordinately regulated in peripheral blood leukocytes. RNA for both receptors is found at high levels in resting neutrophils, but at very low levels in freshly isolated eosinophils and adherent monocytes (less than 1% of the neutrophil level of IL8RA and IL8RB mRNA).[31] Neutrophils express 20,000-40,000 IL-8 binding sites per cell. Radioligand binding experiments with IL-8 and GROα have suggested that IL8RA and IL8RB each account for approximately half of the IL-8 binding activity,[50] and this has been verified by two different sets of antibodies specific for the N-terminal segment of each receptor.[30,61]

Antibody studies have shown that both IL8RA and IL8RB are also coexpressed on monocytes and NK cells from peripheral blood.[30,61] IL-2-stimulated NK cells have been reported to chemotax in response to IL-8;[62] IL-8 treatment induces increased monocyte adhesive functions, but not chemotaxis or degranulation.[47] The functional significance of monocyte IL-8 receptors is not established. Xu et al have reported recently that expression of IL-8 receptors by T lymphocytes is labile, which may account

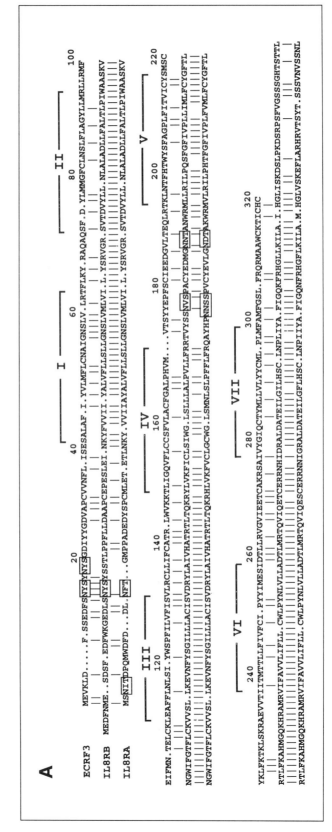

Fig. 3.2. Alignment of the human C-X-C (A, above) and C-C (B, below) chemokine receptors with their viral homologues. In panel A vertical bars indicate identical residues for each adjacent sequence position. In panel B asterisks indicate invariant residues for the human C-C CKRs. Roman numerals demarcate the proposed TMDs. Open boxes, potential sites for N-linked glycosylation; dashes, gaps inserted to optimize the alignment. The arabic numbers above each sequence block enumerate the amino acid sequence for ECRF3 in panel A and C-C CKR1 in panel B.

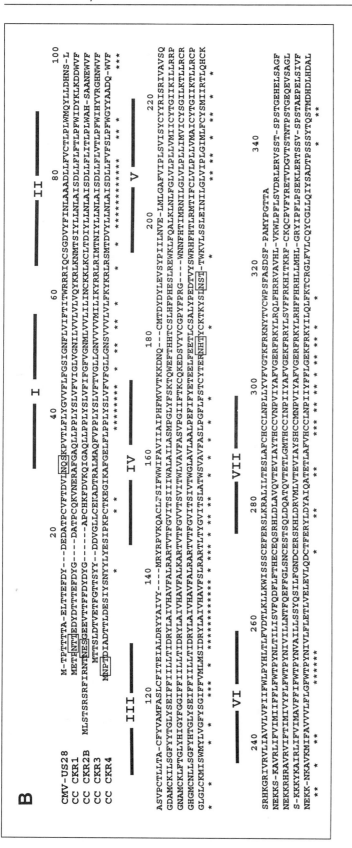

for the failure of the monoclonal antibodies to stain these cells under the conditions tested.[63] Both CD4+ and CD8+ T lymphocytes have been reported to migrate in response to IL-8 in vitro. Moreover, human T cells migrate slowly to sites of IL-8 injection in SCID mice engrafted with human bone marrow.[64] Whether this phenomenon is mediated by activation of T cell IL-8 receptors or by an indirect mechanism has not been established.

Several other cell types, including eosinophils, basophils, fibroblasts and endothelial cells have been reported to respond to IL-8, but the receptors responsible have not been defined.[33,34,65,66] Particularly provocative is the finding that IL-8 and other C-X-C chemokines stimulate neovascularization without inflammation when injected into rat cornea, and regulate angiogenesis in tumors.[34,67] In vitro studies suggest that these effects are due to direct stimulation of endothelial cell proliferation and chemotaxis.[34] In contrast, the ELR-C-X-C chemokine platelet factor 4 is angiostatic, apparently operating in part by blocking heparin-dependent binding of vascular endothelial growth factor-165 to its receptor flk-1.[68,69] Since the ELR+ C-X-C chemokines are heparin binding proteins, they could also mediate their angiogenic effects in part by mechanisms independent of 7TMD receptors. GROα has also been shown to stimulate proliferation of melanoma cells in vitro, accounting for its other widely used name, melanoma growth-stimulatory activity or MGSA;[35] however the receptor responsible appears to be distinct from IL8RB since IL-8 does not displace ^{125}I-GROα from binding sites on these cells.[70]

The factors responsible for the observed distribution of IL-8 receptors have not been defined yet. The genes for both IL8RA and IL8RB have been cloned recently, and genomic regions with promoter activity have been defined.[31,71,72] The genes for IL8RA and IL8RB as well as a pseudogene of IL8RB have been mapped by fluorescence in situ hybridization to human chromosome 2q34-q35, a region that lacks known

human disease susceptibility loci.[73,74] The gene symbols are *IL8RA*, *IL8RB* and *IL8RP*.

Despite being small genes with intronless ORFs, both *IL8RA* and *IL8RB* have surprisingly complex organization of the sequence flanking the ORFs. *IL8RA* is ~3 kb in size. The entire open reading frame, 3'-UTR and 33 bp of the 5'-UTR reside on a single exon. The remainder of the 5'-UTR resides on a single exon separated from the second exon by an 1656 bp intron. There are two polyadenylation signals AATAAA 474 bp apart in the 3'-UTR that are alternatively used, giving rise to similar amounts of 2.0 and 2.4 kb mRNAs with the same ORF in neutrophils. The major transcriptional start point determined by primer extension analysis is located 90 bp upstream from the ATG initiation codon.

The genomic organization of *IL8RB* is even more complicated: 11 exons span ~12 kb of genomic sequence.[31] Like *IL8RA*, the entire ORF, 3'-UTR and 25 bp of the 5'-UTR adjacent to the ORF reside on a single exon. The rest of the 5'-UTR is distributed on the other ten exons. Three sets of exons are adjacent, lacking an intron. Alternative splicing leads to the production of seven distinct IL8RB mRNAs found in varying amounts in normal human neutrophils. The predominant RNA form is composed of exons 3, 4, 5, 6 and 11, forming an unusually long 382 nt 5'-UTR. The other six forms, including one that contains the 5'-most exon, are found in trace amounts. Primer extension indicates that unlike *IL8RA*, in which transcription is precisely initiated, transcription of *IL8RB* begins at multiple alternative points. Given this complexity, additional exons could also exist. Differential cell type expression and function have not been found for the IL-8 receptor mRNA variants.

Upstream regions of genomic DNA for both *IL8RA* and *IL8RB* have been identified that have strong constitutive promoter activity when fused to a CAT reporter gene and transfected into both transformed lymphoid (Jurkat) and myeloid (U937, HL60) precursor cell lines, as well as into a more physiologically relevant environment, peripheral blood derived CD34+ hematopoietic progenitor cells.[75] For IL8RB, high constitutive promoter activity was found in regions upstream from exon 1 in either orientation relative to a CAT reporter gene. High constitutive promoter activity was also found in an 80 bp region upstream from exon 3. For IL8RA, a 300 bp region upstream from exon 1 is active. Compared to the IL-8 ligand promoter, the receptor promoters respond weakly to pro-inflammatory stimuli such as lipopolysaccharide and G-CSF, which is consistent with the small changes in IL-8 receptor mRNA levels in mature neutrophils induced by the same stimuli.[71,72] Taken together, these data suggest that IL-8 receptor genes may be most actively transcribed during cell differentiation, equipping the mature neutrophil with a full complement of IL-8 receptors ready to bind IL-8 induced at a site of tissue injury.

The region upstream from exon 1 of IL8RA lacks a TATA sequence. In contrast, a TATA sequence is found 47 bp upstream from the 5' end of exon 1 of IL8RB defined by cDNA cloning and primer extension. Sequences that compare favorably with the consensus sequences for a variety of enhancer elements, including the NFkB and NF-ATp elements, are found in the upstream regions of both genes, but transcription factor binding to these sequences has not been tested yet. Additional work will be needed to locate the cis- and transacting factors that permit expression of both genes in leukocytes.

IL-8 Receptors in Other Species

The anatomy of the chemokine system can be quite different between species. For example, despite intensive efforts a mouse form of IL-8 has not been identified. However, a mouse gene encoding a protein 83% identical in sequence to human IL8RB has been cloned by several groups.[76-78] Its physiologic agonist appears to be the mouse equivalent of GROα known as KC.[77]

Whole mouse neutrophils and transfected cells expressing the mouse IL8RB homologue both bind KC, but direct binding of human IL-8 has not been demonstrated to either substrate. A binding interaction of human IL-8 with the mouse receptor can be inferred by the ability of human IL-8 to compete, albeit weakly, for ^{125}I-KC binding sites on mouse neutrophils and COS cells transfected with mouse IL8RB. Moreover, in vitro human IL-8 chemoattracts mouse neutrophils with high potency. Interestingly, a chimeric receptor containing human IL8RB sequence from the first amino acid to the beginning of TMD1 with the remaining sequence from mouse IL8RB binds human IL-8 with high affinity, supporting a role for the N-terminal segment in high affinity binding of IL-8.[78]

Like IL-8, a mouse equivalent of human IL8RA has not been identified.[77] The rat genome contains two IL8R-like genes, but their full sequences and functional properties have not been analyzed (D Sibley, personal communication). Mouse IL8RB maps to a region of conserved synteny with human IL8RB on mouse chromosome 1 near the *bcg/lsh/ity* locus.[76] However, it appears that the gene *nramp* and not mouse IL8RB is the parasite susceptibility gene.[79]

The rabbit IL-8 system more closely resembles that of the human with one surprising twist: rabbit IL-8 binds with high affinity to both rabbit IL8RA and IL8RB, as well as to human IL8RB, but binds weakly to human IL8RA.[80-82] Nevertheless, human IL-8 binds with high affinity to both receptor subtypes in both species.[71] These differences must be kept in mind when attempting to make human inferences about experimental observations obtained in animal models.

Biological Functions of IL-8 Receptors

There is abundant evidence reviewed elsewhere in this volume that IL-8 is a major mediator of acute neutrophil-mediated inflammation in vivo. The in vivo effects of other C-X-C chemokines on acute inflammation are less well-defined. The relative contribution of IL8RA and IL8RB in mediating IL-8 action in vivo has not yet been defined. In vitro, IL8RA and IL8RB appear to mediate most, if not all, of the chemotactic responses of human neutrophils to ELR+ C-X-C chemokines: (1) specific immunoreactivity and RNA for both receptors are found in neutrophils, at comparable levels of expression;[30,61] (2) Jurkat cells transfected with the receptors acquire chemotactic responsiveness to appropriate ELR+ C-X-C chemokines[56] and (3) the biochemical properties of the cloned receptors are consistent with radioligand competition studies of human neutrophils.[50-52] At least one specialized role for IL8RB is not shared by IL8RA, the ability to relay signals to the neutrophil by GROα, GROβ, GROγ, ENA-78 and NAP-2. IL8RA may be needed to maintain the sensitivity of the neutrophil to IL-8 when IL8RB has been desensitized by GROα or one of the other ELR+ C-X-C chemokines.

Alternatively, the two receptors could mediate different phases of the inflammatory response. In this regard, Chuntharapai and Kim have recently reported differences in the rate and IL-8 concentration dependence for up- and down-modulation of IL8RA and IL8RB on neutrophils. In particular, higher concentrations of IL-8 are required to induce internalization of IL8RA than IL8RB.[83] They have proposed that IL8RB may be most important in initiation of chemotaxis whereas IL8RA may be most important in signal transduction at the site of inflammation.

Genetic tests of function in experimental animals will be important for confirming old suspicions and for gaining new insights about the biological roles played by individual receptors. Moore and colleagues described a mouse lacking IL8RB created by gene disruption using homologous recombination technology.[84] Two important phenotypes were found: (1) neutrophil accumulation in the peritoneal cavity during chemical irritation was severely depressed and (2) neutrophil and B cell numbers were massively expanded in the bone marrow, lymphoid tissue and peripheral blood. Neutrophils from the "knockout" mice failed to migrate in response to IL-8 or KC in chemotaxis assays in vitro. This experiment supported a role for IL8RB in acute inflammation, and suggested a previously unsuspected role for IL8RB as a negative regulator of hematopoiesis. So far, a host defense or repair defect in these animals has not been reported.

Structure-Activity Relationships for IL-8 Receptors

Chemotactic receptors, like other G protein-coupled receptors appear to have two basic functions, to bind ligand and to activate bound G protein. In the absence of direct structural information, one can use mutant receptors exhibiting gain or loss of wild type functions, and the general structural model for G protein-coupled receptors, to make inferences about the nature of the ligand and G protein binding sites with the aim of designing clinically useful receptor antagonists. Since G protein-coupled receptors probably lack independently folding domains, allosteric effects of mutation are very likely to occur, and probably account for the complex properties that have been observed in mutant receptors. Two major mutagenesis strategies have been used, creation of chimeric receptors and point mutagenesis, and several useful insights have been obtained.

Most of the residues that differ between IL8RA and IL8RB lie in three small receptor regions: the N-terminal segment prior to TMD1, the region from the middle of TMD4 to the end of the e2 loop and the C-terminal cytoplasmic extension. The contribution of these differences to receptor subtype determination has been extensively analyzed using chimeric receptors made by switching homologous but divergent domains of rabbit IL8RA, mouse IL8RB, human IL8RA, human IL8RB or human C-C chemokine receptor 1 (MIP-1α/RANTES receptor).[54,55,57,78,85] All of the chimeric receptors tested so far have binding sites for C-X-C chemokines that differ from those of IL8RA and IL8RB. Moreover, reciprocal chimeras do not have reciprocal ligand binding or agonist selectivity. This supports the idea that IL-8 receptors do not have independently folding domains. The results suggest that the sets of binding determinants on IL8RB for IL-8, GROα and NAP-2 are overlapping but distinct, and that multiple regions on the extracellular face bind chemokine and contribute to receptor subtype selectivity. The N-terminal segment may be important for high affinity IL-8 binding as suggested by C-C CKR1/IL8RB and rabbit IL8RA/mouse IL8RB chimeras, but its importance in receptor activation has not been shown.[78,85] The divergent region from TMD4 to the end of the e2 loop appears to be particularly important for GROα selectivity, whereas determinants of NAP-2 selectivity appear to reside in the e3 loop. Several of the chimeras display markedly reduced affinity for one or another ligand with no change in the corresponding agonist activity relative to wild type IL8RB, suggesting that the determinants necessary for high affinity binding differ from those necessary for agonist activity. Mutants of IL8RB with truncations of the C-terminal cytoplasmic tail bind ligand normally, but fail to transduce signals. The loss of function determinants have been mapped to a region adjacent to TMD7 between aa 317 and 324.[86] Like other 7TMD receptors,[87] the C-terminal cytoplasmic domain of the IL-8 receptors and other chemokine receptors is rich in serine and threonine residues that may be phosphorylation sites for kinases that regulate receptor function. However, receptor phosphorylation studies have not been reported yet.

Exhaustive alanine scanning mutagenesis of all of the extracellular residues of human IL8RA has been reported.[88] Mutants bearing substitutions for any one of the four cysteines in the ectodomains are expressed in transiently transfected 293 cells, but they do not bind IL-8 nor do they exhibit a calcium flux in response to IL-8. It has been proposed that the cysteines form two disulfide bonds bridging the N-terminal segment and e3 loop and the e1 and e2 loops.[2] Disruption of one of these bonds could seriously perturb receptor folding. Mutants bearing alanine substitutions at five residues in the ectodomain, all of which are charged, fail to bind IL-8. Mutants E275A and R280A have reduced signal transduction capacity, whereas mutants R199A, R203A and D265A lack signal transduction capacity. Whether these mutation-sensitive residues actually make contact with IL-8 has not yet been determined. Alanine scanning mutagenesis has also been performed for the intracellular loops of IL8RA.[89] Loss of function occurred when mutations were made in the i2 and i3 loops but not the i1 loop, as assessed by calcium mobilization in transfected cells. Synthetic peptides corresponding to the sequences of these loops disrupted formation of receptor-Giα2 protein complexes, as assessed physically by coimmunoprecipitation experiments and functionally by IL-8 stimulation of permeabilized neutrophils loaded with peptide.

Model for IL-8 Receptor Activation

The model for IL-8 receptor insertion in the membrane introduced earlier is based largely on sequence analysis and analogy with rhodopsin.[38,39] The close proximity of the four ectodomains in this model, and their relatively small combined size relative to that of chemokines[43] suggest that each of them is likely to contact ligand. A corollary to this is that the TMDs are unlikely to be available for binding to the bulky ordered portion of the chemokine, which forms the major part of the ligand structure.

While it is clear from the mutagenesis data reviewed above that for IL8RB the specific contacts must differ in detail for IL-8, GROα and NAP-2, there are likely to be general features of the ligand binding pocket that are shared. One of these may be a charge interaction between C-X-C chemokines, which are basic, and the N-terminal segments of IL8RA and IL8RB, which are acidic. A second may be an interaction of the unordered ELR+

N-terminal segment of the chemokine with a binding site made up of one or more determinants in the TMDs. Binding of the ordered chemokine domain to the receptor ectodomains could create a conformational change exposing the TMDs which may then bind the unordered ELR domain of the chemokine, causing receptor and then G protein activation. A similar model has been proposed and substantially validated by Siciliano et al for the C5a receptor, which is quite similar in sequence to the chemokine receptors and binds a ligand analogous in size, charge and structure to chemokines.[90] Additional mutagenesis, biochemical and structural studies will be required to judge the validity of this model for IL-8 and other chemokine receptors.

C-C Chemokine Receptors

C-C Chemokines

The most widely used names for the known human C-C chemokines are MIP-1α, MIP-1β, MCP-1, MCP-2, MCP-3, RANTES and I-309. Sequence variants of these proteins in human and other species have been reviewed.[91] The sets of leukocyte subtypes that are targeted by these molecules are quite distinct. All of them chemoattract monocytes, although the efficacy varies considerably both in vitro and in vivo.

Additional C-C chemokines have been identified in other species, and at least eleven novel human C-C chemokines have been identified by analysis of expressed sequence tags by Li and co-workers at Human Genome Sciences.[92] In contrast, only one previously unknown C-X-C chemokine has been identified by Li's group by random cDNA sequencing. This suggests that the number of C-C chemokine receptors is likely to be large and their functional properties complex.

Human C-C Chemokine Receptors

Like C-X-C chemokines, the actions of C-C chemokines on leukocytes (chemotaxis, regulation of adhesion, degranulation, calcium mobilization, etc.) are highly sensitive to pertussis toxin, suggesting that Gi-coupled receptors are involved.[93] ^{125}I-labeled MIP-1α, MIP-1β, RANTES and MCP-1 bind specifically to peripheral blood monocytes.[94-97] Like the C-X-C chemokine binding sites on neutrophils, distinct patterns of crosscompetition by unlabeled C-C chemokines have been reported for binding by each C-C chemokine radioligand, suggesting multiple sets of shared 7TMD receptors. C-C chemokine binding sites on peripheral blood basophils, eosinophils and neutrophils have not been described yet, although these cell types can clearly respond to C-C chemokines.[98-100] Several C-C chemokines, most notably MIP-1α, have been shown to act as negative regulators of hematopoietic stem cells, but the nature of the putative receptors involved has not been defined.[101,102]

So far, six functional human C-C chemokine receptor cDNAs have been cloned, all of them by homology hybridization using conserved sequence motifs found in other chemoattractant receptors (Fig. 3.2B).[8,14-18] Since the number of distinct C-C chemokine receptors is large and growing, and since their agonist selectivities extensively overlap, it is reasonable to assign the receptors numerical rather than function-based names. The properties of these complicated receptors are given in Table 3.1. Since they have been identified only recently, relatively little is known about their relative functional importance.

The amino acid sequences of the C-C chemokine receptors are similar in length (355-373 amino acids), and they are 40-60% identical to each other for all pairwise comparisons, but only 25-30% identical to the IL-8 receptors. The gene for C-C CKR1 has been mapped to human chromosome 3p21.[14] Since two C-C CKR-like orphan receptor genes, CMKBRL1 and GPR5, also map to this region,[24,25] it is likely that the other functional chemokine receptor genes are clustered at 3p21. C-C CKR2A and C-C CKR2B appear to be alternatively spliced products of the same gene, differing only in the amino acid sequence beyond residue 313 in the C-terminal cytoplasmic tail.[16,103] The other cloned C-C CKRs are the products of distinct genes.[14,17,18] The gene for C-C CKR2 is the only known chemokine receptor gene that has an intron in the open reading frame. MCP-2 and I-309 are the only known human chemokines that have not been connected functionally to one of these cloned receptors.

C-C Chemokine Receptor Expression

RNA analysis has suggested that the expression of C-C CKRs is highly regulated in peripheral blood leukocytes and solid organs.[14,15,17,18,24] RNA for C-C CKR2A and C-C CKR2B is detectable by Northern blot analysis in monocytes, but not in neutrophil or eosinophil samples. C-C CKR3 is eosinophil selective. C-C CKR4 RNA has been detected in T lymphocyte, monocyte and basophil samples, but the relative levels of expression have not been defined. C-C CKR1 RNA is detectable at highest levels in monocytes; its RNA is also detectable in neutrophils and lymphocytes however, and in much smaller amounts in eosinophils. C-C CKR1 RNA is found in all of eight solid organs that have so far been tested (placenta, brain, lung, liver, spleen, kidney, heart, skeletal muscle), with highest expression in placenta, lung and spleen. In contrast, C-C CKR2 RNA has been detected only in lung and liver. C-C CKR3 RNA was not detectable in any of these solid organs. The specific cell types accounting for these hybridization signals in human organs have not been defined.

Based on the RNA analysis, it is evident that monocytes express at least two receptors selective for MIP-1α and RANTES (C-C CKR1, C-C CKR4 and C-C CKR5),[14,18,24] two receptors selective for MCP-3 (C-C CKR1 and C-C CKR2B)[103,104] and three receptors selective for MCP-1 (C-C CKR2A, C-C CKR2B and C-C CKR4).[16,24,103] It is likely that C-C CKR2A is also an MCP-3 receptor, although it has not been tested yet. The agonists for C-C CKR5, MIP-1α, RANTES and IP-1β, were

mistakenly attributed to C-C CKR3, owing to a mislabeled DNA sample.[17] The cloning of C-C CKR5 cDNA has been submitted for publications. We subsequently showed that C-C CKR3 is slelective for the novel human chemokine, eotaxin.[103a]

Comparison of Native and Cloned C-C Chemokine Receptors

Given the shear numbers of known C-C CKRs and their broadly overlapping tissue and cell type distributions and sets of agonists, sorting out signaling specificity is going to be a challenging and complex problem that will require receptor subtype-specific neutralizing antibodies and antagonists, and genetically manipulated leukocytes for its solution. At the present time, one can only make inferences about the functional role of each cloned C-C chemokine receptor based on the concordance of binding, signal transduction and RNA data for native leukocytes and cloned receptors. There is a large amount of conflicting data that needs to be reconciled, as reviewed below.

In the case of monocytes, unlabeled MCP-1 and MCP-3 compete for monocyte ^{125}I-MCP-1 binding sites, just as they do for C-C CKR2B, yet the rank orders of competition are inverted: MCP-3 > MCP-1 for monocytes and MCP-1 > MCP-3 for C-C CKR2B.[103-105] Furthermore, MCP-1 and MCP-3 completely crossdesensitize monocyte $[Ca^{2+}]_i$ transients elicited by each other, whereas asymmetric desensitization is found for MCP-1 and MCP-3 for C-C CKR2B, which is selectively expressed in monocytes. Wang et al have shown that binding of ^{125}I-MIP-1α and ^{125}I-MIP-1β to monocytes can be competed equally effectively by unlabeled MIP-1α and MIP-1β, whereas ^{125}I-MIP-1α but not ^{125}I-MIP-1β binds to C-C CKR1 and unlabeled MIP-1β very weakly competes for the binding.[8,97] None of the cloned C-C CKRs appears to be the monocyte MIP-1β receptor. Wang et al and Van Riper et al also characterized a THP-1 cell RANTES receptor.[95,96] MCP-1 was able to completely desensitize

THP-1 cell $[Ca^{2+}]_i$ transients elicited by RANTES, whereas MCP-1 has no effect on C-C CKR1 RANTES responses. Moreover, MCP-1 effectively competes for ^{125}I-RANTES binding to THP-1 cells, but poorly competes for the C-C CKR1 binding site for ^{125}I-RANTES.

In the case of eosinophils and basophils, MCP-3 binding has not yet been evaluated. In the case of eosinophils, MIP-1α has little effect on the RANTES-induced calcium response, whereas it is able to completely desensitize the C-C CKR1 RANTES response.[8,98] Like C-C CKR2B expressed in HEK 293 cells, basophil $[Ca^{2+}]_i$ transients elicited by MCP-1 and MCP-3 are asymmetrically crossdesensitized; however, the asymmetries are inverted: for basophils, MCP-1 partially affects the response to MCP-3 and MCP-3 completely desensitizes the response to MCP-1, whereas for C-C CKR2B, the converse is true.[100,103] Since C-C CKR4 is expressed in basophils, it is a good candidate to mediate basophil responses to MIP-1α, RANTES and MCP-1, its known agonists.[18] The ability of MCP-3 to activate C-C CKR4 has not been reported yet.

The most concordant response pattern for a cloned C-C chemokine receptor and a native leukocyte receptor is found in lymphocytes. Crossdesensitization of $[Ca^{2+}]_i$ transients induced by MCP-1 and MCP-3 for CD4$^+$ and CD8$^+$ human lymphocytes resembles that observed for C-C CKR2B.[106] Chemotactic activity is relatively weak and is restricted to specific subsets that in some cases require a prior cell activation step. RNA for C-C CKR1 is present in peripheral blood-derived lymphocytes,[15] but its expression in subsets has not yet been delineated. RANTES specifically attracts both resting and anti-CD3-stimulated CD45RO$^+$ T cells, also known as "memory" cells.[107] Two reports have shown that MIP-1α attracts anti-CD3-stimulated, but not unstimulated, T cells, preferentially the CD8$^+$ subset.[108,109] MIP-1β preferentially attracts activated CD4$^+$ cells in vitro. These results differed from those of Tanaka et al who reported that MIP-1β, but not MIP-1α, could attract "resting" T cells.[109,110]

The leukocyte targets defined in vitro have not yet all been shown to respond to C-C chemokine challenges in vivo. For example, recombinant human MCP-1 can be injected intradermally into dogs with little if any inflammatory cell infiltration of the injected site, despite the fact that canine monocytes bind MCP-1 with high affinity.[111] In contrast, intradermal injection of dogs with human RANTES causes monocyte and eosinophil infiltration.

In neutrophils, two pieces of evidence indicate that C-C CKR1 may play a functional role: (1) RNA for the cloned receptor is present and (2) both MIP-1α and RANTES activate a calcium flux. However, the number of receptors per cell must be very low or of low affinity in the neutrophil environment, as direct ligand binding has not been demonstrated. Moreover, the precise function that is performed is unknown: neither chemokine stimulates neutrophil chemotaxis, degranulation or superoxide production.[112] Recent information suggests that the other agonist for C-C CKR1, MCP-3, does induce neutrophil chemotaxis perhaps operating through C-C CKR1.[113]

The differences summarized above for cloned and native leukocyte C-C chemokine receptors could be due to the presence of additional as yet undiscovered C-C chemokine receptors on leukocytes, or else to different properties of the cloned receptors in leukocytes relative to their properties when expressed in heterologous cell types. Two chemokine receptor examples of the latter are known. First, the native Duffy antigen (see below) on erythrocytes binds ^{125}I-IL-8 with high affinity, whereas binding of ^{125}I-IL-8 to the cloned Duffy antigen expressed in HEK 293 cells is not detectable. IL-8 binding can be inferred by the ability of unlabeled IL-8 to compete for ^{125}I-GROα to Duffy-transfected cells.[21] Second, the agonist rank order for IL8RB expressed in HEK 293 cells is IL-8 =

GROα = NAP-2, whereas when it is expressed in *Xenopus* oocytes it is IL-8>>GROα=NAP-2.[13,57]

C-C Chemokine Receptors in Other Species

Three C-C chemokine receptor-like genes have been cloned from the mouse.[37,114] They have been provisionally designated the mouse MIP-1α receptor (MIP-1αR) and mouse MIP-1α receptor-like 1 and 2 receptors (MIP-1αRL1 and 2). MIP-1αR is the mouse orthologue of C-C CKR1. It has 83% amino acid identity with C-C CKR1 and binds both human MIP-1α and human RANTES with high affinity; however MIP-1α is a much more potent agonist than human RANTES. Mouse RANTES has not been tested yet. RNA for all three genes is expressed in mouse leukocytes, but in solid organs distinct tissue specific expression is observed: skeletal muscle only (MIP-1αRL1), vs. lung, heart and spleen (MIP-1αRL2), vs. lung, liver and spleen (MIP-1αR). These genes will be useful for performing genetic tests of function in knockout mice.

THE DUFFY ANTIGEN/ RECEPTOR FOR CHEMOKINES: A C-C AND C-X-C CHEMOKINE BINDING PROTEIN

Only one 7TMD protein is presently known that binds both C-C and C-X-C chemokines. Horuk and co-workers have given this protein the name DARC for Duffy antigen/receptor for chemokines which summarizes its known functional properties. While the Duffy blood group antigen has been known for many years, its relationship to chemokines is a recent discovery made from the synthesis of several serendipitous observations and astute insights. Darbonne and co-workers first made the surprising observation that red blood cells possess high affinity binding sites for IL-8.[115] Binding could be competed by some but not all C-X-C and C-C chemokines (IL-8, GROα, RANTES and MCP-1, but not MIP-1α or MIP-1β) distinguishing it from the leukocyte chemokine receptors.[116,117] Horuk then noted that red cells from most African-American donors did not bind chemokines. The only other known red cell protein with this property is the Duffy blood group antigen. Miller had shown in 1975 that Duffy is missing in most black Africans and African-Americans, proved that it functions pathologically as an invasion receptor for the malaria-causing simian parasite *Plasmodium knowlesi* and the related human parasite *Plasmodium vivax*, and proposed that in Africa the form of malaria caused by *P. vivax* selected against Duffy.[118,119] This suggested to Horuk that the Duffy antigen and the chemokine binding protein on red cells might be identical. He proved this in a collaborative study with Miller's group, showing that a monoclonal antibody to the Duffy antigen could block chemokine binding to red cells and vice versa, and that chemokines could block invasion of Duffy positive red cells by *P. knowlesi*.[120]

Independently and almost simultaneously, Chaudhuri and colleagues reported the cloning of a cDNA encoding a 7TMD protein that bears the Duffy antigen on its N-terminal segment before TMD1.[20,22] This is a rare example of a 7TMD protein whose DNA cloning involved prior purification and sequencing of the native protein. The deduced sequence of this protein is ~25% identical to those of the C-C and C-X-C chemokine receptors reviewed above. When it is expressed in 293 or K562 cells, DARC binds ^{125}I-GROα and several other CXC and CC chemokines in the transfected cells.[21] Two DARC haplotypes, Fy^a and Fy^b, have been defined serologically that arise from a single base difference in codon 44 [Fy^a = GAT(Asp44); Fy^b = GGT (Gly44)]. This residue is located in the N-terminal segment of DARC.

DARC mRNA is detectable in normal human bone marrow, but not in bone marrow samples from individuals whose erythrocytes lack DARC. Nevertheless, individuals whose red cells lack DARC express it in other body sites such as lung, spleen, kidney and brain.[122,123] Surveys with monoclonal antibodies to DARC indicate that it is normally expressed not only on erythrocytes, but also on endothelial cells of postcapillary venules.[122,124] DARC has evidently been silenced in a tissue-specific manner in a geographically restricted population by the selective pressure imposed by malaria. Tissue-specific inactivation strongly suggests a mutation in a regulatory region of the gene.

The physiologic function of DARC is not known. Since it lacks a known signaling function, a chemokine clearance function was originally proposed for red cell DARC. This would keep the concentration of chemokines in plasma at low levels, and perhaps maximize the sensitivity of circulating leukocytes to changes in the concentration of chemokines in the tissues. Other than susceptibility to *vivax* malaria, however, DARC status has not been linked either positively or negatively to any diseases. Moreover, infusion of large doses of IL-8 is well-tolerated in nonhuman primates.[125] Even if DARC expression on red cells is not physiologically important, it may still play an important role, perhaps in chemokine clearance or chemokine presentation to signaling chemokine receptors in one or another of the tissues where it has been detected. However, the nature of that role is presently totally unknown.

The ability of IL-8 to bind to red cells in vivo has been shown in human subjects undergoing experimental IL-1α therapy for cancer.[126] If red cell DARC is physiologically important, a difference in clinical course might be detectable in DARC negative as compared to DARC positive individuals when circulating IL-8 levels become elevated for long periods of time, as occurs during endotoxic shock, and IL-1α or IL-2 cytokine therapy. Regardless of the physiologic function of DARC, the fact that chemokines bind to it and block invasion of red cells by *P. knowlesi* in vitro, establishes them as reasonable parent structures for the development of drugs for *vivax* malaria.

VIRAL CHEMOKINE RECEPTORS

After their complete genomes were sequenced, data base searches identified ORF US28 of human cytomegalovirus (HCMV) and ORF ECRF3 of Herpesvirus saimiri as having low amino acid sequence similarity to rhodopsin-like receptors (Figs. 3.2A and 3.2B).[7,127] The highest similarity was to C-C CKR1 and IL8RB, respectively, but was still at the level of only 30% amino acid identity.[1,14] Closer inspection indicated that the N-terminal segments of the viral sequences were surprisingly well-conserved with the corresponding sequences of the chemokine receptors. This suggested a closer evolutionary relationship than was otherwise apparent from comparing the entire sequences, since this region is the least well-conserved for even closely related G protein-coupled receptors such as IL8RA and IL8RB. Based on this observation, both viral ORFs were studied and were shown to encode functional receptors for human chemokines.[8,9,11]

Two other viral ORFs have subsequently been identified that have interesting sequence relationships to the chemokine receptors: ORF K2R of swinepox virus is most like that of IL8RB (30% aa identity),[128] and ORF E1 of equine herpesvirus-2 is most related to C-C CKR1 (55% aa identity).[129] Direct binding to chemokines has not yet been reported for these predicted proteins, however. The very existence of viral chemokine receptor mimics strongly attests to the general biological importance of chemokines; however the specific roles of the viral receptors in viral life cycles are not yet known.

OPEN READING FRAME US28 OF HUMAN CYTOMEGALOVIRUS

Human cytomegalovirus (HCMV) is a species-restricted β herpesvirus that infects epithelial, endothelial, myeloid, lymphoid and smooth muscle cells in vivo causing acute, latent and chronic infections.[130] HCMV infection is often asymptomatic but can cause a mononucleosis syndrome in normal hosts and severe retinal, pulmonary and gastrointestinal inflammation in immunocompromised hosts, particularly in transplant patients undergoing immunosuppressive therapy and patients with AIDS. HCMV grows slowly in vitro and is highly species-restricted. Because of these obstacles, its molecular pathogenesis has been hard to study and is poorly understood.

ORF US28 is found at the right end of the HCMV genome in the unique short region. It is expressed in the late phase during lytic infection of human fibroblasts in vitro as two 3' coterminal mRNAs, one that contains only US28 and another that contains in addition ORF US27 which encodes an orphan G protein-coupled receptor sequence.[131] A third HCMV ORF encoding another orphan G protein-coupled receptor homologue known as *UL33* is found at the left end of HCMV DNA in the unique long region of the genome.[7]

US28 Binds C-C Chemokines

Direct evidence that US28 encodes a functional receptor for multiple C-C chemokines came from expression studies in human cell lines transfected with plasmids containing the US28 ORF. Neote et al initially reported that adenovirus-transformed human embryonic kidney 293 cells transiently transfected with the US28 ORF bind ^{125}I-human MIP-1α with high affinity, and the binding can be competed by MIP-1β, MCP-1 and RANTES, but not by IL-8.[8] This result was confirmed and extended by Gao and Murphy who established the ligand selectivity for US28 and showed that it was capable of signal transduction when stably expressed in transfected K562 cells.[9] The suspended cells bind ^{125}I-human MIP-1α with high affinity at 4°C. Binding is competed equally effectively by MIP-1α, MIP-1β, MCP-1 and RANTES with a K_i~5 nM. Neither of the C-X-C chemokines that were tested, IL-8 and γIP-10, compete for the MIP-1α binding site.

US28 Signal Transduction

While the four C-C chemokines appear to bind to the MIP-1α site on US28 with similar affinity, their agonist potencies as assessed by a calcium flux assay differ dramatically. RANTES is a high potency agonist with an EC_{50} = 5 nM, whereas the other high affinity C-C chemokine ligands for US28, MIP-1β, RANTES and MCP-1, all elicit feeble calcium flux responses at best, at threshold concentrations exceeding 100 nM. The strong response induced by RANTES could be desensitized by prior stimulation with RANTES, MIP-1α and MCP-1, but not by IL-8. Thus MIP-1α and MCP-1 have partial agonist and partial antagonist activities with respect to RANTES activation of US28.

A virus bearing a disrupted US28 will be useful for assessing the role of US28 in the viral life cycle in vitro and in animal models in vivo. Human cytomegalovirus is highly adapted to humans, and is not found naturally in other species. Good animal models have not been developed; therefore information about US28 obtained in nonhuman hosts must be interpreted cautiously. Nevertheless, any evidence that US28 is an important virulence factor for HCMV would justify a search for antagonists to it that could be tested for therapeutic efficacy during CMV infections in immunocompromised hosts.

OPEN READING FRAME ECRF3 OF HERPESVIRUS SAIMIRI

Herpesvirus saimiri (HVS) is an oncogenic γ herpesvirus that is most closely related to the Epstein-Barr virus (EBV). HVS can infect T lymphocytes of a wide variety of primate hosts, whereas EBV infection is restricted to B lymphocytes.[132] EBV has homologues for most HVS ORFs, but not for ECRF3. In its natural host, the squirrel monkey, HVS does not cause disease, whereas in nonnatural primate hosts, such as common marmosets, HVS causes rapidly fatal lymphomas and leukemias. HVS can transform T lymphocytes from humans and nonhuman primates in vitro. The saimiri-transforming principle has been located by the study of deletion mutants to the right end of HVS L-DNA, whereas ECRF3 is located at the left end of L-DNA.[133] Interestingly, a reciprocal gene copying event is found for EBV. Instead of a host receptor gene, EBV has copied the host gene for the cytokine IL-10, which suppresses the Th2 arm of the immune response. Viral IL-10 mimics the anti-inflammatory and proliferative effects of mammalian IL-10.[134]

ORF 74 of equine herpesvirus-2, which is also a γ herpesvirus, is a positional counterpart of HVS ECRF3. It encodes a putative 7TMD receptor that has only 20% aa identity to ECRF3 and IL8RB.[129]

Comparison of ECRF3 Sequence to Mammalian IL-8 Receptors

The sequence of ECRF3 is only 30% identical to those of the mammalian IL-8 receptors (Fig. 3.2A). Moreover, multiple insertions and deletions relative to the mammalian IL-8 receptor sequences are found throughout the alignment. All of these involve single amino acids, with the exception of a four residue deletion at the end of the fourth transmembrane domain. ECRF3 has two potential sites for N-linked glycosylation in the N-terminal segment before TMD1, and none in the e2 loop, whereas both human IL-8 receptor sequences have one or more sites in both the N-terminal segment and the e2 loop. The LRC sequence at the end of TMD3 of ECRF3 is a marked change from the DRY motif present in 80% of other rhodopsin-like receptors and the ERY or ERW sequence present in the remaining 20%. The IL-8 receptors have the DRY motif, which is important for coupling to G proteins.[135] The ECRF3 ORF terminates prematurely relative to the IL-8 receptors. This results in the absence of 26 amino acids including multiple serines and threonines that could be sites for receptor desensitization by phosphorylation, as they are in other G protein-coupled receptors.

ECRF3 Signal Transduction

Despite these substantial differences in sequence, frog oocytes injected with ECRF3 cRNA mobilize intracellular calcium in response to the same C-X-C chemokines that bind to IL8RB, namely IL-8, GROα and NAP-2.[11] C-C chemokines are ineffective. The agonist rank orders determined for calcium mobilization in frog oocytes for human IL-8 receptors and ECRF3 are: ECRF3, GROα~NAP-2>>IL-8; IL8RB, IL-8>GROα~NAP-2; and IL8RA, only IL-8—GROα and NAP-2 are ineffective.

These agonist-receptor relationships are paradoxical, since IL8RB is much more highly related in sequence to IL8RA than to ECRF3, yet its chemokine selectivity is more like that of ECRF3. Most of the residues of ECRF3 that are conserved in IL8RB are also conserved in IL8RA. Of the 16 that are not, 9 are located in the N-terminal segment prior to TMD1.

ORIGINS OF US28 AND ECRF3

The origins of US28 and ECRF3 cannot be proved. Most likely they were copied from the RNA for a mammalian C-C chemokine receptor in an infected cell and inserted into the viral genome, a process known as retroposition. This is plausible since the cell types that are permissive for human CMV and HVS infection overlap with the cell types that express C-C chemokine receptor RNA.

BIOLOGICAL ROLES OF US28 AND ECRF3

Until the viral chemokine receptors are studied in the context of a viral infection in vivo, one can only speculate about their biological roles based on the known properties of human chemokines that bind to them. The major known functions of chemokines are leukocyte chemotaxis and degranulation, but it is hard to imagine how these functions would benefit a virus. Perhaps instead, HCMV and HVS use chemokine receptors to control viral replication by regulating cell cycle progression of the host cell or by inhibiting apoptosis of the host cell. If the chemokine receptor is present on the virion, it could serve as an address label targeting virus for entry into cells with chemokines tethered to their surface. Nevertheless, the preservation of the signaling function of these receptors suggests that it is used by the virus.

FUTURE DIRECTIONS

Large-scale sequencing of expressed human genes has already given an approximate size of the chemokine family and can be expected to do the same for the receptor family soon. Defining ligand:receptor relationships can then be accomplished in a systematic and comprehensive manner. A more difficult long-range challenge will be to determine chemokine signaling specificity, particularly for the C-C chemokines. This can most clearly be accomplished by developing receptor-specific neutralizing monoclonal antibodies and small molecule antagonists, as well as by loss and gain of function genetic tests in transgenic animals and cultured cells. The same approaches can be used to tease out the roles of specific chemokines and receptors in disease processes. Specific areas that merit close attention are the development of agents that block binding of *P. vivax* to DARC, identification of the role of viral chemokine receptors in viral pathogenesis, development of antagonists to IL8RA and IL8RB, and assessment of the role of C-C chemokine receptors in allergy, chronic inflammation and wound repair. Finally, recent information that chemokine receptors are broadly and differentially expressed in human tissues should be followed up to look for specialized functions at specific tissue sites.

REFERENCES

1. Murphy PM. The molecular biology of leukocyte chemoattractant receptors. Annu Rev Immunol 1994; 12:593-633.
2. Horuk R. The interleukin-8 receptor family: from chemokines to malaria. Immunol Today 1994; 15:169-174.
3. Murphy PM. Molecular piracy of chemokine receptors by herpesviruses. Infect Agents Dis 1994; 3:137-154.
4. Probst WB, Snyder LA, Schuster DI et al. Sequence alignment of the G protein-coupled receptor superfamily. DNA Cell Biol 1993; 11:1-20.
5. Libert F, Parmentier M, Lefort A et al. Selective amplification and cloning of four new members of the G protein-coupled receptor family. Science 1989; 244:569-572.
6. Murphy PM. Chemokine receptors: cloning strategies. Immunomethods 1995; (in press).
7. Chee MS, Satchwell SC, Preddie E et al. Human cytomegalovirus encodes three G protein-coupled receptor homologues. Nature 1990; 344:774-777.
8. Neote K, DiGregorio D, Mak JY et al. Molecular cloning, functional expression, and signaling characteristics of a C-C chemokine receptor. Cell 1993; 72:415-425.
9. Gao J-L, Murphy PM. Open reading frame US28 of human cytomegalovirus encodes a functional β chemokine receptor. J Biol Chem 1994; 269:28539-28542.
10. Albrecht J-C, Nicholas J, Biller D et al. Primary structure of the Herpesvirus saimiri genome. J Virol 1992; 66:5047-5058.
11. Ahuja SK, Murphy PM. Molecular piracy of mammalian interleukin-8 receptor type B by Herpesvirus saimiri. J Biol Chem 1993; 268:20691-20694.
12. Holmes WE, Lee J, Kuang W-J et al. Structure and functional expression of a human interleukin-8 receptor. Science 1991; 253:1278-1280.
13. Murphy PM, Tiffany HL. Cloning of complementary DNA encoding a functional interleukin-8 receptor. Science 1991; 253:1280-1283.
14. Gao J-L, Kuhns DB, Tiffany HL et al. Structure and functional expression of the human macrophage inflammatory protein-1α/RANTES receptor. J Exp Med 1993; 177:1421-1427.
15. Nomura H, Nielsen BW, Matsushima K. Molecular cloning of cDNAs encoding a LD78 receptor and putative leukocyte chemotactic peptide receptors. Int Immunol 1993; 5:1239-1249.
16. Charo IF, Myers SJ, Herman A et al. Molecular cloning and functional expression of two monocyte chemoattractant protein 1

receptors reveals alternative splicing of the carboxyl-terminal tails. Proc Natl Acad Sci USA 1994; 91:2752-2756.

17. Combadiere C, Ahuja SK, Murphy PM. Cloning and functional expression of a human eosinophil C-C chemokine receptor. J Biol Chem 1995; 270:16491-16494. [Correction: J Biol Chem 1995; 270:30255].

18. Power CA, Meyer A, Nemeth K et al. Molecular cloning and functional expression of a novel C-C chemokine receptor cDNA from a human basophilic cell line. J Biol Chem 1995; 270:19495-19500.

19. Horuk R, Chitnis C, Darbonne W et al. The erythrocyte chemokine receptor is a receptor for the malarial parasite Plasmodium vivax. Science 1993; 261:1182-1184.

20. Chaudhuri A, Polyakova J, Zbrzezna V et al. Cloning of glycoprotein D cDNA, which encodes the major subunit of the Duffy blood group system and the receptor for the Plasmodium vivax malaria parasite. Proc Natl Acad Sci USA 1993; 90:10793-10797.

21. Neote K, Mak JY, Kolakowski LF Jr et al. Functional and biochemical analysis of the cloned Duffy antigen: identity with the red blood cell chemokine receptor. Blood 1994; 84:44-52.

22. Chaudhuri A, Zbrzezna V, Polyakova J et al. Expression of the Duffy antigen in K562 cells. Evidence that it is the human erythrocyte chemokine receptor. J Biol Chem 1994; 269:7835-7838.

23. Birkenbach M, Josefsen K, Yalamanchili R et al. Epstein-Barr virus-induced genes: first lymphocyte-specific G protein-coupled peptide receptors. J Virol 1993; 67:2209-2220.

24. Combadiere C, Ahuja SK, Murphy PM. Cloning, chromosomal localization and RNA expression of a novel human β chemokine receptor-like gene. DNA Cell Biol 1995; 14:673-680.

25. Heiber M, Doherty JM, Shah G et al. Isolation of three novel human genes encoding G protein-coupled receptors. DNA Cell Biol 1995; 14:25-35.

26. Loetscher M, Geiser T, O'Reilly T et al. Cloning of a human seven-transmembrane domain receptor, LESTR, that is highly expressed in leukocytes. J Biol Chem 1994; 269:232-237.

27. Harrison JK, Barber CM, Lynch KR. cDNA cloning of a G-protein-coupled receptor expressed in rat spinal cord and brain related to chemokine receptors. Neurosci Letts 1994; 169:85-88.

28. Dobner T, Wolf I, Emrich T et al. Differentiation-specific expression of a novel G protein-coupled receptor from Burkitt's lymphoma. Eur J Immunol 1992; 22: 2795-2799.

29. Baggiolini M, Dewald B, Moser B. Interleukin-8 and related chemotactic cytokines—C-X-C and C-C chemokines. Adv Immunol 1994; 55:97-179.

30. Morohashi H, Miyawaki T, Nomura H et al. Expression of both types of human interleukin-8 receptors on mature neutrophils, monocytes, and natural killer cells. J Leukoc Biol 1995; 57:180-187.

31. Ahuja SK, Shetty A, Tiffany HL et al. Comparison of the genomic organization and promoter function for human interleukin-8 receptors A and B. J Biol Chem 1994; 269:26381-26389.

32. L'Heureux GP, Bourgoin S, Jean N et al. Diverging signal transduction pathways activated by interleukin-8 and related chemokines in human neutrophils: interleukin-8, but not NAP-2 or GRO alpha, stimulates phospholipase D activity. Blood 1995; 85:522-531.

33. Unemori EN, Amento EP, Bauer EA et al. Melanoma growth-stimulatory activity/ GRO decreases collagen expression by human fibroblasts. Regulation by C-X-C but not C-C cytokines. J Biol Chem 1993; 268:1338-1342.

34. Koch AE, Polverini PJ, Kunkel SL et al. Interleukin-8 as a macrophage-derived mediator of angiogenesis. Science 1992; 258:1798-1801.

35. Bordoni R, Fine R, Murray D et al. Characterization of the role of melanoma growth stimulatory activity (MGSA) in the growth of normal melanocytes, nevocytes, and malignant melanocytes. J Cell Biochem 1990; 44:207-219.

36. Rot A. Endothelial cell binding of NAP-1/ IL-8: role in neutrophil emigration. Immunol Today 1992; 13:291-294.

37. Gao J-L, Murphy PM. Cloning and differ-

ential tissue-specific expression of three mouse β chemokine receptor-like genes, including the gene for a functional MIP-1α receptor. J Biol Chem 1995; 270:17494-17501.

38. Baldwin JM. The probable arrangement of the helices in G protein-coupled receptors. EMBO J 1993; 12:1693-1703.

39. Schertler GF, Villa C, Henderson R. Projection structure of rhodopsin. Nature 1993; 362:770-772.

40. Parker EM, Kameyama K, Higashijima T et al. Reconstitutively active G protein-coupled receptors purified from baculovirus-infected insect cells. J Biol Chem 1991; 266:519-527.

41. Samanta AK, Dutta S, Ali E. Modification of sulfhydryl groups of interleukin-8 (IL-8) receptor impairs binding of IL-8 and IL-8-mediated chemotactic response of human polymorphonuclear neutrophils. J Biol Chem 1993; 268:6147-6153.

42. Lodi PJ, Garrett DS, Kuszewski J et al. High-resolution solution structure of the beta chemokine hMIP-1 beta by multidimensional NMR. Science 1994; 263: 1762-1767.

43. Clore GM, Gronenborn AM. Comparison of the solution nuclear magnetic resonance and crystal structures of interleukin-8. Possible implications for the mechanism of receptor binding. J Mol Biol 1992; 217:611-620.

44. Clark-Lewis I, Kim K-S, Rajarathnam K et al. Structure-activity relationships of chemokines. J Leukocyte Biol 1995; 57:703-711.

45. Walz A, Peveri P, Aschauer H et al. Purification and amino acid sequencing of NAF, a novel neutrophil-activating factor produced by monocytes. Biochem Biophys Res Commun 1987; 149:755-761.

46. Yoshimura T, Matsushima K, Tanaka S et al. Purification of a human monocyte-derived neutrophil chemotactic factor that has peptide sequence similarity to other host defense cytokines. Proc Natl Acad Sci U S A 1987; 84:9233-9237.

47. Thelen M, Peveri P, Kernen P et al. Mechanism of neutrophil activation by NAF, a novel monocyte-derived peptide agonist.

FASEB J 1988; 2:2702-2706.

48. Leonard EJ, Skeel A, Yoshimura T et al. Leukocyte specificity and binding of human neutrophil attractant/activation protein-1. J Immunol 1990; 144:1323-1330.

49. Leonard EJ, Yoshimura T, Rot A et al. Chemotactic activity and receptor binding of neutrophil attractant/activation protein-1 (NAP-1) and structurally related host defense cytokines: interaction of NAP-2 with the NAP-1 receptor. J Leukoc Biol 1991; 49:258-265.

50. Moser B, Schumacher C, von Tscharner V et al. Neutrophil-activating peptide 2 and gro/melanoma growth-stimulatory activity interact with neutrophil-activating peptide 1/interleukin 8 receptors on human neutrophils. J Biol Chem 1991; 266:10666-10671.

51. Cerretti DP, Kozlosky CJ, Vanden Bos T et al. Molecular characterization of receptors for human interleukin-8, GRO/melanoma growth-stimulatory activity and neutrophil activating peptide-2. Mol Immunol 1993; 30:359-367.

52. Lee J, Horuk R, Rice GC et al. Characterization of two high affinity human interleukin-8 receptors. J Biol Chem 1992; 267:16283-16287.

53. Kozak M. An analysis of 5'-noncoding sequences from 699 vertebrate messenger RNAs. Nucleic Acids Res 1987; 15: 8125-8148.

54. LaRosa GJ, Thomas KM, Kaufmann ME et al. Amino terminus of the interleukin-8 receptor is a major determinant of receptor subtype specificity. J Biol Chem 1992; 267:25402-25406.

55. Gayle RB III, Sleath PR, Srinivason S. Importance of the amino terminus of the interleukin-8 receptor in ligand interactions. J Biol Chem 1993; 268:7283-7289.

56. Loetscher P, Seitz M, Clark-Lewis I et al. Both interleukin-8 receptors independently mediate chemotaxis. Jurkat cells transfected with IL-8R1 or IL-8R2 migrate in response to IL-8, GRO alpha and NAP-2. FEBS Lett 1994; 341:187-192.

57. Ahuja SK, Murphy PM. Reassessment of the role of the extracellular N-terminal segment of the human interleukin-8 receptors in determining subtype selectivity. (submitted).

58. Hebert CA, Vitangcol RV, Baker JB. Scanning mutagenesis of interleukin-8 identifies a cluster of residues required for receptor binding. J Biol Chem 1991; 266: 18989-18994.

59. Clark-Lewis I, Schumacher C, Baggiolini M et al. Structure-activity relationships of interleukin-8 determined using chemically synthesized analogs. Critical role of NH2-terminal residues and evidence for uncoupling of neutrophil chemotaxis, exocytosis, and receptor binding activities. J Biol Chem 1991; 266:23128-23134.

60. Schraufstatter IU, Barritt DS, Ma M et al. Multiple sites on IL-8 responsible for binding to α and β IL-8 receptors. J Immunol 1993; 151:6418-6428.

61. Chuntharapai A, Lee J, Hebert CA et al. Monoclonal antibodies detect different distribution patterns of IL-8 receptor A and IL-8 receptor B on human peripheral blood leukocytes. J Immunol 1994; 153:5682-5688.

62. Sebok K, Woodside D, al-Aoukaty A et al. IL-8 induces the locomotion of human IL-2-activated natural killer cells. Involvement of a guanine nucleotide binding (Go) protein. J Immunol 1993; 150:1524-1534.

63. Xu L, Kelvin DJ, Ye GQ et al. Modulation of IL-8 receptor expression on purified human T lymphocytes is associated with changed chemotactic responses to IL-8. J Leukoc Biol 1995; 57:335-342.

64. Murphy WJ, Taub DD, Anver M et al. Human RANTES induces the migration of human T lymphocytes into the peripheral tissues of mice with severe combined immune deficiency. Eur J Immunol 1994; 24:1823-1827.

65. Krieger M, Brunner T, Bischoff SC et al. Activation of human basophils through the IL-8 receptor. J Immunol 1992; 149: 2662-2667.

66. Kernen P, Wymann MP, von Tscharner V et al. Shape changes, exocytosis, and cytosolic free calcium changes in stimulated human eosinophils. J Clin Invest 1991; 87:2012-2017.

67. Strieter RM, Polverini PJ, Arenberg DA et al. Role of C-X-C chemokines as regulators of angiogenesis in lung cancer. J Leukoc Biol 1995; 57:752-762.

68. Maione TE, Gray GS, Petro J et al. Inhibition of angiogenesis by recombinant platelet factor 4 and related peptides. Science 1990; 247:77-79.

69. Gengrinovitch S, Greenberg SM, Cohen T et al. Platelet factor-4 inhibits the mitogenic activity of VEGF121 and VEGF165 using several concurrent mechanisms. J Biol Chem 1995; 270:15059-15065.

70. Horuk R, Yansura DG, Reilly D et al. Purification, receptor binding analysis, and biological characterization of human melanoma growth stimulating activity (MGSA). Evidence for a novel MGSA receptor. J Biol Chem 1993; 268:541-546.

71. Sprenger H, Lloyd AR, Meyer RG et al. Genomic structure, characterization, and identification of the promoter of the human IL-8 receptor A gene. J Immunol 1994; 153:2524-2532.

72. Sprenger H, Lloyd AR, Lautens LL et al. Structure, genomic organization, and expression of the human interleukin-8 receptor B gene. J Biol Chem 1994; 269:11065-11072.

73. Ahuja SK, Ozcelik T, Milatovich A et al. Molecular evolution of the human interleukin-8 receptor gene cluster. Nature Genet 1992; 2:31-36.

74. White JK, Shaw MA, Barton CH et al. Genetic and physical mapping of 2q35 in the region of the NRAMP and IL8R genes: identification of a polymorphic repeat in exon 2 of NRAMP. Genomics 1994; 24:295-302.

75. Ahuja SK, Shetty A, Tiffany HL et al. Characterization of the promoters for human IL-8 receptors A and B in myeloid and lymphoid cell lines, and CD34+ peripheral blood hematopoietic progenitor cells. Mol Biol Cell 1994; 5:122a.

76. Cerretti DP, Nelson N, Kozlosky CJ et al. The murine homologue of the human interleukin-8 receptor type B maps near the Ity-Lsh-Bcg disease resistance locus. Genomics 1993; 18:410-413.

77. Bozic CR, Gerard NP, von Uexkull-Guldenband C et al. The murine interleukin-8 type B receptor homologue and its ligands. J Biol Chem 1994; 269:29355-29358.

78. Suzuki H, Prado GN, Wilkinson N et al. The N terminus of interleukin-8 (IL-8) receptor confers high affinity binding to human IL-8. J Biol Chem 1994; 269: 18263-18266.

79. Vidal SM, Malo D, Vogan K et al. Natural resistance to infection with intracellular parasites: isolation of a candidate for Bcg. Cell 1993; 73:469-485.

80. Thomas KM, Taylor L, Navarro J. The interleukin-8 receptor is encoded by a neutrophil-specific cDNA clone, F3R. J Biol Chem 1991; 266:14839-14841.

81. Prado GN, Thomas KM, Suzuki H et al. Molecular characterization of a novel rabbit interleukin-8 receptor isotype. J Biol Chem 1994; 269:12391-12394.

82. Schraufstatter IU, Ma M, Oades ZG et al. The role of Tyr13 and Lys15 of interleukin-8 in the high affinity interaction with the interleukin-8 receptor type A. J Biol Chem 1995; 270:10428-10431.

83. Chuntharapai A, Kim KJ. Regulation of the expression of IL-8 receptor A/B by IL-8: possible function(s) of each receptor. 9th Int Congr Immunol 1995; A626.

84. Cacalano G, Lee J, Kikly K et al. Neutrophil and B cell expansion in mice that lack the murine IL-8 receptor homolog. Science 1994; 265:682-685.

85. Ahuja SK, Murphy PM. Mapping of distinct high and low affinity C-X-C chemokine binding sites that mediate human interleukin-8 receptor B activation. (submitted).

86. Ben-Baruch A, Bengali KM, Biragyn A et al. Interleukin-8 receptor beta. The role of the carboxyl terminus in signal transduction. J Biol Chem 1995; 270:9121-9128.

87. Lefkowitz RJ. G protein-coupled receptor kinases. Cell 1994; 74:409.

88. Leong SR, Kabakoff RC, Hebert CA. Complete mutagenesis of the extracellular domain of interleukin-8 (IL-8) type A receptor identifies charged residues mediating IL-8 binding and signal transduction. J Biol Chem 1994; 269:19343-19348.

89. Damaj BB, Neote K, McColl SR, Naccache P. Functional maping of the intracellular loops of the human interleukin-8 type A receptor: identification of the G protein binding sites to the IL-8RA receptor. 9th Int Congr Immunol 1995; A628.

90. Siciliano SJ, DeMartino J, Konteatis Z et al. Two-site binding of C5a by its receptor: a new binding paradigm for G protein-coupled receptors. Proc Natl Acad Sci USA 1993; 91:1214-1218.

91. Michiel D. Chemokines: the missing link. Bio/Technol. 1993; 11:739.

92. Li H. Discovery and characterization of novel human chemokines. In: Chemotactic Cytokines. Targets for Novel Therapeutic Development. Philadelphia: IBC., 1995.

93. Sozzani S, Zhou D, Locati M et al. Receptors and transduction pathways for monocyte chemotactic protein-2 and monocyte chemotactic protein-3. J Immunol 1994: 7:3615-3622.

94. Napolitano M, Seamon KB, Leonard WJ. Identification of cell surface receptors for the Act-2 cytokine. J Exp Med 1990; 172:285-289.

95. Van Riper G, Siciliano S, Fischer PA et al. Characterization and species distribution of high affinity GTP-coupled receptors for human rantes and monocyte chemoattractant protein 1. J Exp Med 1993; 177:851-856.

96. Wang JM, McVicar DW, Oppenheim JJ et al. Identification of RANTES receptors on human monocytic cells: competition for binding and desensitization by homologous chemotactic cytokines. J Exp Med 1993; 177:699-705.

97. Wang JM, Sherry B, Fivash MJ et al. Human recombinant macrophage inflammatory protein-1α andβ and monocyte chemotactic and activating factor utilize common and unique receptors on human monocytes. J Immunol 1993; 150:3022-3029.

98. Baggiolini M, Dahinden CA. C-C chemokines and allergic inflammation. Immunol Today 1994; 15:127-133.

99. Bischoff SC, Krieger M, Brunner T et al. RANTES and related chemokines activate human basophil granulocytes through different G protein-coupled receptors. Eur J Immunol 1993; 23:761-767.

100. Dahinden CA, Geiser T, Brunner T et al. Monocyte chemotactic protein 3 is a most effective basophil-and eosinophil-activating chemokine. J Exp Med 1994; 179:751-756.

101. Dunlop DJ, Wright EG, Lorimore S et al. Demonstration of stem cell inhibition and myeloprotective effects of SCI/rhMIP1α in vivo. Blood 1992; 79:2221-2225.

102. Graham GJ, Wright EG, Hewick R et al. Identification and characterization of an inhibitor of haemopoietic stem cell proliferation. Nature 1990; 344:442-444.

103. Combadiere C, Ahuja SK, Van Damme J et al. Monocyte chemoattractant protein-3 is a functional ligand for C-C chemokine receptors 1 and 2B. J Biol Chem. 1995; 270:(in press).

103a Kitaura M, Nakajima T, Imai T et al. Molecular cloning of human eotaxin, an eosinophil eotaxin receptor, CC chemokine receptor 3. J Biol Chem 1996; 27: 7725-7730.

104. Franci C, Wong LM, Van Damme J et al. Monocyte chemoattractant protein-3, but not monocyte chemoattractant protein-2, is a functional ligand of the human monocyte chemoattractant protein-1 receptor. J Immunol 1995; 154:6511-6517.

105. Uguccioni M, D'Apuzzo M, Loestcher M et al. Actions of the chemotactic cytokines MCP-1, MCP-2, MCP-3, RANTES, MIP-1α, and MIP-1β on human monocytes. Eur J Immunol 1995; 25:64-68.

106. Loetscher P, Seitz M, Clark-Lewis I et al. Monocyte chemotactic proteins MCP-1, MCP-2, and MCP-3 are major attractants for human CD4+ and CD8+ T lymphocytes. FASEB Journal 1994; 8:1055-1060.

107. Schall TJ, Bacon K, Toy KJ et al. Selective attraction of monocytes and T lymphocytes of the memory phenotype by cytokine RANTES. Nature 1990; 347:669-671.

108. Schall TJ, Bacon K, Camp RD et al. Human macrophage inflammatory protein α (MIP-1α) and MIP-1β chemokines attract distinct populations of lymphocytes. J Exp Med 1993; 177:1821-1826.

109. Taub DD, Conlon K, Lloyd AR et al. Preferential migration of activated CD4+ and CD8+ T cells in response to MIP-1α and MIP-1β. Science 1993; 260:355-358.

110. Tanaka Y, Adams DH, Hubscher S et al. T cell adhesion induced by proteoglycan-immobilized cytokine MIP-1β. Nature 1993; 361:79-82.

111. Meurer R, Van Riper G, Feeney W et al. Rapid formation of eosinophilic intradermal inflammatory sites in the dog by injection of human RANTES but not hMCP-1, hMIP-1α or hIL-8. J Exp Med 1993; 178:1913-1921.

112. McColl SR, Hachicha M, Levasseur S et al. Uncoupling of early signal transduction events from effector function in human peripheral blood neutrophils in response to recombinant macrophage inflammatory proteins-1 alpha and -1 beta. J Immunol 1993; 150:4550-4560.

113. Xu LL, McVicar D, BenBaruch A et al. Human neutrophils express functional receptor(s) for monocyte chemoattractant protein-3 (MCP3). 9th Int. Congr. Immunol 1995; A659.

114. Kozak C, Gao J-L, Murphy PM. Mapping of the mouse macrophage inflammatory protein-1α receptor gene Scya3r and two related mouse β chemokine receptor-like genes to chromosome 9. Genomics 1995; (in press).

115. Darbonne WC, Rice GC, Mohler MA et al. Red blood cells are a sink for interleukin 8, a leukocyte chemotaxin. J Clin Invest 1991; 88:1362-1369.

116. Horuk R, Colby TJ, Darbonne WC et al. The human erythrocyte inflammatory peptide (chemokine) receptor. Biochemical characterization, solubilization, and development of a binding assay for the soluble receptor. Biochemistry 1993; 32:5733-5738.

117. Neote K, Darbonne W, Ogez J et al. Identification of a promiscuous inflammatory peptide receptor on the surface of red blood cells. J Biol Chem 1993; 268:12247-12249.

118. Miller LH, Mason SJ, Clyde DF et al. The resistance factor to Plasmodium vivax in blacks. The Duffy-blood-group genotype, FyFy. N Engl J Med 1976; 295:302-304.

119. Miller LH, Mason SJ, Dvorak JA et al. Erythrocyte receptors for (Plasmodium knowlesi) malaria: Duffy blood group determinants. Science 1976; 189:561-564.

120. Hesselgesser J, Chitnis CE, Miller LH et al. A mutant of melanoma growth stimulating activity does not activate neutrophils but blocks erythrocyte invasion by malaria. J Biol Chem 1995; 270:11472-11476.

121. Iwamoto S, Omi T, Kajii E et al. Genomic

organization of the glycoprotein D gene: Duffy blood group Fya/Fyb alloantigen system is associated with a polymorphism at the 44-amino acid residue. Blood 1995; 85:622-626.

122. Peiper SC, Wang ZX, Neote K et al. The Duffy antigen/receptor for chemokines (DARC) is expressed in endothelial cells of Duffy negative individuals who lack the erythrocyte receptor. J Exp Med 1995; 181:1311-1317.

123. Chaudhuri A, Polyakova J, Zbrzezna V et al. The coding sequence of Duffy blood group gene in humans and simians: restriction fragment length polymorphism, antibody and malarial parasite specificities, and expression in nonerythroid tissues in Duffy-negative individuals. Blood 1995; 85: 615-621.

124. Hadley TJ, Lu Z, Wasniowska K et al. Postcapillary venule endothelial cells in kidney express a multispecific chemokine receptor that is structurally and functionally identical to the erythroid isoform, which is the Duffy blood group antigen. J Clin Invest 1994; 94:985-991.

125. Van Zee KJ, Fischer E, Hawes AS et al. Effects of intravenous IL-8 administration in nonhuman primates. J Immunol 1992; 148:1746-1752.

126. Tilg H, Pape D, Trehu E et al. A method for the detection of erythrocyte-bound interleukin-8 in humans during interleukin-1 immunotherapy. J Immunol Methods 1993; 163:253-258.

127. Nicholas J, Cameron KR, Honess RW. Herpesvirus saimiri encodes homologues of G protein-coupled receptors and cyclins. Nature 1992; 355:362-365.

128. Massung RF, Jayarama V, Moyer RW. DNA sequence analysis of conserved and unique regions of swinepox virus: identification of genetic elements supporting phenotypic observations including a novel G protein-coupled receptor homologue. Virology 1993; 197:511-528.

129. Davison AJ. The DNA sequence of equine herpesvirus 2. J Mol Biol 1995; 249: 520-528.

130. Alford CA, Britt WJ. Cytomegalovirus. In: Fields BN, ed. Virology. New York: Raven, 1990:1981-2010.

131. Welch AR, McGregor LM, Gibson W. Cytomegalovirus homologs of cellular G protein-coupled receptor genes are transcribed. J Virol 1991; 65:3915-3918.

132. Fleckenstein B, Desrosiers RC. Herpesvirus saimiri and Herpesvirus ateles. In: Roizman B, ed. The Herpesviruses. Vol. I. New York: Plenum Press, 1982:253-332.

133. Jung JU, Trimble JJ, King NW et al. Identification of transforming genes of subgroup A and C strains of Herpesvirus saimiri. Proc Natl Acad Sci USA 1991; 88:7051-7055.

134. Moore KW, Rousset F, Banchereau J. Evolving principles in immunopathology: interleukin 10 and its relationship to Epstein-Barr virus protein BCRF1. Springer Semin Immunopathol 1991; 13:157-166.

135. Savarese TM, Fraser CM. In vitro mutagenesis and the search for structure-function relationships among G protein-coupled receptors. Biochem J 1992; 283:1-19.

136. Marchese A, Docherty JM, Nguyen T et al. Cloning of human genes encoding novel G protein-coupled receptors. Genomics 1995; 23:609-618.

THE ROLE OF CHEMOKINES IN SKIN DISEASE

Kimberly E. Foreman and Brian J. Nickoloff

INTRODUCTION

Due to the accessibility of skin to sampling and cytokine measurements, it has been possible to define cytokine networks in a number of skin disorders. To date, such networks have been determined in the following diseases: psoriasis, atopic dermatitis, cutaneous T cell lymphoma, allergic contact dermatitis, intradermal delayed type hypersensitivity reactions, leprosy (Hansen's disease) and leishmaniasis. In addition to these inflammatory, immunological and infectious diseases, cytokines have been extensively studied as important molecular contributors to the physiological wound healing response, and investigated as contributing to the pathogenic events in chronic nonhealing cutaneous ulcers. In this chapter, the specific pathophysiological role of cytokines (with particular emphasis on chemokines) in these skin diseases will be reviewed.

The skin is the largest organ of the body and is composed of a confederacy of cell types, even under normal conditions. Resident skin cell types include non-migratory cells such as keratinocytes, melanocytes, fibroblasts and endothelial cells. In addition, migratory cells that originate in the bone marrow are consistently found in the normal skin including Langerhans cells, dermal dendritic cells, mast cells, monocyte/macrophages and T lymphocytes. Cytokines, including chemokines, are present in normal skin, and are likely to contribute to the maintenance of cutaneous homeostasis by providing directional signals that coordinate the interplay of indigenous and recruited circulating bone-marrow-derived cells. In the diseased state, there are nonrandom cutaneous patterns of infiltrating leukocytes that are responsible for the distinctive clinical and histopathological features of each specific skin disorder. Once again, it is highly likely that cytokines and chemokines, as well as adhesion

Chemokines in Disease, edited by Alisa E. Koch and Robert M. Strieter.
© 1996 R.G. Landes Company.

molecules and localized immune reactions, play critically important contributing roles to the pathophysiology of these processes. In the following sections, a review of recent research findings that focuses on chemokines in skin diseases will be presented, along with commentary on the therapeutic implication and future research trends to be expected for this rapidly progressing and highly clinically relevant line of inquiry.

PSORIASIS

Psoriasis is a common chronic inflammatory skin disease that affects approximately 2-3% of the population.[1,2] It is characterized by erythematous plaques of various sizes, often covered with silvery white scales, that most often affects, the trunk and extremities, typically at points of trauma in a symmetrical fashion. Histologically, psoriasis is characterized by keratinocyte hyperplasia, abnormal maturation of the keratinocytes, dermal neovascularization and an inflammatory cell infiltrate including T cells, monocytes, macrophages and dendritic cells with variable neutrophil accumulation in the dermis and epidermis.

In recent years, the involvement of cytokines, including chemokines, in development of the psoriatic lesion has become an active area of research. The major abnormalities of psoriatic plaques may be initiated and/or sustained by cytokines produced by resident and/or infiltrating cells. In fact, studies have demonstrated that injection of interferon-gamma (IFN-γ) in clinically symptomless skin of psoriasis patients results in the development of a lesion that is indistinguishable from idiopathic lesions.[3] A model for the generation of psoriatic plaques has been proposed.[4] The lesion is thought to be initiated by an assortment of internal and external stimuli that result in an acute inflammatory response including recruitment of leukocytes into the area. Following the acute inflammatory response, there is an attempt at regenerative wound healing process;

however, in the psoriatic patient, a variety of factors including continued inflammatory cell infiltration and cytokine production results in keratinocyte hyperplasia and neovascularization.

Recent work from a variety of laboratories has begun to unravel the complex cytokine network involved in psoriasis. The inflammatory cell infiltrate, particularly the T cells and mononuclear cells, appears to be critical in the maintenance of the psoriatic lesion. Evidence for this includes the effectiveness of cyclosporin A treatment of psoriasis, which is believed to decrease the infiltration of inflammatory cells resulting in limited cytokine production, as well as therapeutic responses to anti-CD4 monoclonal antibody and IL-2 conjugated to toxins.[5-7] The expression of chemokines and other chemotactic factors that may play a role in the recruitment of these inflammatory cells has become an area of intense interest. Early studies demonstrated that serum from psoriatic patients can serve as a chemoattractant for both normal and psoriatic neutrophils.[8,9] Since then, several chemotactic factors have been identified in psoriatic lesions, including leukotriene B4 (LTB4), the complement cleavage fragment C5a, platelet activating factor (PAF) as well as the chemokines interleukin-8 (IL-8), melanoma growth stimulating activity (MGSA/GROα), monocyte chemotactic protein-1 (MCP-1) and IFN-γ inducible protein-10 (γIP-10) (Table 4.1).[10] Both the protein and mRNA for IL-8 have been identified in psoriasis.[10-12] There is also a small, but significant increase in the number of IL-8 receptors on psoriatic neutrophils compared with normal controls.[13] IL-8 is produced by a variety of cells in the skin following stimulation with mediators such as tumor necrosis factor-alpha (TNF-α) and IL-1 which have both been identified in psoriasis. In vitro studies have shown that isolated keratinocytes can be stimulated with TNF-α to produce biologically active IL-8.[14] TNF-α is produced by the dermal dendritic cells in the papillary dermis as well as by keratinocytes and

Table 4.1. Chemokines involved in psoriasis

Chemokine	Produced by	Function	Ref.
IL-8	Keratinocytes Fibroblasts Monocytes T lymphocytes Endothelial cells Dermal dendritic cells	Neutrophil migration Stimulate keratinocyte growth Lymphocyte migration Basophil migration Neovascularization	4, 11, 12, 14 23, 24, 34
γIP-10	Keratinocytes	Neutrophil migration	28
GRO	Fibroblasts	Neutrophil migration Neutrophil enzyme release	10, 25-27
MCP-1	T lymphocytes Fibroblasts Endothelial cells Smooth muscle cells Keratinocytes	Monocyte migration	14

intraepidermal Langerhans cells.[12,15] As expected, IL-8 has been localized to the suprabasal keratinocytes located immediately above the TNF-α expressing dendrocytes and in the upper layers of the epidermis.[12,16] IL-8 is a potent chemoattractant for neutrophils and is able to induce keratinocyte growth.[17,18] This chemokine is thought to be crucial to the influx of neutrophils into the epidermis resulting in the formation of microabcesses that are characteristic of psoriasis.[19] IL-8 has been shown to induce lymphocyte chemotaxis in vitro, indicating that this chemokine may be involved in the influx of the T lymphocytes into psoriatic lesions.[20,21] However, it is controversial as to whether this occurs in vivo as injection of IL-8 into human skin did not result in lymphocyte infiltration.[22] IL-8 has also been previously shown to mediate angiogenesis.[23] Conditioned media from psoriatic keratinocytes is able to induce angiogenesis in a rat corneal bioassay and to induce endothelial cell chemotaxis in vitro.[24] Under these experimental conditions, it was shown that IL-8 was increased 10- to 20-fold

while the angiogenesis inhibitor thrombospondin-1 was decreased 7-fold.[24]

In addition to IL-8, there is evidence for the production of two other C-X-C chemokines, MGSA/GROα and γIP-10, as well as the C-C chemokine MCP-1. High levels of immunoreactivity for MGSA/GROα, a neutrophil chemoattractant, have been identified in psoriasis.[25,26] GROα was found to be 6 times more abundant than GROβ and 25 times more abundant than Groγ in psoriasis.[27] It has been suggested by Tettelbach and co-workers that differentiated keratinocytes in the stratum spinosum and the stratum granulosum harbor GROα protein as a reservoir so that, upon stimulation, GROα can be readily released and initiate the inflammatory response by recruiting neutrophils and lymphocytes.[25] γIP-10 is a neutrophil chemoattractant that is produced by keratinocytes following stimulation with IFN-γ. Both the protein and the mRNA for this chemokine have been found in psoriatic tissue, but not in the uninvolved skin in psoriasis patients.[28] Staining for γIP-10 was predominantly localized in the basal keratinocytes and may play a role in the migration of neutrophils into the area and the subsequent development of microabcesses. Successful treatment of psoriatic plaques with topical tar or ultraviolet light significantly reduced the expression of γIP-10 as determined by immunostaining.[28] MCP-1 can be produced by a variety of cells including T cells, endothelial cells and keratinocytes following stimulation with TNF-α, IL-1 and transforming growth factor-beta (TGF-β). Using in situ hybridization to evaluate MCP-1 mRNA expression in lesional psoriatic skin, Gillitzer et al found MCP was produced predominantly by the basal keratinocytes.[19] Production of MCP-1 in this area correlates with the presence of mobile dermal dendritic cells.

As expected following the identification of so many chemotactic factors in psoriatic lesion, several studies have addressed the relative importance of each of these chemotactic factors in the development of the psoriasis. One study suggests that the noncytokine member of the complement factor family, C5a, is of great importance, as the chemotactic activity correlates significantly with levels of C5a in lesional scales.[29] However, the in vivo stability of each of the compounds must be considered to accurately determine which mediator has a more profound effect in psoriasis. It has been shown that IL-8 and related proteins are resistant to inactivation and have slow clearance times once they are produced.[30,31] On the other hand, chemoattractant peptides such as C5a and LTB4 are rapidly inactivated, indicating that they may not be as important in vivo in lesion development as the longer acting chemokines.[30]

In addition to the chemokines listed above, a variety of cytokines have been found to be upregulated at the mRNA and/or protein level in psoriasis including IL-1β, IL-2, transforming growth factor-alpha (TGF-α), IL-6, granulocyte-monocyte-colony stimulating factor (GM-CSF), IFN-γ and TNF-α.[32-34] These cytokines follow the classification system initially described for mouse T cell clones dividing

CD4+ T cells into distinct functional subsets based upon cytokine production.[35] Th1 type cells produce IL-2 and IFN-γ which are important in T cell proliferation and macrophage activation while Th2 type cells produce IL-4, IL-5 and IL-10 and are involved in B cell stimulation. These cytokine profiles are particularly interesting as they are self-regulating. That is, the IFN-γ in the Th1 response inhibits production of Th2 type cytokines while the Th2 type cytokine IL-10 can inhibit IFN-γ production and suppress cell-mediated reactions.[36,37] In psoriasis, studies have found there is predominantly a Th1 type response which is accompanied by a significant decrease in the IL-10 protein production.[38-40] This imbalance between the pro-inflammatory Th1 cytokines and the anti-inflammatory cytokine IL-10 may be involved in lesion development.[40] It has been suggested that increasing IL-10 in the lesion may be useful therapeutically as dermal dendrocytes incubated with IL-10 have a reduced capacity to stimulate T cells because the IL-10 can inhibit expression of T cell costimulatory molecules such as CD86.[39]

It is controversial whether or not IL-1 plays a role in psoriasis. Studies have found upregulation of IL-1β and a decrease in IL-1α, but the presence of an IL-1 inhibitor has also been shown, indicating that any IL-1 produced may not be biologically active due to the concomitant presence of the inhibitor.[41,42] IL-6 has been found to be increased in psoriasis. It is produced by psoriatic keratinocytes as well as T cells and mononuclear cells following stimulation with IL-1 or TNF-α and IL-6 has been shown to stimulate keratinocyte proliferation and lymphocyte chemotaxis.[12,43] TGF-α is increased in psoriatic tissue based on the presence of both mRNA and protein in epidermal extract; however, TGF-β is found at similar levels in both psoriatic and normal skin.[44] TGF-α is produced by keratinocytes and binds to the epidermal growth factor (EGF) receptor resulting in autostimulated growth of the keratinocytes. Studies have shown that EGF receptor on keratinocytes is increased in psoriasis, indicating a possible role for TGF-α in keratinocyte hyperplasia.[45] IFN-γ mRNA has been identified in psoriatic lesions using polymerase chain reaction (PCR), and it appears that there may be an altered response to IFN-γ by the keratinocytes.[46] IFN-γ is know to inhibit keratinocyte growth; however, psoriatic keratinocytes are not inhibited by IFN-γ. Furthermore, IFN-γ induces HLA-DR expression on normal keratinocytes, but this is rarely observed in psoriatic tissue. The identification of IFN-γ in psoriasis is supported, however, by the induction of γIP-10 and intercellular adhesion molecule-1 (ICAM-1, CD54) expression on keratinocytes.

TNF-α is postulated to be the center of the cytokine network of psoriasis.[4] Several TNF-α inducible proteins have been identified in psoriasis including TGF-α, IL-6, IL-8 and ICAM-1, vascular cell adhesion molecule-1 (VCAM-1) and E-selectin.[4,10] The TNF-α is produced by the dermal dendritic cells in the papillary dermis and the TNF-α inducible proteins such as IL-8 and ICAM have been found in the surrounding keratinocytes.[12] Keratinocyte ICAM-1 expression is important, as there is strong evidence that LFA-1 positive T cells are retained in the epidermis via ICAM-1 expression induced on keratinocytes.[14]

To facilitate our further understanding of the pathophysiology of psoriasis, we have developed a novel animal model experimental system in which human skin is transplanted onto severe combined immunodeficient (SCID) mice.[47] Psoriatic plaques retained their phenotype for 6 weeks after transplantation and many different human cell types persisted in their typical anatomic configuration within the plaque. Moreover, cytokine levels such as IL-8 were also found to remain elevated after transplantation indicating that relevant T cell activation events were still on-going inside the transplanted human tissue. This model should allow us to introduce into transplanted symptomless psoriatic skin T cells, dendritic cells, etc. alone and in combination with various cytokines/chemokines to explore the specific and unique contribution these cells/mediators make to the development of a psoriatic plaque. Such a complex multicellular conspiracy is likely to be required for the underlying genetic abnormality to become phenotypically manifest.

CUTANEOUS T CELL LYMPHOMA

Mycosis fungoides is a type of cutaneous T cell lymphoma (CTCL) characterized clinically by erythematous patches that progress into raised, scaling plaques and development of large, tumor nodules. The disease may remain relatively indolent for years/decades or may disseminate and involve the lymph nodes, visceral organs and blood with generalized erythroderma (Sézary syndrome).[48,49] Histologically, lesions show infiltration of the papillary dermis and epidermis by a clonal proliferation of neoplastic CD4+ T cells. It is currently unknown why the lymphocytes compartmentalize to the skin of these patients or how the malignant clone of T cells gains a selective growth advantage once they enter the immunological domain of the skin.

Studies have implicated various cytokines in the trafficking of T cells and other leukocytes to the epidermis in mycosis fungoides. IL-1, IL-6, IL-8 and IFN-γ have all been identified as potential cytokines that may either directly influence chemotaxis of the lymphocytes (IL-8, IL-1, IL-2 and IL-6) or indirectly influence their migration by induction of chemotactic cytokines or upregulation of adhesion molecules (IL-1, IFN-γ). Recent studies have identified increased levels of the C-X-C chemokine IL-8 in the epidermis of CTCL patients compared to normal controls.[50,51] IL-8 has been shown to be chemotactic not only for neutrophils, but also for lymphocytes in vitro; however, as already mentioned it is controversial as to whether or not this occurs in vivo.[14,20-22,52] The identification of IL-8 in CTCL patients is in contrast to other studies which could not identify IL-8 in exudate fluid from suction blisters of skin or production of IL-8 by phytohemagglutinin (PHA)-stimulated peripheral blood mononuclear cells.[53] However, the difference in results could be explained by the different detection methods used. While the functional activity of lesion associated IL-8 was not addressed in the studies, others have indicated that lymphocyte chemotactic activity associated with mycosis fungoides is partially inhibited by anti-IL-8 antibodies.[53]

Studies have also demonstrated the presence of other cytokines in CTCL patients that are associated with lymphocyte migration. Using a cell proliferation assay, a significant increase in levels of biologically active IL-6 in mycosis fungoides has been shown.[54] IL-6 is produced by epidermal cells, fibroblasts and endothelial cells and has also been shown to activate T cells and induce lymphocyte chemotaxis in vitro.[54,55] IL-1 is a potentially important cytokine in CTCL as it has been shown to function in the migration of lymphocytes directly as a chemotactic factor, indirectly through induction of IL-8 and through the upregulate of adhesion molecules, particularly ICAM-1, VCAM-1 and E-selectin.[56-58] Recent studies have demonstrated using immunohistochemistry, enzyme linked immunosorbant assays (ELISAs) and thymocyte costimulation assays that a small but significant increase in biologically active IL-1α protein is detected in lesions from CTCL patients.[50] IL-1β was not detected in the samples.[50] However, other investigators have indicated that IL-1 may be decreased in CTCL, as exudate fluids from suction blisters in mycosis fungoides patients contained significantly less IL-1 than exudate fluids from normal controls.[54,59]

Reverse transcriptase-polymerase chain reaction (RT-PCR) and Southern blot analysis were used in recent studies to demonstrate that cytokines expressed in mycosis fungoides are a Th1 type response characterized by IL-2 and IFN-γ in the epidermis with no evidence of IL-4, IL-5 or IL-10.[60,68] Sézary syndrome on the other hand was characterized by a Th2 type response with IL-4, IL-5 and IL-10 production.[60] It is currently unknown why there is a different cytokine profile in these related diseases, but it may involve the patient prognosis as a Th2 response correlates with a loss of cell-mediated immunity and Sézary syndrome (with the Th2 response) represents advanced CTCL disease. Both IL-2 and IFN-γ have been implicated in T cell migration. IL-2 has been shown to directly mediate lymphocyte migration while IFN-γ is known to upregulate adhesion molecules.[61,62] Studies using immunoscanning electron microscopy and immunohistochemistry have shown that LFA-1 expressing T cells are localized with ICAM-1 expressing keratinocytes in mycosis fungoides.[63-65] ICAM-1 may be involved in limiting the infiltration to the epidermis in CTCL, because there is evidence for the loss of ICAM-1 in Sézary syndrome while ICAM-1 is present in mycosis fungoides.[66] This is supported by recent studies indicating shedding of ICAM-1 in both mycosis fungoides and Sézary syndrome, but with a marked increase in shedding in Sézary syndrome from Sézary cells.[67] It is of interest that TNF-α, which is known to upregulate adhesion molecule expression, has not been identified in mycosis fungoides.[54]

We currently believe that the malignant CD4+ T cells belong to the Th2 type subset, and can produce high levels of IL-10 which can suppress the T cell mediated immune response.[39,60] Thus, in patch/plaque stage CTCL, when there are only a few malignant T cells, the effective host reaction of infiltrating Th1 cells predominates and keeps the clonal expansion of malignant T cells in check. However, as the malignant clonal population of Th2 type T cells accumulate and overcome the host response, the Th2 type profile dominates. Obviously, much more work remains to validate this hypothesis but it is clear that cytokines/chemokines play an important and dynamic role in the pathophysiology of this common group of non-Hodgkin's lymphomas.

ATOPIC DERMATITIS

Atopic dermatitis is a chronic inflammatory skin disease that affects approximately 2% of the population.[69] Current data indicates that this disease is not primarily a skin defect, but instead is an allergic disorder which is believed to result from an altered immune response.[70] Atopic dermatitis is frequently associated with allergies and extracutaneous involvement such as asthma and hay fever, and the majority of patients (over 80%) have elevated levels of serum IgE with specificity to environmental allergens.[71] While the pathogenesis of this disease is poorly understood it is thought that the primary defect is in the dysfunction of a bone marrow derived cell. Studies have shown that bone marrow transplantation from an atopic donor to a nonatopic recipient results in the development of atopic dermatitis.[72]

The lesions of atopic dermatitis are intensely pruritic. In fact, it has been stated that in atopic dermatitis it is the itch that causes the rash and not the rash that happens to itch. Indeed, subsequent studies have shown that skin trauma from scratching plays an important role in initiating the lesion. Histologically, the lesions are characterized by mild epidermal thickening, intercellular edema and an inflammatory cell infiltrate consisting of T cells (predominantly memory T cells positive for CD3, CD4 and CD45 RO with only occasional CD8+ cells), Langerhans cells, dermal dendrocytes and occasional mast cells and eosinophils.[73,74] It is interesting that eosinophils are not a prominent feature of the skin histology as there are large amounts of eosinophil major basic protein present in the lesion indicating degranulation of eosinophils.[75]

T cells are thought to play a key role in atopic dermatitis. The majority of the T cells found in the lesion are allergen-specific CD4+ T cells.[76-79] Using a variety of assays to detect both protein and mRNA, cytokine production by T cells in atopic dermatitis has been evaluated, and it has been shown that the T cells produce IL-4, IL-5, IL-10 and GM-CSF, but not IL-2 or IFN-γ, indicating a Th2 type response.[76,78,80-82] From a functional point of view, the lesional sites show decreased cell-mediated immune response. This has been shown in the reduced responsiveness of atopic dermatitis patients to the poison ivy antigen urushiol and impaired reactivity to skin tests with various antigens including *Candida* and *Streptococcus*.[83-86] It is known that several cytokines, including IL-4 and IL-5, inhibit cell-mediated immune reactions and promote humoral responses. Thus the cytokine profile found in atopic dermatitis could be directly responsible for the localized reduction in the cell-mediated immune response. In addition to the cytokines mentioned above, several studies have evaluated the production of a number of other cytokines. It has been determined that TNF-α is increased in the plasma of these patients, while IL-6 and IL-1β were barely detectable.[87,88] It has also been found that mononuclear cells from atopic dermatitis patients produced less IL-1 and IL-2 than normal controls.[89] This indicates that mononuclear cells in atopic dermatitis have a decreased capacity to produce some cytokines even when stimulated. Levels of IL-12 and IL-12 receptors were normal in patients. This is interesting as IL-12 is known to induce Th1 responses including IFN-γ production. Inhibition of IL-4 or IL-10 with specific antibodies has been shown to augment IFN-γ production in atopic dermatitis.[90]

The majority of studies have focused on the production of cytokines by migratory and resident cells in the skin of atopic dermatitis, but the molecular mechanism for the recruitment of the T cells and other inflammatory cells into the area has only recently been evaluated. A few groups have recently demonstrated the production of both C-C and C-X-C chemokines in atopic dermatitis. Using immunohistochemistry and in situ hybridization techniques, Ying et al have recently described the production of both RANTES and MCP-3 in atopic dermatitis.[91] Patients were stimulated with allergen, and mRNA and protein for

MCP-3 and RANTES was evaluated at various time points. MCP-3 mRNA was increased at 6 hours poststimulation and had declined by 24 and 48 hours. This expression of MCP-3 correlates with eosinophil migration into the area which was shown to peak at 6 hours. In contrast, mRNA for RANTES, while increased at 6 hours, did not peak until after 24 hours and was just declining at 48 hours. This time course of expression correlates with T cell infiltration, but not with macrophage infiltration which is still increasing at 48 hours. The results presented in this study are in agreement with other studies that have shown a role for RANTES in the migration of eosinophils, basophils, monocytes/macrophages and CD4[+] T cells and a role for MCP-3 in the migration of eosinophils and basophils.[92]

IL-8 has also been recently detected in the plasma of approximately 80% atopic dermatitis patients, and the concentration of IL-8 correlated with the severity of the disease.[88,101] There was no indication of IL-8 in any of the normal control plasma samples or in patients with contact dermatitis indicating that the presence of IL-8 was not due to nonspecific inflammation. It is of interest that there was no increase in the number of IL-8 receptors on the neutrophils of atopic dermatitis patients, while the cells of psoriasis patients do express significantly more of these receptors.[93] In addition to the presence of chemokines, LTB4 has been detected in atopic dermatitis.[94] Neutrophils from patients with atopic dermatitis produce some LTB4 without stimulation; when stimulated with inflammatory mediators such as C5a significantly more LTB4 was released than by normal control cells.[95] Once the inflammatory cells are in the skin, it is likely that adhesion molecules play a role in keeping them in the area. T cells in atopic dermatitis have been shown to express CLA, a ligand for E-selectin that may function as a skin lymphocyte homing receptor in skin lesions. Endothelial cells in the lesion have been shown to express ICAM-1 and E-selectin, which is likely due to

TNF-α stimulation.[87] Keratinocytes in atopic dermatitis also express ICAM-1, as well as CD36 and CD1a, indicating that they are activated. As keratinocytes are a source of many cytokines including IL-8, TNF-α and GM-CSF, injury to the cells, such as may occur with scratching, may result in a release of cytokines that initiate inflammation.[96]

As mentioned earlier, eosinophils are not a major component of the inflammatory infiltrate in atopic dermatitis; however, the accumulation of eosinophil major basic protein indicates the presence and degranulation of these cells. Eosinophils from atopic dermatitis patients have been shown to have increased migratory responses toward N-formyl-methionyl-leucyl-phenylalanine (FMLP), IL-8, platelet activating factor and platelet factor 4 compared to those isolated from normal donors indicating that the eosinophils are present in an activated state.[97] While eosinophils are known to migrate in response to C5a, LTB4 and platelet activating factor, these are not specific chemotactic factors for eosinophils. IL-5, which is produced by the T cell in the lesions of atopic dermatitis, is an eosinophil selective chemotaxin.[98,99]

Recently, clinicians have taken advantage of the dissection of cytokine networks by administering IFN-γ (a Th1 type cytokine) to the atopic dermatitis patients in which Th2 profiles predominanted.[100] Because cytokine profiles are self-reinforcing but mutually antagonistic it should not be too surprising that the presence of IFN-γ (which was previously absent) had beneficial effects on the treated atopic dermatitis patients.

ALLERGIC CONTACT DERMATITIS

When the skin comes into contact with a foreign low molecular weight molecule such as pentadecylcatechol (or urushiol, the poison ivy allergen), the molecule is transferred to the skin. The molecule is recognized as foreign, which results in the induction of a T cell mediated and immunological inflammatory reaction at the points of contact in previously sensitized individuals. There are two distinct phases of allergic contact dermatitis. The inductive phase, which is also called sensitization, occurs during contact of the skin with an allergen. Upon re-exposure to the same allergen, the skin reacts with an immune response which is referred to as the challenge or elicitation phase.[102] Allergic contact dermatitis is characterized clinically by intensely pruritic, erythematous eruptions that are frequently accompanied by edema and vesiculation. The symptoms are evident 1-2 days following exposure to the allergen and generally resolve spontaneously after removal of the allergen within 3-4 weeks. Histologically, allergic contact dermatitis is characterized by edema and a mixed inflammatory infiltrate consisting primarily of CD4+ T cells in the epidermis.

To further characterize the molecular events involved in allergic contact dermatitis, studies have taken the approach of applying allergen to the skin of previously sensitized individuals and performing serial biopsies.[103,104] The skin samples are taken at various time points including prior to the development of clinical symptoms and before infiltration of leukocytes (4-8 hours after exposure), at the peak of inflammation (48-168 hours after exposure) and at the time of resolution (2-3 weeks after exposure). At the earliest time points measured, the skin showed no significant light microscopic changes. However, immunohistochemistry demonstrated that the keratinocytes express TNF-α and ICAM-1 while the endothelial cells in the area express E-selectin, VCAM-1 and ICAM-1.[103-106] The keratinocyte is believed to be the most important cell type in the initiation of allergic contact dermatitis.[103,105] Urushiol has been shown to directly activate keratinocytes, resulting in rapid production of TNF-α which plays a crucial role in autoinduction of ICAM-1 expression and IL-8 production leading to the subsequent inflammatory cell infiltrate.[104,107] Rapid production of TNF-α by keratinocytes has been confirmed both in vitro and in a mouse model of allergic contact dermatitis

at the protein and/or mRNA levels.[107,108] At the peak of inflammation (48-168 hours following allergen exposure), the keratinocytes still express TNF-α and ICAM-1; however, they also express IL-8 which correlates with the onset of epidermal T cell infiltration.[104] The ICAM-1 expressing keratinocytes were found to be colocalized with lymphocyte function-associated antigen-1 (LFA-1) expressing T cells.[103] The importance of IL-8 in delayed hypersensitivity reactions has recently been demonstrated. Studies by Larsen et al showed that neutralizing monoclonal antibodies to IL-8 were able to suppress the development of skin reactions in rabbits.[109] At the time of resolution (2-3 weeks following allergen exposure), there is decreased adhesion molecule expression by both the keratinocytes and the endothelial cells along with a decrease in inflammation.

A variety of cytokines have been found in allergic contact dermatitis including IL-1, IL-4, IL-8, IL-10 and TNF-α indicating primarily a Th2 type response.[39,82,104] Several of these cytokines may be involved directly or indirectly in the emigration of T cells into the epidermis. For example, production of IL-8 mRNA and protein has been shown both in vivo in allergic contact dermatitis and in vitro by TNF-α stimulated keratinocytes.[14,104,110,111] IL-8 is a T cell chemotactic factor, and the expression of IL-8 by the epidermal keratinocytes in allergic contact dermatitis coincides with the T cell infiltration into the area.[104] IL-1 is also a lymphocyte chemotactic factor and is able to induce IL-8 production. Low levels of IFN-γ expression have been identified in allergic contact dermatitis.[82] The production of this cytokine is supported by the expression of HLA-DR by surrounding keratinocytes and the identification of γIP-10 in models of allergic contact dermatitis as described below.[112,113]

The data on chemokine and cytokine production in allergic contact dermatitis has been confirmed and extended through the use of murine models. A series of studies by Enk and colleagues have evaluated cytokine mRNA expression in mice sensitized and challenged with the contact allergen trinitrochlorobenzene.[114-118] Similar to the results found in the human subjects, mRNA for IL-1, IL-10, GM-CSF, IFN-γ and TNF-α has been identified in this mouse model.[115,116] In addition, these studies have identified significant increases in macrophage inflammatory protein-2 (MIP-2) (10- to 50-fold increase), MCP-1 and γIP-10 (10-fold increase).[115-118] Upregulation of γIP-10 as well as IFN-γ was noted within 1.5 hours while increased mRNA for TNF and IL-1β was much more rapid with increases noted in 15-30 minutes.[116]

Further studies of this classical model system and foundation for immunodermatology has revealed some additional new insights. Previously it was believed that allergic contact dermatitis and intradermal delayed type hypersensitivity were similar; however, it is now clear that they are different.[82] For example, allergic contact dermatitis reactions have a predominantly Th2 type cytokine production profile, whereas the intradermal allergic reaction is predominantly Th1 in nature.

Thus many new issues have arisen regarding the basis for this marked dichotomy in T cell responses with the skin. Future work aimed at elucidating the role of keratinocytes versus dendritic cells and the interplay of cytokines in these complex cutaneous reactions is indicated.

LEPROSY

Leprosy, or Hansen's disease, is a chronic inflammatory disease involving primarily the skin and the peripheral nerves. It is caused by an obligate intracellular bacteria, *Mycobacterium leprae*, which multiplies within macrophages and Schwann cells. A broad range of clinical and immunological manifestations is found in leprosy, which seems to reflect the ability of the patient to mount an effective cell-mediated immune response specific for *M. leprae*.[119,120] At one end of the spectrum is tuberculoid leprosy which is characterized by a few well-marginated anesthetic plaques. The plaques are well-organized dermal granulomas containing a core of activated macrophages along with some lymphocytes surrounded by a layer of predominantly CD4+ T cells. The epidermis contains Langerhans cells which could play an important role in cytokine expression in this form of leprosy.[121-123] As these patients are able to mount an effective cellular immune response and limit the growth of the mycobacterium, *M. leprae* is rarely seen in the lesion. At the other end of the spectrum is lepromatous leprosy which is characterized by widespread, poorly defined plaques and nodules which consist of disorganized granulomas containing immature macrophages along with a some CD8+ lymphocytes. There is no surrounding layer of T lymphocytes in this type of lesion. As the patients have a selective deficiency in cell-mediated immunity to *M. leprae*, they are unable to control the infection and the mycobacteria multiply to high levels within the macrophages.

The cytokine patterns in both tuberculoid leprosy and lepromatous leprosy have been studied by a variety of groups.[121-141] Initial evidence for the importance of cytokines in leprosy came from studies examining supernatants from monocytes isolated from leprosy patients which were stimulated with *M. leprae*.[142] Cell supernatants from both normal individuals and tuberculoid leprosy patients were able to inhibit replication of the intracellular pathogen *Legionella pneumophila* in monocytes, whereas cell supernatants from patients with lepromatous leprosy were unable to inhibit *L. pneumophila* replication. These studies indicated that infected cells from patients at the ends of the clinical disease spectrum secrete different cytokines. These studies were extended by Yamamura and colleagues who identified the cytokines produced in leprosy lesions using PCR and Southern blot.[124,125] These studies demonstrated that in the tuberculoid form of the disease, mRNA for IL-2 and IFN-γ predominated, indicating a Th1 type response whereas a Th2 type pattern (IL-4, IL-5 and IL-10 mRNA) was seen in lepromatous leprosy lesions. Other cytokine mRNAs, including IL-1β, TNF-α, TGF-β, GM-CSF, IFN-γ, IL-6, lymphotoxin (TNF-β) and IL-7, were found to be more abundant in lesions of tuberculoid than in lepromatous leprosy.[124] Similarly, Salgame et al used ELISA assays to show that CD4$^+$ T cell clones from tuberculoid leprosy patients produced IL-2, IFN-γ, GM-CSF and TNF-α with virtually no IL-4, IL-6 or IL-5.[126] CD8$^+$ T cell clones from lepromatous leprosy patients produced predominantly IL-4 along with some IFN-γ, IL-5, GM-CSF and TNF-α. No IL-6 was detected in the lepromatous leprosy.

Other groups have shown a Th1 response in tuberculoid leprosy; however, they argue that there is little IL-4 secretion in lepromatous leprosy, suggesting that there is not a major role for typical Th2 cytokines in controlling the nonresponsiveness of patients with lepromatous leprosy to M. leprae antigens.[134,135] Similar contradictory evidence has been found in the use of neutralizing antibodies to IL-4 in leprosy. Salgame et al showed anti-IL-4 antibodies were effective in limiting the Th2 response; others have found no effect of IL-4 neutralizing antibodies.[126,135,143] It is currently unknown why the data on cytokine expression in lepromatous leprosy differs; however, it may be the result of the different methodologies used by the various groups. The involvement of IL-10 in lepromatous leprosy is more certain as several groups have used neutralizing antibodies to IL-10 and demonstrated effective limitation of the Th2 response.[129,135,143]

Despite these differences, the majority of studies indicate that resistance and susceptibility to M. leprae infection correlates with cytokine production. This has lead to several studies evaluating cytokines as potential therapeutic agents in leprosy. Studies have examined the effect of therapy, particularly chemotherapy and multidrug therapy, on cytokine expression in lepromatous leprosy patients. While the cytokine patterns themselves did not change, the number of cells in the lesions positive for IL-1β, TNF-α and IFN-γ by immunohistochemistry increased in treatment groups compared to untreated controls.[121,136] Studies have also evaluated the therapeutic benefit of cytokine administration. Injection of IFN-γ has been shown to improve lepromatous leprosy.[135,143-145] IFN-γ resulted in a local accumulation of mononuclear cells and in killing of M. leprae infected macrophages. However, the administration of IFN-γ resulted in excessive production of TNF-α and development of erythema nodosum leprosum. Administration of IL-2 into patients with lepromatous leprosy resulted in accumulation of CD4$^+$ T cells in the area.[146] IL-2 reduced the levels of M. leprae antigens in the serum and reduced the bacterial load in patients 5-fold over a 2 month period.

The majority of studies have focused on the cytokines produced in leprosy; however, few studies have addressed the questions of the chemotactic factors in leprosy that result in the infiltration of lymphocytes and mononuclear cells. The earliest studies examined patient serum for chemotactic properties. These studies demonstrated the presence of inhibitors in serum of leprosy patients that prevent the migration of normal peripheral blood monocytes.[147] The production of cytokines such as IL-6, IL-2 and IFN-γ, which are either directly or indirectly chemotactic, may be important to the T cell, macrophage and Langerhans cell migration to the skin in leprosy. Higher levels of these cytokines in tuberculoid leprosy in comparison with lepromatous leprosy are consistent with the greater inflammatory infiltrate seen in the tuberculoid leprosy lesion. Messenger RNA for the C-X-C chemokine IL-8 has been detected in both lepromatous and tuberculoid leprosy using PCR and Southern blot analysis. Significantly higher levels of IL-8 was found in lepromatous lesions.[124,125] To date, studies have not addressed the involvement of other C-X-C or C-C chemokines in production of the cellular infiltrate in leprosy. This lack of information may be due in part to the lack of a suitable animal model for leprosy. Only humans and the nine-banded armadillo are naturally susceptible to leprosy, and the organism can not be currently grown in culture.

As can be appreciated from this section, many new insights into the molecular basis for the clinical phenotypes of patients with leprosy have emerged by focusing on cytokine networks. Hopefully, in the future new therapeutic strategies will emerge as a greater understanding of the cellular immunological basis of the response of humans to infection by *M. leprae* is accomplished by continuing to dissect the interaction of the pathogen with T cells, antigen presenting cells, etc.

LEISHMANIASIS

American cutaneous leishmaniasis is a chronic granulomatous disease caused by intracellular parasite, *Leishmania major, L. brazilinesis* or *L. mexicana*, with a broad range of clinical manifestations. There are three distinct forms of the disease including localized, mucocutaneous and diffuse. Localized cutaneous leishmaniasis (LCL) is a self-limiting form of the disease in which an adequate cell-mediated immune response is mounted against the parasite, and the disease is restricted to well-defined skin lesions containing few parasites. The lesions begin as a papule, slowly develop into an ulcer and generally heal within 6 months. At the other end of the spectrum, diffuse cutaneous leishmaniasis (DCL) begins as a single skin papule that continues to spread resulting in bizarre nodular lesions covering the body and subsequent involvement of lymph nodes and nasopharyngeal mucous tissue. DCL is characterized by abundant macrophages filled with organisms and selective anergy of cell-mediated immunity specific for *Leishmania*.[148-150] In mucocutaneous leishmaniasis (MCL), there is a mixed inflammatory cell infiltrate with parasite containing macrophages, lymphocytes and plasma cells. There is eventual granuloma formation and a decrease in the number of parasites, but MCL is resistant to treatment and may be a persistent or recurrent problem. Kala-azar or visceral leishmaniasis is another form of the disease which results from *L. donovani* infection. Visceral and cutaneous leishmaniasis are different diseases immunologically; therefore, the discussion here will be limited to the cutaneous form of the disease.[151]

Resistance and susceptibility to leishmania infection depends on cell-mediated immunity. Macrophages are able to resist and control leishmania infection if activated by the appropriate T cell cytokines. It has been demonstrated that in vitro stimulation of macrophages with recombinant cytokines or supernatants from activated T cells results in decreased binding and ingestion of leishmania promastigotes to macrophages and enhanced intracellular killing of the organism once ingested.[152-158] The cytokines involved in resistance and susceptibility to cutaneous leishmaniasis have been identified using RT-PCR.[151,159-161] These studies have found that IFN-γ, TNF-β and IL-8 were expressed in all three forms of the disease. Messenger RNA was detected for IL-2, IL-6, IL-1β and TNF-α in MCL and LCL, but was virtually absent from DCL. In contrast, IL-4, IL-5 and IL-10 mRNA was predominant in DCL. The data indicates that the CD4+ T cells in cutaneous leishmaniasis secrete a mixture of Th1 and Th2 type cytokines, but the Th2 type cytokines predominate in disseminated form of the disease. This correlates with the known suppressive effects of Th2 cytokines on cell-mediated immune reactions.[161,163]

The clinical spectrum of leishmaniasis seen in humans can be virtually reconstructed in experimental models using inbred strains of mice.[164] Studies have demonstrated that BALB/c mice are susceptible to *L. major* infection resulting in cutaneous disease which progresses to an eventually fatal disease, while C57BL/6 and C3H mice are resistant to infection and develop self-limiting, defined cutaneous lesions.[165,166] Cell-mediated immunity has been shown to be important in controlling *L. major* infection in these animal models. In these studies, mice normally resistant to *Leishmania* infection were coinfected with a murine leukemia virus that significantly reduces cell-mediated immune responses.[167] The animals developed persistent lesions characterized by decreased lymphocyte infiltrate and abundant infected macrophages. In addition, SCID mice and nude mice are susceptible to uncontrolled leishmania infection; however, if T cells are given to the animals, they develop resistance to the infection.[168-170]

C57BL/6 mice have been shown to respond to infection with *L. major* with a Th1 type cytokine response resulting in the production of macrophage activating cytokines, such as IFN-γ.[171] IFN-γ is thought to be one of the most important cytokines in host defense against leishmania. Injection of IFN-γ in BALB/c mice reduces the production of Th2 cytokines and removal of IFN-γ from mice (either with neutralizing antibodies or disruption of the IFN-γ gene) results in uncontrolled growth of the organism in otherwise resistant animals.[172,173] Nitric oxide has been shown to be the final pathway of destruction of *Leishmania*. It is thought that IFN-γ acts by enhancing nitric oxide release from macrophages.[174] In both BALB/c and C57BL/6 mice, IFN-γ as well as IL-2, IL-4 and IL-13 are produced within 4 days of infection; however, resistant mice like C57BL/6 down regulate IL-4 production.[151,175] In contrast, susceptible mice maintain or increase expression of IL-4 and studies have shown that production of IL-4 after 9 weeks of infection correlates with progressive disease.[171,176,177] Susceptible mice also reduced production of IL-2 and IFN-γ with progression of the disease.[176,178, 179]

Few studies have addressed the question of chemotactic factors produced in leishmaniasis that result in macrophage and lymphocyte influx. As already mentioned, IL-8 has been shown to be produced in all forms of human cutaneous leishmaniasis. IL-8, which is chemotactic for lymphocytes, may play a role in bringing the Th1 and Th2 responsive lymphocytes into the area of infection. Production of IL-6, IL-2 and IL-1 may also be indirectly involved in the production of the inflammatory infiltrate.

In addition, it has been shown that *Leishmania* promastigotes are able to directly activate the complement cascade resulting in the production of the chemotactic factor C5a.[180] C5a is chemotactic for macrophages and may be involved in the recruitment of macrophages into the area resulting in their infection by the organism. Studies have also found production of biologically active TGF-β in both in vitro and in vivo *Leishmania* infections.[181] Among its many functions, TGF-β has been shown to be a chemoattractant for monocytes and T cells.[182-186] Few studies have evaluated the role of chemokines other than IL-8 in *Leishmania*. One study examined MIP-1α mRNA levels in murine macrophages challenged with *Leishmania* promastigotes, and found no increase in production after 24 hours compared to baseline levels.[164,175]

SUMMARY AND CONCLUSIONS

It should be clear from reading this chapter that chemokines make a significant contribution to a wide variety of skin diseases. The pathological cutaneous states include autoimmune, inflammatory, immunological and infectious, underscoring the pleiotropic effects of cytokines. It should be noted that investigators outside of dermatology have used similar approaches to dissecting cytokine networks, with investigative skin biologists leading the way in areas involving psoriasis and allergic contact dermatitis reactions, to mention a few. Many new molecules have been discovered with cytokine/chemokine properties and can be identified within diseased skin samples. A major challenge remaining is to understand the genesis of these diverse inflammatory and immunological reactions. We need to identify the relevant antigens, which types of antigen presenting cells are present, which set of costimulatory molecules are involved, and what part of the overall cascade of cytokines is therapeutic versus pathogenic. Some insights into this latter notion have been derived from studies of normal wound healing and by studying chronic nonhealing ulcerations of the skin. This topic is extensively reviewed elsewhere.[187] Even though we do not have a complete understanding as to how cytokine networks are formed, we can begin to consider using our knowledge as to their composition in the maintenance phase of skin diseases, by devising strategies to reverse or negate the disease-associated networks. Specific examples were provided in this chapter, such as the use of IFN-γ in atopic dermatitis patients. We are optimistic that more selective and efficacious treatment protocols will emerge to treat our dermatological patients afflicted by these and many other skin diseases.

REFERENCES

1. Farber EM, Bright RD, Nall ML. Psoriasis. A questionnaire survey of 2,144 patients. Arch Dermatol 1968; 98:248-253.

2. Krueger GG, Bergstresser PR, Lowe NJ et al. Psoriasis. J Am Acad Dermatol 1984; 11:937-947.

3. Fierlbeck G, Rasner G, Maler G. Psoriasis induced at injection site by recombinant gamma interferon. Arch Dermatol 1990; 126:345-355.

4. Nickoloff BJ. The cytokine network in psoriasis. Arch Dermatol 1991; 127:871-884.

5. Ho V, Griffiths CEM, Ellis CN et al. Intralesional cyclosporin A. The treatment of psoriasis: a clinical, immunologic and pharmacokinetic study. J Am Acad Dermatol 1990; 22:94-110.

6. Thivolet J, Nicolas JF. Immunointervention in psoriasis with anti-CD4 antibodies. Int J Dermatol 1994; 33:327-332.

7. Gottlieb SL, Gilleaudeau P, Johnson R et al. Response of psoriasis to a lymphocyte-selective toxin (DAB389IL-2) suggests a primary immune, but not keratinocyte, pathogenic basis. Nature Medicine 1995; 1:442-447.

8. Ellis CN, Kang S, Grekin RC et al. Etretinate therapy reduces polymorphonuclear leukocyte chemotaxis-enhancing properties of psoriatic serum. J Am Acad Dermatol 1985; 13:437-443.

9. Gearing AJH, Fincham NJ, Bird CR et al. Cytokines in skin lesions of psoriasis. Cytokine 1990; 2:68-75.

10. Schroder, JM. Biochemical and biological characterization of NAP-1/IL-8-related cytokines in lesional psoriatic scale. Adv Exp Med Biol 1991; 305:97-107.

11. Sticherling M, Bornscheuer E, Schroder JM et al. Localization of neutrophil activating peptide-1/interleukin-8 immunoreactivity in normal and psoriatic skin. J Invest Dermatol 1991; 96:26-30.

12. Nickoloff BJ, Karabin GD, Barker JN et al. Cellular localization of interleukin-8 and its inducer, tumor necrosis factor-alpha in psoriasis. Am J Pathol 1991; 138:129-140.

13. Arenberger P, Kemeny L, Suss R et al. Interleukin-8 receptors in normal and psoriatic polymorphonuclear leukocytes. Acta Derm Venereol 1992; 72:334-336.

14. Barker JN, Jones ML, Mitra RS et al. Modulation of keratinocyte-derived interleukin-8 which is chemotactic for neutrophils and T lymphocytes. Am J Pathol 1991; 139:869-876.

15. Nestle FO, Nickoloff BJ. Role of dendritic cells in benign and malignant lymphocytic infiltrates of the skin. Cutaneous Lymphomas 1994; 2:271-282.

16. Gillitzer R, Berger R, Mielke V et al. Upper keratinocytes of psoriatic skin lesions express high levels of NAP-1/IL-8 mRNA in situ. J Invest Dermatol 1991; 97:73-79.

17. Krueger G, Jorgenson C, Miller C et al. Effects of IL-8 on epidermal proliferation. J Invest Dermatol 1990; 94:545 (abstract).

18. Tuschil A, Lam C, Haslberger A et al. Interleukin-8 stimulates calcium transients and promotes epidermal cell proliferation. J Invest Dermatol 1992; 99:294-298.

19. Gillitzer R, Wolff K, Tong D et al. MCP-1 mRNA expression in basal keratinocytes of psoriatic lesions. J Invest Dermatol 1993; 101:127-131.

20. Larsen CG, Anderson AO, Appella E et al. The neutrophil activating protein NAP-1 is also chemotactic for T lymphocytes. Science 1989; 243:1464-1466.

21. Bacon KB, Westwick J, Camp RDR. Potent and specific inhibition of IL-8, IL-1α, and IL-1β-induced lymphocyte migration by calcium channel antagonists. Biochem Biophys Res Commun 1989; 165:349-354.

22. Leonard E, Yoshimura T, Tanaka S et al. Neutrophil infiltration caused by intrader-

mal injection of neutrophil attractant protein-1 (NAP-1/IL-8) into human skin. Cytokine 1989; 1:151 (abstract).

23. Koch AE, Polverini PJ, Kunkel SL et al. Interleukin-8 as a macrophage-derived mediator of angiogenesis. Science 1992; 258:1798-1801.

24. Nickoloff BJ, Mitra RS, Varani J et al. Aberrant production of interleukin-8 and thrombospondin-1 by psoriatic keratinocytes mediates angiogenesis. Am J Pathol 1994; 144:820-828.

25. Tettelbach W, Nanney L, Ellis D et al. Localization of MGSA/GRO protein in cutaneous lesions. J Cutan Pathol 1993; 20:259-266.

26. Schroder JM, Gregory H, Young J et al. Neutrophil-activating proteins in psoriasis. J Invest Dermatol 1992; 98:241-247.

27. Kojima T, Cromie MA, Fisher GJ et al. GRO-alpha mRNA is selectively overexpressed in psoriatic epidermis and is reduced by cyclosporin A in vivo, but not in cultured keratinocytes. J Invest Dermatol 1993; 101:767-772.

28. Gottlieb AB, Luster AD, Posnett DN et al. Detection of a gamma interferon-induced protein IP-10 in psoriatic plaques. J Exp Med 1988; 168:941-948.

29. Takematsu H, Tagami H. Quantification of chemotactic peptides (C5a anaphylatoxin and IL-8) in psoriatic lesional skin. Arch Dermatol 1993; 129:74-80.

30. Colditz IG, Zwahlen RD, Baggiolini M. Neutrophil accumulation and plasma leakage induced in vivo by neutrophil activating peptide-1. J Leukocyte Biol 1990; 48:129-137.

31. Zwahlen R, Walz A, Rot A. In vitro and in vivo activity and pathophysiology of human interleukin-8 and related peptides. Int Rev Exp Pathol 1993; 34B:27-42.

32. Castells-Rodellas A, Castell JV, Ramirez-Bosca A et al. Interleukin-6 in normal skin and psoriasis. Acta Derm Venereol 1992; 72:165-168.

33. Bonifati C, Carducci M, Cordiali-Fei P et al. Correlated increases of tumour necrosis factor-α, interleukin-6 and granulocyte monocyte-colony stimulated factor levels in suction blister fluids and sera of psoriatic patients—relationships with disease severity. Clin Exp Dermatol 1994; 19:383-387.

34. Schmid P, Cox D, McMaster GK et al. In situ hybridization analysis of cytokine, proto-oncogene and tumour suppressor gene expression in psoriasis. Arch Dermatol Res 1993; 285:334-340.

35. Mosmann TR, Cherwinski H, Bond MW et al. Two types of murine helper T cell clones. I. Definition according to profiles of lymphokine activities and secretory protein. J Immunol 1986; 136:2348-2357.

36. Gajewski TF, Fitch FW. Antiproliferative effect of IFN-γ in immune regulation. I. IFN-γ inhibits the proliferation of Th2 but not Th1 murine helper T lymphocyte clones. J Immunol 1988; 140:4245-4253.

37. Fiorentino DF, Zlotnik A, Vieira P et al. IL-10 acts on the antigen-presenting cell to inhibit cytokine production by Th1 cells. J Immunol 1991; 146:3444-3451.

38. Uyemura K, Yamamura M, Fivenson DP et al. The cytokine network in lesional and lesion-free psoriatic skin is characterized by a T-helper type 1 cell-mediated response. J Invest Dermatol 1993; 101:701-705.

39. Nickoloff BJ, Fivenson DP, Kunkel SL et al. Keratinocyte interleukin-10 expression is upregulated in tape-stripped skin, poison ivy dermatitis and Sezary syndrome, but not in psoriatic plaques. Clin Immunol Immunopathol 1994; 73:63-68.

40. Mussi A, Bonifati C, Carducci M et al. IL-10 levels are decreased in psoriatic lesional skin as compared to the psoriatic lesion-free and normal skin suction blister fluids. J Biol Regul Homeost Agents 1994; 8:177-120.

41. Cooper KD, Hammerberg C, Baadsgaard O et al. IL-1 activity is reduced in psoriatic skin. Decreased IL-1 alpha and increased nonfunctional IL-1 beta. J Immunol 1990; 144:4593-4603.

42. Cooper KD, Hammerberg C, Baadsgaard O et al. Interleukin-1 in human skin: dysregulation in psoriasis. J Invest Dermatol 1990; 95:24S-26S.

43. Grossman RM, Krueger J, Yourish D et al. Interleukin 6 is expressed in high levels in psoriatic skin and stimulates proliferation of cultured human keratinocytes. Proc Natl Acad Sci USA 1989; 86:6367-6371.

44. Elder JT, Fisher GJ, Lindquist PB et al. Overexpression of transforming growth factor alpha in psoriatic epidermis. Science 1989; 243:811-814.

45. Nanney LB, Stoscheck CM, Magid M et al. Altered [^{125}I]epidermal growth factor binding and receptor distribution in psoriasis. J Invest Dermatol 1986; 86:260-265.

46. Barker JNWN, Karabin GD, Stoof TJ et al. Detection of interferon-gamma mRNA in psoriatic epidermis by polymerase chain reaction. J Dermatol Sci 1991; 2:106-111.

47. Nickoloff BJ, Kunkel SL, Burdick M et al. Severe combined immunodeficiency mouse and human psoriatic skin chimeras. Validation of a new animal model. Am J Pathol 1995; 146:580-588.

48. Lutzner M, Edelson R, Schein P et al. Cutaneous T cell lymphomas: the Sezary syndrome, mycosis fungoides and related disorders. Ann Intern Med 1975; 83:534-552.

49. Knobler RM, Edelson RL. Cutaneous T cell lymphoma. Med Clin North Am 1986; 70:109-138.

50. Hansen ER, Vejlsgaard GL, Lisby S et al. Epidermal interleukin 1α functional activity and interleukin 8 immunoreactivity are increased in patients with cutaneous T cell lymphoma. J Invest Dermatol 1991; 97:818-823.

51. Wismer JM, McKenzie RC, Sauder DN. Interleukin-8 immunoreactivity in epidermis of cutaneous T cell lymphoma patients. Lymphokine Cytokine Res 1994; 13:21-27.

52. Jinquan T, Deleuran B, Gesser B et al. Regulation of human T lymphocyte chemotaxis in vitro by T cell derived cytokines IL-2, IFN-γ, IL-4, IL-10 and IL-13. J Immunol 1995; 154:3742-3752.

53. Zachariae C, Larsen CS, Kaltoft K et al. Soluble IL2 receptor serum levels and epidermal cytokines in mycosis fungoides and related disorders. Acta Derm Venereol 1991; 71:465-470.

54. Lawlor F, Smith NP, Camp RD et al. Skin exudate levels of IL-6, IL-1, and other cytokines in mycosis fungoides. Br J Dermatol 1990; 123:297-304.

55. Van Damme J. Biochemical and biological properties of human HPGF/IL-6. Ann N Y Acad Sci 1989; 557:104-112.

56. Miossec P, Yu CL, Ziff M. Lymphocyte chemotactic activity of human interleukin 1. J Immunol 1984; 133:2007-2011.

57. Sica A, Matsushima K, Van Damme J et al. IL-1 transcriptionally activates the neutrophil chemotactic factor/IL-8 gene in endothelial cells. Immunology 1990; 69:548-553.

58. Camp R, Finchham N, Ross J et al. Potent inflammatory properties in human skin of interleukin-1α like material isolated from normal skin. J Invest Dermatol 1990; 94:735-741.

59. Camp R, Bacon K, Fincham N et al. Chemotactic cytokines in inflammatory skin disease. Adv Exp Med Biol 1991; 305:109-118.

60. Saed G, Fivenson DP, Naidu Y et al. Mycosis fungoides exhibits a Th1-type cell mediated cytokine profile whereas Sezary syndrome expresses a Th2-type profile. J Invest Dermatol 1994; 103:29-33.

61. Robbins RA, Klassen L, Rassmussen J et al. Interleukin-2-induced chemotaxis of human T lymphocytes. J Lab Clin Med 1986; 108:340-345.

62. Kornfeld H, Berman JS, Beer DJ et al. Induction of human T lymphocyte motility by interleukin 2. J Immunol 1985; 134:3887-3890.

63. Simon M Jr, Hunyadi J, Dobozy A. Expression of beta-2 integrin molecules on human keratinocytes in cytokine mediated skin diseases. Acta Derm Venereol 1992; 72:169-171.

64. Imayama S. Differential cell surface distribution of adhesion molecules by immuno-scanning electron microscopy. J Dermatol 1994; 21:855-859.

65. Sterry W, Mielke V, Konter U et al. Role of β1-integrins in epidermotropism of malignant T cells. Am J Pathol 1992; 141:855-860.

66. Nickoloff BJ, Griffiths CEM, Baadsgaard O et al. Markedly diminished epidermal keratinocyte expression of ICAM-1 in Sezary Syndrome. JAMA 1989; 261:2217-2221.

67. Dummer R, Sigg-Zemann S, Kalthof K et al. Various cytokines modulate ICAM-1 shedding on melanoma- and CTCL-derived cell lines: inverse regulation of ICAM-1 shedding in a Sezary cell line by interferon-γ.

Dermatology 1994; 189:120-124.

68. Fivenson DP, Douglass MC, Nickoloff BJ. Cutaneous expression of Thy-1 in mycosis fungoides. Am J Pathol 1992; 141: 1373-1380.

69. Hanifin JM, Rajka G. Diagnostic features of atopic dermatitis. Acta Derm Venereol 1980; 92:44-47.

70. Leung DY. Immunopathology of atopic dermatitis. Springer Semin Immunopathol 1992; 13:427-440.

71. Hanifin JM. Atopic dermatitis. J Am Acad Dermatol 1982; 6:1-13.

72. Agosti JM, Sprenger JD, Lum LG et al. Transfer of allergen-specific IgE-mediated hypersensitivity with allogenic bone marrow transplantation. N Engl J Med 1988; 319:1623-1628.

73. Zachary CB, MacDonald DM. Quantitative analysis of T lymphocyte subsets in atopic eczema, using monoclonal antibodies and flow cytometry. Br J Dermatol 1983; 108:411-422.

74. Sillvis Smitt JH, Bos JD, Hulsebosch HG et al. In situ immunophenotyping of antigen presenting cells and T cell subsets in atopic dermatitis. Clin Exp Dermatol 1986; 11:159-168.

75. Leiferman KM, Ackerman SJ, Sampson HA et al. Dermal deposition of eosinophil granule major basic protein in atopic dermatitis: comparison with onchocerciasis. N Engl J Med 1985; 313:282-285.

76. Wierenga EA, Snoek M, de Groot C et al. Evidence for compartmentalization of functional subsets of $CD4^+$ T lymphocytes in atopic patients. J Immunol 1990; 144: 4651-4656.

77. Wierenga EA, Snoek M, Bos JD et al. Comparison of diversity and function of the house dust mite—specific T lymphocyte clones from atopic and nonatopic donors. Eur J Immunol 1990; 20:1519-1526.

78. Van der Heijden FL, Wierenga EA, Bos JD et al. High frequency of IL-4 producing $CD4^+$ allergen specific T lymphocytes in atopic dermatitis lesional skin. J Invest Dermatol 1991; 97:389-394.

79. Kay AB, Ying S, Varney V et al. Messenger RNA expression of the cytokine gene cluster interleukin-3 (IL-3), IL-4, IL-5, and granulocyte/macrophage colony stimulating factor in allergen-induced late-phase cutaneous reactions in atopic subjects. J Exp Med 1991; 173:775-783.

80. Van Reijsen FC, Bruijnzeel-Koomen CA, Kalthoff FS et al. Skin derived aeroallergen specific T cell clones of Th2 phenotype in patients with atopic dermatitis. J Allergy Clin Immunol 1992; 90:184-192.

81. Hamid Q, Boguniewicz M, Leung DY. Differential in situ cytokine gene expression in acute versus chronic atopic dermatitis. J Clin Invest 1994; 94:870-876.

82. Ohmen JD, Hanifin JM, Nickoloff BJ et al. Overexpression of IL-10 in atopic dermatitis. Contrasting cytokine patterns with delayed-type hypersensitivity reactions. J Immunol 1995; 154:1956-1963.

83. Cronin E, Bandman JH, Calnan CD. Contact dermatitis in the atopic. Acta Dermatol Venereol 1970; 50:183-187.

84. Eliot ST, Hanifin JM. Delayed cutaneous hypersensitivity and lymphocyte transformation: dissociation in atopic dermatitis. Arch Dermatol 1979; 115:36-39.

85. Rogge JL, Hanifin JM. Immunodeficiencies in severe atopic dermatitis: depressed chemotaxis, and lymphocyte transformation. Arch Dermatol 1976; 112:1391.

86. Ogawa H, Yoshiike T. A speculative view of atopic dermatitis: barrier dysfunction in pathogenesis. J Dermatol Sci 1993; 5: 197-204.

87. Sumimoto S, Kawai M. Kasajima Y, Hamamoto T. Increased plasma tumor necrosis factor-alpha concentration in atopic dermatitis. Arch Dis Child 1992; 67: 277-279.

88. Kimata H, Lindley I. Detection of plasma interleukin-8 in atopic dermatitis. Arch Dis Child 1994; 70:119-122.

89. Kapp A, Kirnbauer R, Luger TA et al. Altered production of immunomodulating cytokines in patients with atopic dermatitis. Acta Derm Venereol 1989; 144:97-99.

90. Lester MR, Hofer MF, Gately M et al. Downregulating effects of IL-4 and IL-10 on the IFN-γ response in atopic dermatitis. J Immunol 1995; 154:6174-6181.

91. Ying S, Taborda-Barata L, Meng Q et al. The kinetics of allergen induced transcrip-

tion of messenger RNA for monocyte chemotactic protein-3 and RANTES in the skin of human atopic subjects: relationship to eosinophil, T cell and macrophage recruitment. J Exp Med 1995; 2153-2159.

92. Kapp A, Zeck-Kapp G, Czech W et al. The chemokine RANTES is more than a chemoattractant: characterization of its effect on human eosinophil oxidative metabolism and morphology in comparison with IL-5 and GM-CSF. J Invest Dermatol 1994; 102:906-914.

93. Arenberger P, Kemeny L, Suss R et al. Interleukin-8 receptors in normal and psoriatic polymorphonuclear leukocytes. Acta Derm Venereol 1992; 72:334-336.

94. Ruzicka T, Simmet T, Peskar BA et al. Skin levels of arachidonic acid derived inflammatory mediators and histamine in atopic dermatitis and psoriasis. J Invest Dermatol 1986; 86:105-108.

95. Neuber K, Hilger RA, Konig W. Interleukin-3, interleukin-8, FMLP and C5a enhance the release of leukotrienes from neutrophils of patients with atopic dermatitis. Immunology 1991; 73:83-87.

96. Leung DYM. The immunologic basis of atopic dermatitis. Clin Rev Allergy 1993; 11:447-469.

97. Bruijnzeel PLB, Kuijper PHM, Rihs S et al. Eosinophil migration in atopic dermatitis I: increased migratory responses to N-formyl-methionyl-leucyl-phenylalanine, neutrophil activating factor, platelet activating factor and platelet factor 4. J Invest Dermatol 1993; 100:137-142.

98. Yamaguchi Y, Hayashi Y, Sugama Y et al. Highly purified murine interleukin-5 (IL-5) stimulated eosinophil function and prolongs in vitro survival. IL-5 is an eosinophil chemotactic factor. J Exp Med 1988; 167:1737-1743.

99. Ming Wang J, Rambaldi A, Biondi A et al. Recombinant human interleukin 5 is a selective eosinophil chemoattractant. Eur J Immunol 1989; 19:701-705.

100. Hanifin JM, Schneider LC, Leung DY et al. Recombinant interferon gamma therapy for atopic dermatitis. J Am Acad Dermatol 1993; 28:189-197.

101. Sticherling M, Bornscheuer E, Schroder JM et al. Immunohistochemical studies on NAP-1/IL-8 in contact eczema and atopic dermatitis. Arch Dermatol Res 1992; 284:82-85.

102. Baer RL. The mechanism of allergic contact dermatitis. In: Fisher AA, ed. Contact Dermatitis. 3rd ed. Philadelphia: Lea and Febiger, 1986:1-8.

103. Griffiths CEM, Nickoloff BJ. Keratinocyte intercellular adhesion molecule-1 (ICAM-1) expression precedes dermal T lymphocytic infiltration in allergic contact dermatitis (rhus dermatitis). Am J Pathol 1989; 135:1045-1053.

104. Griffiths CEM, Barker JN, Kunkel S et al. Modulation of leucocyte adhesion molecules, a T cell chemotaxin (IL-8) and a regulatory cytokine (TNF-α) in allergic contact dermatitis (rhus dermatitis). Br J Dermatol 1991; 124:519-526.

105. Nickoloff BJ, Griffiths CE, Barker JN. The role of adhesion molecules, chemotactic factors, and cytokines in inflammatory and neoplastic skin disease—1990 update. J Invest Dermatol 1990; 94:151S-157S.

106. Friedmann PS, Strickland I, Memon AA et al. Early time course of recruitment of immune surveillance in human skin after chemical provocation. Clin Exp Immunol 1993; 91:351-356.

107. Barker JN, Mitra RS, Griffiths CE et al. Keratinocytes as initiators of inflammation. Lancet 1991; 337:211-214.

108. Piguet PF, Grau GE, Hauser C et al. Tumor necrosis factor is a critical mediator in hapten induced irritant and contact hypersensitivity reactions. J Exp Med 1991; 173:673-679.

109. Larsen CG, Thomsen MK, Gesser B et al. The delayed-type hypersensitivity reaction is dependent on IL-8. Inhibition of a tuberculin skin reaction by an anti-IL-8 monoclonal antibody. J Immunol 1995; 155: 2151-2157.

110. Larsen CG, Anderson AO, Oppenheim JJ et al. Production of interleukin-8 by human dermal fibroblasts and keratinocytes in response to interleukin-1 or tumour necrosis factor. Immunology 1989; 68:31-36.

111. Barker JN, Sarma V, Mitra RS et al. Marked synergism between tumor necrosis factor-

alpha and interferon-gamma in regulation of keratinocyte-derived adhesion molecules and chemotactic factors. J Clin Invest 1990; 85:605-608.

112. Barker JN, Ophir J, MacDonald DM. Products of class II major histocompatibility complex gene subregions are differentially expressed on keratinocytes in cutaneous diseases. J Am Acad Dermatol 1988; 19:667-672.

113. Wood GS, Volterra AS, Abel EA et al. Allergic contact dermatitis: novel immuno-histologic features. J Invest Dermatol 1986; 87:688-693.

114. Kondo S, Pastore S, Shivji GM et al. Characterization of epidermal cytokine profiles in sensitization and elicitation phases of allergic contact dermatitis as well as irritant contact dermatitis in mouse skin. Lymphokine Cytokine Res 1994; 13:367-375.

115. Enk AH, Angeloni VL, Udey MC et al. An essential role for Langerhans cell-derived IL-1 beta in the initiation of primary immune responses in skin. J Immunol 1993; 150:3698-3704.

116. Enk AH, Katz SI. Early events in the induction phase of contact sensitivity. J Invest Dermatol 1992; 99:39S-41S.

117. Gautam S, Battisto J, Major JA et al. Chemokine expression in trinitrochlorobenzene-mediated contact hypersensitivity. J Leukoc Biol 1994; 55:452-460.

118. Enk AH, Katz SI. Early molecular events in the induction phase of contact sensitivity. Proc Natl Acad Sci USA 1992; 89: 1398-1402.

119. Kaplan G, Cohn ZA. Leprosy and cell-mediated immunity. Curr Opin Immunol 1991; 3:91-96.

120. Modlin RL, Bloom BR. Immune regulation: learning from leprosy. Hosp Pract (Off Ed) 1993; 28:71-84.

121. Arnoldi J, Gerdes J, Flad HD. Immunohistologic assessment of cytokine production of infiltrating cells in various forms of leprosy. Am J Pathol 1990; 137:749-753.

122. Modlin RL, Hofman FM, Taylor CR et al. T lymphocyte subsets in the skin lesions of patients with leprosy. J Am Acad Dermatol 1983; 8:182-189.

123. Rea TH, Shen JY, Modlin RL. Epidermal keratinocyte Ia expression, Langerhans cell hyperplasia and lymphocytic infiltration in skin lesions of leprosy. Clin Exp Immunol 1986; 65:253-259.

124. Yamamura M, Uyemura K, Deans RJ et al. Defining protective responses to pathogens: cytokine profiles in leprosy lesions. Science 1991; 254:277-279.

125. Yamamura M, Wang XH, Ohmen JD et al. Cytokine patterns of immunologically mediated tissue damage. J Immunol 1992; 149:1470-1475.

126. Salgame P, Abrams JS, Clayberger C et al. Differing lymphokine profiles of functional subsets of human CD4 and CD8 T cell clones. Science 1991; 254:279-282.

127. Parida SK, Grau GE, Zaheer SA et al. Serum tumor necrosis factor and interleukin-1 in leprosy and during lepra reactions. Clin Immunol Immunopathol 1992; 63:23-27.

128. Cooper CL, Mueller C, Sinchaisri TA et al. Analysis of naturally occurring delayed type hypersensitivity reactions in leprosy by in situ hybridization. J Exp Med 1989; 169:1565-1581.

129. Sieling PA, Abrams JS, Yamamura M et al. Immunosuppressive roles for interleukin-10 and interleukin-4 in human infection: in vitro modulation of T cell responses in leprosy. J Immunol 1993; 150:5501-5510.

130. Sieling PA, Sakimura L, Uyemura K et al. IL-7 in the cell-mediated immune response to a human pathogen. J Immunol 1995; 154:2775-2783.

131. Volc-Platzer B, Stemberger H, Luger T et al. Defective intralesional interferon-gamma activity in patients with lepromatous leprosy. Clin Exp Immunol 1988; 71:235-240.

132. Modlin RL, Hofman FM, Horwitz DA et al. In situ identification of cells in human leprosy granulomas with monoclonal antibodies to interleukin 2 and its receptor. J Immunol 1984; 132:3085-3090.

133. Longley J, Haregewoin A, Yemaneberhan T et al. In vivo responses to Mycobacterium leprae: antigen presentation, interleukin 2 production, and immune cell phenotypes in naturally occurring leprosy lesions. Int J Lepr 1985; 53:385-394.

134. Howe RC, Wondimu A, Demissee A et al. Functional heterogeneity among CD4+

T cell clones from blood and skin lesions of leprosy patients. Identification of T cell clones distinct from Th0, Th1 and Th2. Immunology 1995; 84:585-594.

135. Mutis T, Kraakman EM, Cornelisse YE et al. Analysis of cytokine production by Mycobacterium-reactive T cells. Failure to explain Mycobacterium leprae-specific nonresponsiveness of peripheral blood T cells from lepromatous leprosy patients. J Immunol 1993; 150:4641-4651.

136. Flad HD, Richter E, Schluter C et al. Mycobacterium leprae DNA content, cellular and cytokine patterns in skin lesions of leprosy patients undergoing multidrug therapy (MDT). Immunobiology 1994; 191:388-394.

137. Kamradt T. T cell unresponsiveness in lepromatous leprosy. J Rheumatol 1993; 20:904-906.

138. Parida SK, Grau GE. Role of TNF in immunopathology of leprosy. Res Immunol 1993; 144:376-384.

139. Sieling PA, Modlin RL. Regulation of cytokine patterns in leprosy. Ann N Y Acad Sci 1994; 730:42-52.

140. Modlin RL. Th1-Th2 paradigm: insights from leprosy. J Invest Dermatol 1994; 102:828-832.

141. Sieling PA, Modlin RL. Cytokine patterns at the site of mycobacterial infection. Immunobiology 1994; 191:378-387.

142. Horwitz MA, Levis WR, Cohn ZA. Defective production of monocyte-activating cytokines in lepromatous leprosy. J Exp Med 1984; 159:666-678.

143. Kaplan G. Cytokine regulation of disease progression in leprosy and tuberculosis. Immunobiology 1994; 191:564-568.

144. Nathan CF, Kaplan G, Levis WR et al. Local and systemic effects of intradermal recombinant IFN-γ in patients with lepromatous leprosy. N Engl J Med 1986; 315:6-15.

145. Nathan CF, Squires K, Griffo W et al. Widespread intradermal accumulation of mononuclear leukocytes in lepromatous leprosy patients treated systematically with recombinant interferon-γ. J Exp Med 1990; 172:1509-1512.

146. Kaplan G. Recent advances in cytokine therapy in leprosy. J Infect Dis 1993;

167:S18-22.

147. Campbell PB, Tolson TA, Yoder L et al. Lesional modulation of peripheral monocyte leucotactic responsiveness in leprosy. Clin Exp Immunol 1987; 70:289-297.

148. Convit J, Pinardi ME, Rondon AJ. Diffuse cutaneous leishmaniasis: a disease due to an immunological defect of the host. Trans R Soc Trop Med Hyg 1972; 66:603-610.

149. Castes M, Cabrera M, Trujillo D et al. T cell subpopulations, expression of interleukin-2 receptor, and production of interleukin-2 and gamma interferon in human American cutaneous leishmaniasis. J Clin Microbiol 1988; 26:1207-1213.

150. Castes M, Agnelli A, Verde O et al. Characterization of the cellular immune response in American cutaneous leishmaniasis. Clin Immunol Immunopathol 1983; 27:176-186.

151. Reed SG, Scott P. T cell and cytokine responses in leishmaniasis. Curr Opin Immunol 1993; 5:524-531.

152. Mosser DM, Handman E. Treatment of murine macrophages with interferon-gamma inhibits their ability to bind leishmania promastigotes. J Leukoc Biol 1992; 52: 369-376.

153. Nacy CA, Meltzer MS, Leonard EJ et al. Intracellular replication and lymphokine-induced destruction of Leishmania tropica in C3H/HeN mouse macrophages. J Immunol 1981; 127:2381-2386

154. Panosian CB, Wyler DJ. Acquired macrophage resistance to in vitro infection with Leishmania. J Infect Dis 1983; 148: 1049-1054.

155. Titus RG, Kelso A, Louis JA. Intracellular destruction of Leishmania tropica by macrophages activated with macrophage activating factor/interferon. Clin Exp Immunol 1984; 55:157-165.

156. Murray HW, Rubin BY, Rothermel CD. Killing of intracellular Leishmania donovani by lymphokine-stimulated human mononuclear phagocytes. Evidence that interferon-gamma is the activating lymphokine. J Clin Invest 1983; 72:1506-1510.

157. Buchmuller Y, Mauel J. Studies on the mechanisms of macrophage activation. II. Parasite destruction in macrophages activated by supernatants from concanavalin A-

stimulated lymphocytes. J Exp Med 1979; 150:359-370.

158. Bogdan C, Gessner A, Rollinghoff M. Cytokines in leishmaniasis: a complex network of stimulatory and inhibitory interactions. Immunobiology 1993; 189:356-396.

159. Caceres-Dittmar G, Tapia FJ, Sanchez MA et al. Determination of the cytokine profile in American cutaneous leishmaniasis using the polymerase chain reaction. Clin Exp Immunol 1993; 91:500-505.

160. Pirmez C, Yamamura M, Uyemura K et al. Cytokine patterns in the pathogenesis of human leishmaniasis. J Clin Invest 1993; 91:1390-1395.

161. Melby PC, Andrade-Narvaez FJ, Darnell BJ et al. Increased expression of proinflammatory cytokines in chronic lesions of human cutaneous leishmaniasis. Infect Immun 1994; 62:837-842.

162. Gajewski TF, Fitch FW. Antiproliferative effect of IFN-γ in immune regulation. I. IFN-γ inhibits the proliferation of Th2 but not Th1 murine helper T lymphocyte clones. J Immunol 1988; 140:4245-4253.

163. Fiorentino DF, Zlotnik A, Vieira P et al. IL-10 acts on the antigen-presenting cell to inhibit cytokine production by Th1 cells. J Immunol 1991; 146:3444-3451.

164. Reiner SL, Locksley RM. The regulation of immunity to Leishmania major. Annu Rev Immunol 1995; 13:151-177.

165. Behin R, Mauel J, Sordat B. Leishmania tropica: pathogenicity and in vitro macrophage function in strains of inbred mice. Exp Parasitol 1979; 48:81-91.

166. Handman E, Ceredig R, Mitchell GF. Murine cutaneous leishmaniasis: disease patterns in intact and nude mice of various genotypes and examination of some differences between normal and infected macrophages. Aust J Exp Biol Med Sci 1979; 57:9-29.

167. Barral-Netto M, da Silva JS, Barral A et al. Upregulation of T helper 2 and downregulation of T helper 1 cytokines during murine retrovirus-induced immunodeficiency syndrome enhances susceptibility of a resistant mouse strain to Leishmania amazonensis. Am J Pathol 1995; 146:635-642.

168. Varkila K, Chatelain R, Leal LM et al. Reconstitution of C.B-17 SCID mice with BALB/c T cells initiates a T helper type-1 response and renders them capable of healing Leishmania major infection. Eur J Immunol 1993; 23:262-268.

169. Mitchell GF. Murine cutaneous leishmaniasis: resistance in reconstituted nude mice and several F1 hybrids infected with Leishmania tropica major. J Immunogenet 1983; 10:395-412.

170. Holaday BJ, Sadick MD, Wang ZE et al. Reconstitution of Leishmania immunity in severe combined immunodeficient mice using Th1 and Th2-like cell lines. J Immunol 1991; 147:1653-1658.

171. Locksley RM, Heinzel FP, Sadick MD et al. Murine cutaneous leishmaniasis. Susceptibility correlates with differential expansion of helper T cells subsets. Ann Inst Pasteur/Immunol 1987; 138:744-749.

172. Swihart K, Fruth U, Messmer N et al. Mice from a genetically resistant background lacking the interferon gamma receptor are susceptible to infection with Leishmania major but mount a polarized T helper cell 1-type CD4+ T cell response. J Exp Med 1995; 181:961-971.

173. Wang ZE, Reiner SL, Zheng S et al. CD4+ effector cells default to the Th2 pathway in interferon gamma-deficient mice infected with Leishmania major. J Exp Med 1994; 179:1367-1371.

174. Ding AH, Nathan CF, Stuehr DJ. Release of reactive nitrogen intermediates and reactive oxygen intermediates from mouse peritoneal macrophages. Comparison of activating cytokines and evidence for independent production. J Immunol 1988; 141:2407-2412.

175. Reiner SL, Zheng S, Wang ZE et al. Leishmania promastigotes evade IL-12 induction by macrophages and stimulate a broad range of cytokines from CD4+ T cells during initiation of infection. J Exp Med 1994; 179:447-456.

176. Heinzel FP, Sadick MD, Holaday BJ et al. Reciprocal expression of interferon-γ or interleukin 4 during the resolution or progression of murine leishmaniasis. Evidence for expansion of distinct helper T cell sub-

sets. J Exp Med 1989; 169:59-72.

177. Morris L, Troutt AB, McLeod KS et al. Interleukin 4 but not gamma interferon production correlates with the severity of murine cutaneous Leishmaniasis. Infect Immun 1993; 61:3459-3465.

178. Sadick MD, Locksley RM, Tubbs C et al. Murine cutaneous leishmaniasis: resistance correlated with the capacity to generate interferon-γ in response to Leishmania antigens in vitro. J Immunol 1986; 136: 655-661.

179. Solbach W, Lohoff M, Streck H et al. Kinetics of cell mediated immunity developing during the course of Leishmania major infection in healer and nonhealer mice: progressive impairment of response to and generation of interleukin-2. Immunology 1987; 62:485-492.

180. Bray RS. Leishmania: chemotaxic responses of promastigotes and macrophages in vitro. J Protozool 1983; 30:322-329.

181. Barral-Netto M, Barral A, Brownell CE et al. Transforming growth factor-β in leishmanial infections: a parasite escape mecha-nism. Science 1992; 257:545-548.

182. Wahl SM, Hunt DA, Wakefield L et al. Transforming growth factor-beta (TGF-β) induces monocyte chemotaxis and growth factor productions. Proc Natl Acad Sci USA 1987; 84:5788-5792.

183. Adams DH, Hathaway M, Shaw J et al. Transforming growth factor-β induces human T lymphocyte migration in vitro. J Immunol 1991; 147:609-612.

184. Tsunawaki S, Sporn MB, Ding A et al. Deactivation of macrophages by transforming growth factor beta. Nature 1988; 334:260-262.

185. Ding A, Nathan CF, Graycar J et al. Macrophage deactivating factor and transforming growth factor beta1,-beta2, and -beta3 inhibit induction of macrophage nitrogen oxide synthesis by IFN-gamma. J Immunol 1990; 145:940-944.

186. Barral-Netto M, Barral A. Transforming growth factor-beta in tegumentary leishmaniasis. Braz J Med Biol Res 1994; 27:1-9.

187. Fivenson DP, Strieter RM, Nickoloff BJ. Cytokine networks in skin disease. In: Remick DG, ed. Cytokines in Health and Disease. 2nd ed. New York: Marcel Dekker, Inc., 1995: (in press).

═══ CHAPTER 5 ═══

CHEMOKINES IN ARTHRITIS

Alisa E. Koch, Steven L. Kunkel and Robert M. Strieter

INTRODUCTION

Rheumatoid arthritis is a systemic chronic inflammatory disease which
has a prevalence of 1.8 to 3% of the population.[1,2] This disease predominantly involves the joints, but may also result in inflammation of
the eye, lung and blood vessels. In the inflamed joint, leukocytes migrate from the peripheral blood to the synovial tissue lining the joint
and the surrounding synovial fluid. The synovial pannus containing inflamed synovial tissue has been likened to a benign tumor, invading cartilage and bone and resulting in destruction of the surrounding tissues.[3]
Though these events are multifactorial, cytokines have emerged as key
players in mediating joint destruction.[4] Cytokines are released by cells
and can in turn function in an autocrine and paracrine manner on cells
of the joint.

It has become clear that a number of cytokines and growth factors
are involved in the immunopathogenesis of rheumatoid arthritis. These
include: interleukin-1 (IL-1), -6, -8; tumor necrosis factor-α (TNF-α),
leukemia inhibitory factor, tumor necrosis factor stimulated gene-6, the
colony stimulating factors, and leukemia inhibitory factor, fibroblast
growth factors (FGF), endothelins, platelet derived endothelial cell growth
factor/gliostatin, platelet derived growth factor (PDGF), transforming
growth factor-β (TGF-β), and hepatocyte growth factor (HGF) have all
been found in the inflamed rheumatoid joint, suggesting their role in
joint destruction.[4-39]

The chemokines are chemotactic cytokines which appear to play a
particularly important role in both the destructive and the fibrovas-
culoproliferative phase of rheumatoid arthritis. The purpose of this ar-
ticle is to review some of the chemokines present in the arthritic joint,
paying special attention to their potential role in perpetuating rheumatoid inflammation. The chemokine IL-8 will serve as the prototype, since
it has been studied more extensively in arthritis than the other
chemokines.

Chemokines in Disease, edited by Alisa E. Koch and Robert M. Strieter.
© 1996 R.G. Landes Company.

IL-8

IL-8 in the Pathogenesis of Arthritis

IL-8 is a member of the C-X-C family of chemokines.[40] There are a variety of potential triggers for IL-8 production in the joint. Neutrophils which phagocytose particulates can produce large quantities of IL-8.[41] This is perhaps the case in diseases, such as rheumatoid arthritis, in which large aggregates of inflammatory debris may be present. Monosodium urate crystals, such as are present in gouty inflammation, induce monocytes to release IL-8.[42]

The concept that IL-8 induced synovial inflammation was first demonstrated by Endo, Matsushima and colleagues.[43] These investigators injected recombinant IL-8 into the normal rabbit knee joint. Following a single 5 µg intraarticular injection of IL-8, the animals developed joint erythema and a limp after 4 hours. Concomitant with these events, inflammatory leukocytes entered the joint, peaking at 4 hours post-IL-8 injection and persisting until 24 hours postinjection. While neutrophils were the main synovial exudate cells at 4 hours postinjection, subsequently mononuclear cells accumulated and became the main infiltrating cells after 8 hours postinjection. Mirroring the events in the synovial fluid, at 4 hours post-IL-8 injection, a large number of neutrophils infiltrated the synovial lining and were also found perivascularly. However, at 24 hours post-IL-8 injection the synovial tissue lining cells, which are composed of macrophages and fibroblasts, became ovoid, pleomorphic and multilayered, as is often seen in synovial biopsies from patients with rheumatoid arthritis. This study indicates that in principal IL-8 can induce joint inflammation and synovial changes similar to those found in patients with rheumatoid arthritis.

Early Demonstrations of Neutrophil Chemotactic Activity in the Joint

Early investigation by Watson, Westwick and co-workers showed that human synovial cells stimulated with IL-1 in vitro released a low molecular weight factor which stimulated neutrophil locomotion and elevated neutrophil Ca^{2+}.[44,45] It is likely that these workers noted the effects of IL-8 or one of the IL-8 related chemokines.

IL-8 is Found in Human Synovial Fluids

Several investigative groups, including our own, found increased levels of synovial fluid IL-8 in rheumatoid arthritis compared to other rheumatic diseases.[43,46-53] In these studies, levels of rheumatoid synovial fluid IL-8 were generally in the range of 1-18 ng/ml. Interestingly, though other forms of arthritis, including gonococcal arthritis were accompanied by a massive influx of neutrophils into the joint, these patients appeared to have an absence of detectable IL-8.[53] As might be expected, noninflammatory forms of arthritis, such as osteoarthritis, exhibited virtually no synovial fluid IL-8.[43,46,52]

Since antigenic demonstration of a cytokine does not necessarily constitute functional bioactivity, we demonstrated that the IL-8 present in rheumatoid synovial fluids was bioactive. When rheumatoid synovial fluid IL-8 is immunodepleted, this results in a significant drop in the synovial fluid chemotactic activity for neutrophils in vitro.[46] These results suggest that IL-8 is bioactive in the joint.

Rheumatoid Serum Contains IL-8

IL-8, unlike many cytokines, is detectable in the serum of rheumatoid patients.[46] Moreover, serum IL-8 levels are strongly positively correlated with synovial fluid IL-8 levels (r = 0.9, p < 0.05), suggesting that serum IL-8 levels may serve as a useful diagnostic test to indicate intraarticular IL-8 levels.

Rheumatoid Bone Marrow Cells Produce IL-8

In contrast to many other cytokines, including IL-1, -2, -3, -4, -7, granulocyte-macrophage colony stimulating factor

(GM-CSF), granulocyte colony stimulating factor (G-CSF) or TNF-α and -β, IL-8 is increased in rheumatoid bone marrow aspirates compared to normal.[54] Moreover, the levels of IL-8 correlated with the degree of synovitis in these patients. Thus, the bone marrow may be an important site for the production or accumulation of IL-8 in rheumatoid arthritis.

Synovial Fibroblasts Produce IL-8

In addition to the synovial fluid cells, synovial tissue cells also produce IL-8.[55-57] Synovial fibroblasts do not produce IL-8 mRNA or protein constitutively. However, when incubated in the presence of agonists in vitro, they are a rich source of IL-8. Agonists include IL-1β, TNF-α and lipopolysaccharide. In one study, pretreatment of rheumatoid fibroblasts with both IL-1 and TNF-α induced a synergistic effect compared to incubation with either cytokine alone.[56] Pretreatment of synovial fibroblast supernatants resulted in inhibition of IL-1 or TNF-α induced rheumatoid fibroblast IL-8 production.[56] These results indicate that IL-8 may be one of the more important chemokines in rheumatoid arthritis. In another study, inhibition of protein synthesis resulted in superinduction of IL-8 mRNAs in IL-1, but not TNF-α stimulated fibroblasts, indicating that IL-1 and TNF-α are likely to regulate the expression of these mRNAs by different mechanisms.[57]

Of note, bacterial superantigens, upon engagement of MHC class II antigens, can serve as triggers for synovial fibroblast IL-8.[58] One may envision these as possible activating signals for synovial fibroblasts in vivo. Thus, it appears that while synovial fibroblasts are capable of producing IL-8, they require exogenous stimulation to do so.

Identification of Synovial Tissue Macrophages as a Source of IL-8

We have shown that macrophages isolated from synovial tissues are a potent source of IL-8 mRNA and protein in vitro.[46] Unlike synovial tissue fibroblasts, these cells constitutively produce IL-8. Moreover, we have shown that stimuli such as IL-1 do not increase the production of this chemokine. These results indicate that macrophages are likely maximally stimulated in vivo to produce IL-8.

We have described a novel function for IL-8 as a mediator of new blood vessel growth or angiogenesis.[59] IL-8 is both chemotactic and mitogenic for endothelial cells in vitro. Moreover, it is a potent angiogenic factor in the in vivo rat corneal bioassay for angiogenesis. Anti-IL-8 neutralizes the majority of angiogenic activity found in activated peripheral blood monocyte supernatants or in the supernatants from synovial tissue macrophages. Additionally, IL-8 antisense oligonucleotides inhibit the production of monocyte-derived angiogenic activity. Thus, IL-8 is an important chemotactic cytokine which not only participates in the inflammatory phase of rheumatoid arthritis, but also participates in the vasculoproliferative phase of this disease.

Cartilage and Articular Chondrocytes Release IL-8

In addition to synovial fluid and synovial tissue, cartilage explants and cultured chondrocytes release IL-8 upon exposure to IL-1.[60-62] While primary chondrocytes continue to secrete prostromelysin and procollagenase after removal of an IL-1 stimulus, IL-8 synthesis by these cells requires the continuous presence of IL-1.[60] These results are consistent with the suggested instability of cytokine mRNAs and also suggest that there is no significant accumulation of biologically active IL-1 in the cartilage matrix of normal cartilage.

While one of the major known functions of IL-8 is neutrophil chemotaxis, the contribution of neutrophil-mediated destruction has been difficult to determine, since it has not been possible to demonstrate the presence of neutrophils on articular surfaces. Yet, chondrocytes produce sufficient quantities of IL-8 to allow for the establishment of a transient chemotactic gradient towards the cartilage surface. Additionally, the in vitro neutrophil, cartilage and IL-8 coculture experiments described above suggest that neutrophil-mediated cartilage destruction is indeed feasible in vivo.

LOCALIZATION OF IL-8 IN VIVO

Since a number of cell types appear to produce IL-8 in vivo, it becomes important to discern which are the major cell types which produce IL-8 in situ. We performed immunohistochemistry on synovial tissues from patients with rheumatoid and osteoarthritis.[46] We found immunoreactive IL-8 localized to macrophages and the macrophage-derived synovial lining layer. Deleuran and co-workers found a similar pattern of reactivity, but additionally described synovial tissue endothelial reactivity.[48] These results suggest that the macrophage is among the principal producers of IL-8 in the synovial tissue.

RELATIONSHIP OF IL-8 AND CLINICAL MARKERS OF DISEASE ACTIVITY

Various studies suggested different relationships between clinical disease markers and serum or synovial fluid IL-8 levels. Brennan and co-workers were unable to show a correlation between synovial fluid neutrophil counts and synovial fluid IL-8 levels.[51] On the other hand, Peichel and colleagues found a direct correlation between RA synovial fluid IL-8 levels and the number of joint leukocytes or circulating C-reactive protein levels.[53] In the study by Rampart and co-workers, no correlation was demonstrated between synovial fluid IL-8 and disease markers, erythrocyte sedimentation rate or C-reactive protein levels.[47] However, these workers found that synovial fluids from patients with rheumatoid arthritis seropositive for rheumatoid factor contained significantly higher concentrations of IL-8 than synovial fluids from seronegative rheumatoid patients and patients with nonrheumatoid joint inflammation. There was a significant correlation between serum IL-8 levels and serum rheumatoid factor titers. Thus, it appears that it is difficult to show a consistent relationship between IL-8 levels and clinical disease activity. This may be due to several factors, including the small number of patients examined in most studies as well as the insensitivity of most conventional markers of rheumatoid disease activity.

Interestingly, in another study, Peichel and co-workers found that circulating antibodies to IL-8 were present in rheumatoid serum, and these correlated with C-reactive protein and the number of arthritic joints.[49] Additionally, levels of anti-IL-8 correlated with disease activity and were associated with a lack of clinical improvement upon treatment of patients with systemic steroids. Thus, it may be that serum anti-IL-8 will provide a useful diagnostic marker for disease activity in rheumatoid arthritis.

EFFECTS OF IMMUNE MODULATORS ON IL-8 PRODUCTION

IL-8 production may be modulated by a number of factors. Colchicine, which is used to treat acute gout, is a potent suppressor of neutrophil activation by IL-8.[39] Among the most potent suppressors of IL-8 production are corticosteroids. Seitz and co-workers have shown that rheumatoid synovial fluid mononuclear cell production of IL-8 was inhibited upon exposure to dexamethasone (10^{-9} to 10^{-5} M).[50] Dexamethasone inhibited the production of rheumatoid synoviocyte IL-8 by 60-80%.[63] These authors also found that when rheumatoid patients were given intraarticular bethamethasone-dipropionate (5 mg) or bethamethasone-disodium phosphate (2 mg), their synovial fluid mononuclear cells exhibited decreased spontaneous and LPS-dependent release of mononuclear IL-8. Additionally, the total number of white blood cells and percentage of neutrophils was decreased. van den Brink and colleagues showed that rheumatoid patients given pulse corticosteroid therapy exhibited a decrease in their synovial fluid IL-8 levels.[64] These results suggest that IL-8 production by a number of synovial cells may by modified clinically by antirheumatic drugs, such as corticosteroids.

In contrast to the effects observed with corticosteroids, gold sodium thiomalate inhibited rheumatoid synovial fibroblast IL-8 production only in suboptimally stimulated cells in vitro.[63] Indomethacin treatment of rheumatoid synovial fluid mononuclear cells or synovial fibroblasts in vitro did not decrease the mononuclear IL-8 levels.[50,63] Other nonsteroidal anti-inflammatory compounds such as piroxicam, naproxen and tiaprofenic acid were also unable to decrease rheumatoid fibroblast IL-8 production. The remittive agent methotrexate was also ineffective in inhibiting rheumatoid fibroblast IL-8 production.[63] In sum, these results suggest that part of the antirheumatic action of corticosteroids, but not nonsteroidal anti-inflammatory is due to the prevention of accumulation of IL-8 by cells from the inflamed joint.

IL-8 AND GENE THERAPY

Studies employing IL-8 and gene therapy are still in early phases of development. Chen and co-workers have shown that rabbit IL-8 cDNA can be transduced into rabbit synoviocytes using replication defective adenovirus.[65] This technique may help to study the effects of local and prolonged expression of IL-8 in an experimental model of arthritis.

EPITHELIAL NEUTROPHIL ACTIVATING PEPTIDE-78 (ENA-78)

ENA-78 is a recently described member of the C-X-C chemokine subfamily.[66] ENA-78 is a potent chemotactic and less potent chemokinetic factor for neutrophils. We have recently identified significantly increased levels of ENA-78 in rheumatoid compared to osteoarthritic synovial fluids.[67] Rheumatoid synovial fluid mononuclear cells produce ENA-78. Synovial tissue fibroblasts constitutively produce antigenic ENA-78, which is augmented upon incubation of cells with TNF-α. Using immunohistochemistry, we found that the main cellular source of this chemokine was the synovial lining cell layer, followed by macrophages, endothelial cells and fibroblasts. Immunohistological ENA-78 was present in a greater percentage of macrophages and fibroblasts in rheumatoid compared to normal synovium. Interestingly, ENA-78 was present in significantly greater quantities in the serum from rheumatoid patients compared to normal subjects, suggesting that for diagnostic purposes, this cytokine can be readily measured. ENA-78 is a very abundant protein, with mean levels being approximately 15 times higher than mean IL-8 levels in rheumatoid synovial fluid. Moreover, ENA-78 in synovial fluid was biologically active and accounted for a significant percentage of the chemotactic activity for neutrophils in these fluids. Thus, like IL-8, one of the main actions of ENA-78 in rheumatoid arthritis appears to be the recruitment of neutrophils.

GROWTH-RELATED GENE (GRO) PROTEINS

GRO, or growth-related gene product, is also a member of the C-X-C chemokine subfamily.[68] GRO was originally considered to be an oncogene growth-related peptide, but was soon found to be identical to melanoma growth stimulating activity (MSGA).[68] GRO stimulates the growth of fibroblasts and is a neutrophil chemoattractant.[68] Both synovial fibroblasts and articular chondrocytes respond to IL-1 or TNF-α stimulation to produce mRNA for GRO.[57,60,69]

Hogan and co-workers recently examined the production of GROα (GRO/MSGA), GROβ/(MIP-1α) and GROγ (MIP-2β).[70] Curiously, these authors found that the majority of synovial fibroblast lines derived from osteoarthritic or other noninflammatory synovia showed a relative increase in the constitutive expression of GROα and GROβ when compared to fibroblasts from rheumatoid synovia. These authors were also unable to detect IL-8 production in any of the synovial fibroblast lines they examined by polymerase chain reaction, even after stimulation with IL-1 or TNF-α, in contrast to many other studies. It is unclear whether the discordant results are due to technical differences between studies.

Synovial fluid mononuclear cells are another cellular source of GRO. Hosaka and co-workers showed increased mRNA for GRO in rheumatoid synovial fluid mononuclear cells compared to peripheral blood from the same patients and from normal subjects.[71]

Since rheumatoid synovial fluids have been shown to contain both immunoreactive and bioactive IL-8, ENA-78 and GROα, one may ask which of these chemo-kines plays the greatest role in neutrophil recruitment in the joint. We simultaneously immunodepleted rheumatoid synovial fluids of IL-8, ENA-78 and GROα and measured the chemotactic response of normal neutrophils to these synovial fluids.[72] We found that IL-8 accounted for 36% of the chemotactic activity, while ENA-78 accounted for 34%, and GROα accounted for 28% of the chemotactic activity. These results appear to indicate that all three of these chemokines are important in neutrophil recruitment in the rheumatoid joint, with IL-8 accounting for slightly more of the neutrophil chemotactic activity than the other chemokines. The cellular interactions of a number of C-X-C chemokines is shown in Figure 5.1.

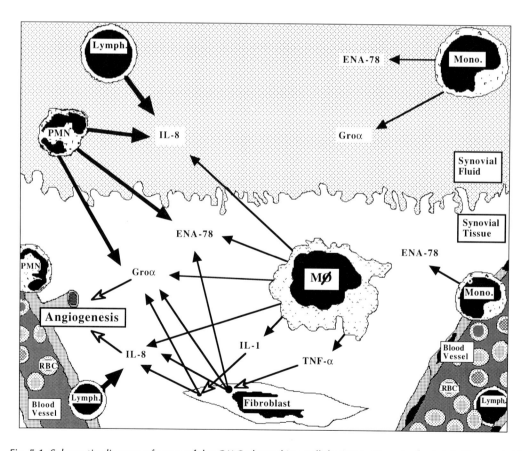

Fig. 5.1. Schematic diagram of some of the C-X-C chemokine cellular interactions in the joint. Rheumatoid synovial fluid is shown by the hatched area adjacent to the synovial tissue, which is shown by the clear area. Narrow, dark arrows represent production of cytokines while wide, dark arrows represent chemoattraction of cells in response to cytokines. IL-1 and TNF-α (clear arrowheads) produced by macrophages induce synovial tissue fibroblast production of cytokines.

It is interesting that GRO is expressed in many proliferative disease tissues, such as psoriasis, melanomas and carcinomas, but not in normal fibroblasts, vascular endothelium, lymphocytes and alveolar macrophages.[73,74] Unemori and associates found that GROα contributes to net collagen loss by inhibiting its synthesis in rheumatoid synovial fibroblasts.[75] Thus, along with promoting inflammation, GROα may be involved in repair of the damaged joint.

CONNECTIVE TISSUE ACTIVATING PEPTIDE-III (CTAP-III) AND ITS CLEAVAGE PRODUCTS

Another member of the C-X-C chemokine subfamily, CTAP-III, is a human platelet α-granule derived growth factor that is more than 100 times as abundant as other growth factors in plasma.[76] Rheumatoid plasma contains elevated levels of CTAP-III but not its cleavage products β-thromboglobulin or neutrophil activating peptide-2.[76] CTAP-III affects many aspects of connective tissue metabolism. It stimulates synthesis of DNA, hyaluronic acid, sulfated glycosaminoglycan chains, proteoglycan monomer and proteoglycan core protein in human synovial fibroblast cultures.[76,77]

MONOCYTE CHEMOATTRACTANT PROTEIN-1 (MCP-1)

MCP-1 is member of the C-C chemokine subfamily. We and others have shown elevated levels of MCP-1 in synovial fluids from rheumatoid arthritis compared to osteoarthritis patients.[78,79] Rheumatoid synovial fibroblasts produce MCP-1 in response to IL-1, TNF-α or interferon-γ.[55,80,81] Synovial tissue macrophages are the major MCP-1 immunopositive cells in the rheumatoid synovium, and these cells constitutively produce MCP-1.[78] Like synovial fibroblasts, chondrocytes produce MCP-1 in response to IL-1, TNF-α, PDGF, lipopolysaccharide or TGF-β.[40] The main function of MCP-1 in the joint appears to be the recruitment of macrophages, since injection of MCP-1 into rabbit joints resulted in marked infiltration of macrophages into the synovial tissue.[79] Like IL-8, MCP-1 production can be altered by antirheumatic drugs and immune modulators. Loetscher and coworkers showed that dexamethasone and gold sodium thiomalate inhibited the production of MCP-1 by rheumatoid synovial fibroblasts.[63] Dexamethasone inhibited the production of MCP-1 by 20-65%. As was the case with IL-8, gold sodium thiomalate inhibited the production of MCP-1 only by suboptimally stimulated fibroblasts in vitro. Again, methotrexate and nonsteroidal anti-inflammatory compounds were inactive in reducing MCP-1 production. Similarly, Villiger showed that dexamethasone blunted the induction of MCP-1 expression by IL-1 and by activators of protein kinase C and protein kinase A in human articular chondrocytes.[40] Glucocorticoids bind to intracellular receptors that recognize glucocorticoid-responsive elements in the promoter regions of genes. It may be that glucocorticoids act in this way to modulate chemokine gene expression. In contrast, retinoic acid strongly increased phorbol myristate acetate-induced MCP-1 expression and potentiated the effects of IL-1 and LPS.

MACROPHAGE INFLAMMATORY PROTEIN-1α (MIP-1α)

MIP-1α is an 8 kDa member of the C-C chemokine subfamily. Murine MIP-1α is an endogenous pyrogen which, unlike other endogenous pyrogens, does not mediate its effects via prostaglandins.[82] MIP-1α is chemotactic for monocytes and T lymphocytes.[83] Murine MIP-1α, but not MIP-1β, activates murine macrophages to secrete IL-1, TNF-α or IL-6.[84,85] Though murine MIP-1α may be chemokinetic for neutrophils, it appears that in the rheumatoid joint, like MCP-1, one of the main functions of MIP-1α appears to be the recruitment of macrophages.[86] We found that rheumatoid synovial fluids contained significantly more MIP-1α than did osteoarthritis synovial fluids. Synovial fluid MIP-1α was biologically active and accounted for a mean of 36% of the chemotactic activity for monocytes in these fluids. Like MCP-1, the main immunopositive cells in rheumatoid synovial tissue are macrophages and fibroblasts. Synovial fibroblasts produce MIP-1α in response to TNF-α. Synovial fluid mononuclear cells also produce MIP-1α. Thus, MIP-1α appears to be a major factor facilitating the extravasation of synovial tissue macrophages in the rheumatoid joint. Some of the C-C chemokine interactions in the joint are shown in Figure 5.2.

MACROPHAGE INFLAMMATORY PROTEIN-1β (MIP-1β)

MIP-1β is a member of the C-C chemokine subfamily. MIP-1 is a term applied originally to LPS-stimulated murine macrophage conditioned medium containing two distinct molecules, MIP-1α and MIP-1β, that copurified.[87] The human counterparts of these two proteins were independently discovered by several groups.[68,88] Murine MIP-1α and β have 60% peptide identity and are 70% homologous to their human counterparts.[87] Interestingly, despite this structural similarity, we found the expression of human MIP-1α and β to be quite different.[87a] In contrast to the other chemokines we have examined, MIP-1β was upregulated in synovial fluids from patients with rheumatoid arthritis compared to osteoarthritis. MIP-1β in these osteoarthritis synovial fluids was bioactive, inducing neutrophil recruitment. Thus, contrary to popular belief, it does not appear that all chemokines are upregulated in rheumatoid inflammation.

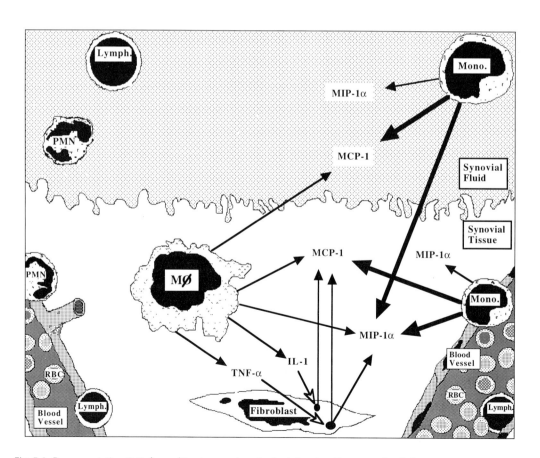

Fig. 5.2. Representative C-C chemokine interactions in the joint. See Figure 5.1 for definitions. Representative chemokine network in the rheumatoid synovial fluid (hatched) and tissue (clear).

RANTES

RANTES, a member of the chemo-kine-β subfamily, is a chemotactic factor for monocytes and memory T lymphocytes.[89] Rheumatoid synovial fibroblasts produce RANTES mRNA in response to TNF-α or IL-1.[90] Interferon-γ enhances the TNF-α or IL-1β induction of fibroblast RANTES mRNA, while IL-4 downregulates this induction. RANTES expression, like that of GRO, is upregulated in rheumatoid synovial fluid mononuclear cells compared to peripheral blood mononuclear cells obtained from rheumatoid patients or normal volunteers.[71]

CYTOKINE INHIBITORS

The net biological effect of cytokines depends on the presence of cytokines relative to specific and nonspecific inhibitory molecules. Future therapeutic strategies of rheumatic diseases may entail inhibition of proinflammatory cytokines, upregulation of anti-inflammatory cytokines, or both. In the case of IL-1, a naturally occurring inhibitor termed IL-1 receptor antagonist protein (IRAP or IL-1ra) has been identified.[91,92] This molecule binds to type I and type II IL-1 receptors with the same affinity as IL-1, but does not activate signal transduction and therefore acts as a competitive inhibitor.[93] IL-1ra is found in the synovial fluids from patients with rheumatoid arthritis and levels correlate with the neutrophil counts in these fluids.[94] Synovial fluid neutrophils are a source of this cytokine.[94] Immunohistologic IL-1ra is present in synovial tissue macrophages and lining cells.[95,96] IL-1ra is produced by synovial fibroblasts in culture, particularly in response to IL-1, TNF-α, lipopolysaccharide or phorbol myristate acetate.[97] When the quantities of IL-1 are compared to those of IL-1ra produced by rheumatoid synovial tissue cells, only a 3-fold excess of IL-1ra is present.[93] This is well below the 10- to 100-fold excess of IL-1ra needed to inhibit IL-1 bioactivity. Hence, in rheumatoid arthritis, an IL-1ra deficiency state may exist, resulting in relative overactivity of IL-1. Clinical trials are in progress examining the effect of IL-1ra or soluble IL-1 receptors in modulating rheumatoid inflammation. It may be that by inhibiting the effects of IL-1 on synovial fibroblast-derived cytokine production, one may mitigate the effects of the variety of chemokines induced by IL-1 in these cells. It is possible that naturally occurring chemokine inhibitors will also be discovered and similar therapeutic avenues may be attempted. Thus, efforts aimed at interrupting the cytokine network involving chemokine production may be beneficial in the therapy of rheumatoid arthritis.

CONCLUSIONS

In this review we have examined the putative role of chemokines in arthritis. We have emphasized the role of IL-8 in rheumatoid inflammation. Some of these proteins are detectable in the serum of rheumatoid patients and may eventually serve as useful laboratory markers of disease activity. Moreover, in the next decade, it is likely that clinically available specific antagonists of chemokines or their receptors will be developed.

Future directions in cytokine research may include somatic cytokine gene therapy. A recent study has shown that direct injection of cDNA expression vectors encoding cytokine genes into murine skeletal muscle induces the biological effects of these cytokines in vivo.[98] Given the sometimes limited efficacy of therapeutic armamentarium currently used to treat rheumatoid patients, it seems prudent to consider alternative therapeutic regimens such as ablation of cytokines, in order to prevent severe joint destruction. Hopefully, the study of cytokines and their networks will lead to specific immunomodulatory therapies that will benefit rheumatoid patients and prevent joint destruction.

ACKNOWLEDGEMENTS

This work was supported by National Institute of Health grants AR30692 and AR41492 (A.E. Koch), HL02401 and HL50057 (R.M. Strieter), HL31693 (S.L. Kunkel), SCOR grant IP50HL46487 (R.M.

Strieter and S.L. Kunkel); The Dr. Ralph and Marion Falk Challenge Prize of the Illinois Chapter Arthritis Foundation (A.E. Koch); and funds from the Veteran's Administration Research Service (A.E. Koch). We wish to thank Ms. Catherine Haskell for her expert artwork.

REFERENCES

1. Harris EDJ. Rheumatoid arthritis: pathophysiology and implications for therapy. N Engl J Med 1990; 332:1277-87.

2. Harris ED. Pathogenesis of rheumatoid arthritis: a disorder associated with dysfunctional immunoregulation. In: Gallin JI, Goldstein IM, Snyderman R, eds. New York: Raven Press Ltd, 1988:751-73.

3. Fassbender HG, Simmling-Annefeld N. The potential aggressiveness of synovial tissue in rheumatoid arthritis. J Pathol 1983; 139:399-406.

4. Koch AE, Kunkel SL, Strieter RM. Cytokines in rheumatoid arthritis. J Invest Med 1995; 43:28-38.

5. Fava R, Olsen N, Keski-Oja J et al. Active and latent forms of transforming growth factor β activity in synovial effusions. J Exp Med 1989; 169:291-96.

6. Fava RA, Olsen NJ, Postlethwaite AE et al. Transforming growth factor β1 (TGF-β1) induced neutrophil recruitment to synovial tissues: Implications for TGF-β-driven synovial inflammation and hyperplasia. J Exp Med 1991; 173:1121-32.

7. Cooper WO, Fava RA, Gates CA et al. Acceleration of onset of collagen-induced arthritis by intra-articular injection of tumour necrosis factor or transforming growth factor-beta. Clin Exp Immunol 1992; 89:244-50.

8. Fava RA, Olsen NJ, Spencer-Green G et al. Vascular permeability factor/endothelial growth factor (VPF/VEGF): accumulation and expression in human synovial fluids and rheumatoid synovial tissue. J Exp Med 1994; 180:341-46.

9. Lotz M, Moats T, Villiger PM. Leukemia inhibitory factor is expressed in cartilage and synovium and can contribute to the pathogenesis of arthritis. J Clin Invest 1992; 90:888-96.

10. Lotz M, Kekow J, Carson DA. Transforming growth factor-β and cellular immune responses in synovial fluids. J Immunol 1990; 144:4189-94.

11. Villiger PM, Geng Y, Lotz M. Induction of cytokine expression by leukemia inhibitory factor. J Clin Invest 1993; 91:1575-81.

12. Wisniewski H-G, Maier R, Lotz M et al. TSG-6: a TNF-, IL-1, and LPS-inducible secreted glycoprotein associated with arthritis. J Immunol 1993; 151:6593-601.

13. Szeckanecz Z, Haines GK, Harlow LA et al. Increased synovial expression of transforming growth factor-beta (TGF-β) receptor endoglin and TgF-β1 in rheumatoid arthritis: possible interactions in the pathogenesis of the disease. Clinical Immunol Immunopathol 1995; 76.187-194.

14. Lafyatis R, Thompson N, Remmers E et al. Demonstration of local production of PDGF and TGF-β by synovial tissue from patients with rheumatoid arthritis (abstract). Arthritis Rheum 1988; 31:S62.

15. Lafyatis R, Thompson NL, Remmers EF et al. Transforming growth factor-β production by synovial tissues from rheumatoid patients and streptococcal cell wall arthritic rats. J Immunol 1989; 143:1142-48.

16. Kumkumian GK, Lafyatis R, Remmers EF et al. Platelet-derived growth factor and IL-1 interactions in rheumatoid arthritis. Regulation of synoviocyte proliferation, prostaglandin production, and collagenase transcription. J Immunol 1989; 143:833-37.

17. Remmers EF, Lafyatis R, Kumkumian GK et al. Cytokines and growth regulation of synoviocytes from patients with rheumatoid arthritis and rats with streptococcal cell wall arthritis. Growth Factors 1990; 2:179-88.

18. Sano H, Forough R, Maier JAM et al. Detection of high levels of heparin binding growth factor-1 (acidic fibroblast growth factor) in inflammatory arthritic joints. J Cell Biol 1990; 110:1417-26.

19. Wilder RL, Lafyatis R, Roberts AB et al. Transforming growth factor-β in rheumatoid arthritis. Ann N Y Acad Sci 1990; 593:197-207.

20. Remmers EF, Sano H, Wilder RL. Platelet-derived growth factors and heparin-binding (fibroblast) growth factors in the synovial

tissue pathology of rheumatoid arthritis. Semin Arthritis Rheum 1991; 21:191-99.

21. Takeuchi M, Otsuka T, Matsui N et al. Aberrant production of gliostatin/platelet-derived endothelial cell growth factor in rheumatoid synovium. Arthritis Rheum 1994; 37:662-72.

22. Arend WP, Dayer J-M. Cytokines and cytokine inhibitors or antagonists in rheumatoid arthritis. Arthritis Rheum 1990; 33:305-15.

23. Firestein GS, Alvaro-Garcia JM, Maki R. Quantitative analysis of cytokine gene expression in rheumatoid arthritis. J Immunol 1990; 144:3347-53.

24. Brennan FM, Chantry D, Turner M et al. Detection of transforming growth factor-beta in rheumatoid arthritis synovial tissue: lack of effect on spontaneous cytokine production in joint cell cultures. Clin Exp Immunol 1990; 81:278-85.

25. Field M, Chu C, Feldmann M et al. IL-6 localisation in the synovial membrane in rhuematoid arthritis. Rheumatol Int 1991; 11:45-50.

26. Chu CQ, Field M, Feldmann M et al. Localization of tumor necrosis factor α in synovial tissues and at the cartilage-pannus junction in patients with rheumatoid arthritis. Arthritis Rheum 1991; 34:1125-32.

27. Chu CQ, Field M, Abney E et al. Transforming growth factor-β1 in rheumatoid synovial membrane and cartilage/pannus junction. Clin Exp Immunol 1991; 86: 380-86.

28. Hirano T, Matsuda T, Turner M et al. Excessive production of interleukin 6/B cell stimulatory factor-2 in rheumatoid arthritis. Eur J Immunol 1988; 18:1797-801.

29. Houssiau FA, Devogelaer J-P, Van Damme J et al. Interleukin-6 in synovial fluid and serum of patients with rheumatoid arthritis and other inflammatory arthritides. Arthritis Rheum 1988; 31:784-88.

30. Helle M, Boeije L, de Groot E et al. Sensitive ELISA for interleukin-6. Detection of IL-6 in biological fluids: synovial fluids and sera. J Immunol Methods 1991; 138:47-56.

31. Waage A, Kaufmann C, Espevik T et al. Interleukin-6 in synovial fluid from patients with arthritis. Clin Immunol Immunopathol 1989; 50:394-98.

32. Brozik M, Rosztoczy I, Meretey K et al. Interleukin 6 levels in synovial fluids of patients with different arthritides: correlation with local IgM rheumatoid factor and systemic acute phase protein production. J Rheumatol 1992; 19:63-68.

33. Cohick CB, Furst DE, Quagliata S et al. Analysis of elevated serum interleukin-6 levels in rheumatoid arthritis: Correlation with erythrocyte sedimentation rate of C-reactive protein. J Lab Clin Med 1994; 123:721-27.

34. Bhardwaj N, Santhanam U, Lau LL et al. IL-6/IFN-β2 in synovial effusions of patients with rheumatoid arthritis and other arthritides. J Immunol 1989; 143:2153-59.

35. Tan PLJ, Farmiloe S, Yeoman S et al. Expression of the interleukin 6 gene in rheumatoid synovial fibroblasts. J Rheumatol 1990; 17:1608-12.

36. Rosenbaum JT, Cugnini R, Tara DC et al. Production and modulation of interleukin 6 synthesis by synoviocytes derived from patients with arthritic disease. Ann Rheum Dis 1992; 51:198-202.

37. Harigai M, Kitani A, Hara M et al. Rheumatoid adherent synovial cells produce B cell differentiation factor activity neutralizable by antibody to B cell stimulatory factor-2/interleukin 6. J Rheumatol 1988; 15:1616-22.

38. Miyasaka N, Sato K, Hashimoto J et al. Constitutive production of interleukin 6/B cell stimulatory factor-2 from inflammatory synovium. Clin Immunol Immunopathol 1989; 52:238-47.

39. Hart PH, Ahern MJ, Smith MD et al. Regulatory effects of IL-13 on synovial fluid macrophages and blood monocytes from patients with inflammatory arthritis. Clin Exp Immunol 1995; 99:331-37.

40. Villiger PM, Terkeltaub R, Lotz M. Monocyte chemoattractant protein-1 (MCP-1) expression in human articular cartilage. J Clin Invest 1992; 90:488-96.

41. Bazzoni F, Castella MA, Rossi F et al. Phagocytosing neutrophils produce and release high amounts of the neutrophil-activating peptide/interleukin-8. J Exp Med 1991; 173:77174.

42. Terkeltaub R, Zachariae C, Santoro D et al. Monocyte-derived neutrophil chemotactic factor/interleukin-8 is a potential mediator of crystal-induced inflammation. Arthritis Rheum 1991; 34:894-903.

43. Endo H, Akahoshi T, Takagishi K et al. Elevation of interleukin-8 (IL-8) levels in joint fluids of patients with rheumatoid arthritis and the induction by IL-8 of leukocyte infiltration and synovitis in rabbit joints. Lymphokine Cytokine Res 1991; 10:245-52.

44. Watson ML, Lewis GP, Westwick J. Neutrophil stimulation by recombinant cytokines and a factor produced by IL-1 treated human synovial cell cultures. Immunology 1988; 65:567-72.

45. Watson ML, Lewis GP, Westwick J. PMN stimulation by factors from IL-1 treated human synovial cell cultures. Agents Actions 1989; 27:448-50.

46. Koch AE, Kunkel SL, Burrows JC et al. Synovial tissue macrophage as a source of the chemotactic cytokine IL-8. J Immunol 1991; 147:2187-95.

47. Rampart M, Herman AG, Grillet B et al. Development and application of a radioimmunoassay for interleukin-8: Detection of interleukin-8 in synovial fluids from patients with inflammatory joint disease. Lab Invest 1992; 66:512-18.

48. Deleuran B, Lemche P, Kristensen M et al. Localisation of interleukin 8 in the synovial membrane, cartilage-pannus junction and chondrocytes in rheumatoid arthritis. Scand J Rheumatol 1994; 23:2-7.

49. Piechel P, Ceska M, Broell H et al. Human neutrophil activating peptide/interleukin 8 acts as an autoantigen in rheumatoid arthritis. Ann Rheum Dis 1992; 51:19-22.

50. Seitz M, Dewald B, Gerber N et al. Enhanced production of neutrophil-activating peptide-1/interleukin-8 in rheumatoid arthritis. J Clin Invest 1991; 87:463-69.

51. Brennan FM, Zachariae CO, Chantry D et al. Detection of interleukin 8 biological activity in synovial fluids from patients with rheumatoid arthritis and production of interleukin 8 mRNA by isolated synovial cells. Eur J Immunol 1990; 20:2141-44.

52. Symons JA, Wong WL, Palladino MA et al. Interleukin 8 in rheumatoid arthritis and osteoarthritis. Scand J Rheumatol 1992; 21:92-94.

53. Peichel P, Ceska M, Effenberger F et al. Presence of NAP-1/IL-8 in synovial fluids indicates a possible pathogenic role in rheumatoid arthritis. Scand J Immunol 1991; 34:333-39.

54. Tanabe M, Ochi T, Tomita T et al. Remarkable elevation of interleukin 6 and interleukin 8 levels in the bone marrow serum of patients with rheumatoid arthritis. J Rheumatol 1994; 21:830-35.

55. DeMarco D, Kunkel SL, Strieter RM et al. Interleukin-1 induced gene expression of neutrophil activating protein (interleukin-8) and monocyte chemotactic peptide in human synovial cells. Biochem Biophys Res Commun 1991; 174:411-16.

56. Rathanaswami P, Hachicha M, Wong WL et al. Synergistic effect of interleukin-1 beta and tumor necrosis factor alpha on interleukin-8 gene expression in synovial fibroblasts. Evidence that interleukin-8 is the major neutrophil-activating chemokine released in response to monokine activation. Arthritis Rheum 1993; 36:1295-304.

57. Bedard PA, Golds EE. Cytokine-induced expression of mRNAs for chemotactic factors in human synovial cells and fibroblasts. J Cell Physiol 1993; 154:433-41.

58. Mourad W, Mehindate K, Schall TJ et al. Engagement of major histocompatibility complex class II molecules by superantigen induces inflammatory cytokine gene expression in human rheumatoid fibroblast-like synoviocytes. J Exp Med 1992; 175:613-16.

59. Koch AE, Polverini PJ, Kunkel SL et al. Interleukin-8 as a macrophage-derived mediator of angiogenesis. Science 1992; 258:1798-801.

60. Recklies AD, Golds EE. Induction of synthesis and release of interleukin-8 from human articular chondrocytes and cartilage explants. Arthritis Rheum 1992; 35:1510-19.

61. Van Damme J, Bunning RAD, Conings R et al. Characterization of granulocyte chemotactic activity from human cytokine-stimulated chondrocytes as interleukin 8. Cytokine 1990; 2:106-11.

62. Lotz M, Terkeltaub R, Villiger PM. Cartilage and joint inflammation: regulation of IL-8 expression by human articular chondrocytes. J Immunol 1991; 148:466-73.

63. Loetscher P, Dewald B, Baggiolini M et al. Monocyte chemoattractant protein 1 and interleukin 8 production by rheumatoid synoviocytes: effects of antirheumatic drugs. Cytokine 1994; 6:162-70.

64. Van Den Brink HR, Van Wijk MJG, Geertzen RGM et al. Influence of corticosteroid pulse therapy on the serum levels of soluble interleukin 2 receptor, interleukin 6 and inteleukin 8 in patients with rheumatoid arthritis. J Rheumatol 1994; 21:430-34.

65. Chen Y, Davidson BL, Marks RM et al. Adenovirus-mediated transduction of the interleukin 8 gene into synoviocytes. Arthritis Rheum 1994; 37:S304.

66. Walz A, Burgener R, Car B et al. Structure and neutrophil-activating properties of a novel inflammatory peptide (ENA-78) with homology to interleukin 8. J Exp Med 1991; 174:1355-62.

67. Koch AE, Kunkel SL, Harlow LA et al. Epithelial neutrophil activating peptide-78: a novel chemotactic cytokine for neutrophils in arthritis. J Clin Invest 1994; 94:1012-18.

68. Oppenheim JJ, Zachariae CO, Mukaida N et al. Properties of the novel proinflammatory supergene "intercrine" cytokine family. Annu Rev Immunol 1991; 9:617-48.

69. Golds EE, Mason P, Nyirkos P. Inflammatory cytokines induce synthesis and secretion of gro protein and a neutrophil chemotactic factor but not beta 2-microglobulin in human synovial cells and fibroblasts. Biochem J 1989; 259:585-88.

70. Hogan M, Sherry B, Ritchlin C et al. Differential expression of the small inducible cytokines GROα and GROβ by synovial fibroblasts in chronic arthritis: possible role in growth regulation. Cytokine 1994; 6:61-69.

71. Hosaka S, Akahoshi T, Wada C et al. Expression of the chemokine superfamily in rheumatoid arthritis. Clin Exp Immunol 1994; 97:451-57.

72. Koch AE, Kunkel SL, Shah MR et al. Growth related gene product α: A chemotactic cytokine for neutrophils in rheumatoid arthritis. J Immunol 1995; 155:3660-3666.

73. Richmond A, Thomas HG. Melanoma growth stimulatory activity: isolation from human melanoma tumors and characterization of tissue distribution. J Cell Biochem 1988; 36:185-98.

74. Schroder JM, Gregory H, Young J et al. Neutrophil-activating proteins in psoriasis. J Invest Dermatol 1992; 98:241-47.

75. Unemori EN, Amento EP, Bauer EA et al. Melanoma growth-stimulatory activity/ GRO decreases collagen expression by human fibroblasts. Regulation by C-X-C but not C-C cytokines. J Biol Chem 1993; 268:1338-42.

76. Castor CW, Andrews PC, Swartz RD et al. The origin, variety, distribution, and biologic fate of connective tissue activating peptide-III isoforms: characteristics in patients with rheumatic, renal, and arterial disease. Arthritis Rheum 1993; 36:1142-53.

77. Castor CW, Smith EM, Hossler PA et al. Detection of connective tissue activating peptide-III isoforms in synovium from osteoarthritis and rheumatoid arthritis patients: patterns of interaction with other synovial cytokines in cell culture. Arthritis Rheum 1992; 35:783-93.

78. Koch AE, Kunkel SL, Harlow LA et al. Enhanced production of monocyte chemoattractant protein-1 in rheumatoid arthritis. J Clin Invest 1992; 90:772-79.

79. Akahoshi T, Wada C, Endo H et al. Expression of monocyte chemotactic and activating factor in rheumatoid arthritis. Arthritis Rheum 1993; 36:762-71.

80. Hachicha M, Rathanaswami P, Schall TJ et al. Production of monocyte chemotactic protein-1 in human type B synoviocytes. Arthritis Rheum 1993; 36:26-34.

81. Villiger PM, Terkeltaub R, Lotz M. Production of monocyte chemoattractant protein-1 by inflamed synovial tissue and cultured synoviocytes. J Immunol 1992; 149:722-27.

82. Davatelis G, Wolpe SD, Sherry B et al. Macrophage inflammatory protein-1: a prostaglandin-independent endogenous pyrogen. Science 1989; 243:1066-68.

83. Taub DD, Conlon K, Lloyd AR et al. Preferential migration of activated CD4[+] and CD8[+] T cells in response to MIP-1α and MIP-1β. Science 1993; 260:355-58.

84. Fahey TJ III, Tracey KJ, Tekamp-Olson P et al. Macrophage inflammatory protein 1 modulates macrophage function. J Immunol 1991; 148:2764-69.

85. Martin CA, Dorf ME. Differential regulation of interleukin-6, macrophage inflammatory protein-1, and JE/MCP-1 cytokine expression in macrophage cell lines. Cell Immunol 1991; 135:245-58.

86. Koch AE, Kunkel SL, Harlow LA et al. Macrophage inflammatory protein-1 alpha. A novel chemotactic cytokine for macrophages in rheumatoid arthritis. J Clin Invest 1994; 93:921-28.

87. Wolpe SD, Cerami A. Macrophage inflammatory proteins 1 and 2: members of a novel superfamily of cytokines. FASEB J 1989; 3:2565-73.

87a. Koch AE, Kunkel SL, Shah MR et al. Macrophage inflammatory protein-1 beta: a C-C chemokine in osteoarthritis. Clin Immunol Immunopathol 1995; 77:307-314.

88. Schall TJ. Biology of the RANTES/SIS cytokine family. Cytokine 1991; 3:165-83.

89. Schall TJ, Bacon K, Toy KJ et al. Selective attraction of monocytes and T lymphocytes of the memory phenotype by cytokine RANTES. Nature 1990; 347:669-71.

90. Rathanaswami P, Hachicha M, Sadick M et al. Expression of the cytokine RANTES in human rheumatoid synovial fibroblasts. J Biol Chem 1993; 268:5834-39.

91. Carter DB, Deibel MR Jr, Dunn CJ et al. Purification, cloning, expression and biological characterization of an interleukin-1 receptor antagonist protein. Nature 1990; 344:633-38.

92. Eisenberg SP, Evans RJ, Arend WP et al. Primary structure and functional expression from complementary DNA of a human interleukin-1 receptor antagonist. Nature 1990; 343:341-46.

93. Firestein GS, Boyle DL, Yu C et al. Synovial interleukin-1 receptor antagonist and interleukin-1 balance in rheumatoid arthritis. Arthritis Rheum 1994; 37:644-52.

94. Malyak M, Swaney RE, Arend WP. Levels of synovial fluid interleukin-1 receptor antagonist in rheumatoid arthritis and other arthropathies. Arthritis Rheum 1993; 36:781-89.

95. Koch AE, Kunkel SL, Chensue SW et al. Expression of interleukin-1 and interleukin-1 receptor antagonist by human rheumatoid synovial tissue macrophages. Clin Immunol Immunopathol 1992; 65:23-29.

96. Deleuran BW, Chu CQ, Field M et al. Localization of interleukin-1 alpha, type 1 interleukin-1 receptor and interleukin-1 receptor antagonist in the synovial membrane and cartilage/pannus junction in rheumatoid arthritis. Br J Rheumatol 1992; 31:801-09.

97. Krzesicki RF, Hatfield CA, Bienkowski MJ et al. Regulation of expression of IL-1 receptor antagonist protein in human synovial and dermal fibroblasts. J Immunol 1993; 150:4008-18.

98. Raz E, Watanabe A, Baird SM et al. Systemic immunological effects of cytokine genes injected into skeletal muscle. Proc Natl Acad Sci USA 1993; 90:4523-27.

====== CHAPTER 6 ======

THE ROLE OF CHEMOKINES IN RENAL DISEASE

Xiaobo Wu, Gregory J. Dolecki and James B. Lefkowith

INTRODUCTION

Almost as rapidly as our knowledge of chemokines has evolved over the past several years, this knowledge has been applied specifically to renal pathobiology. Because of the pleotrophic properties of chemokines, complexities regarding their synthesis, and overlapping activities, the importance of chemokines to renal disease will, of necessity, come from the specific study of these mediators in systems relevant to the kidney.

The goal of this chapter is to summarize current knowledge regarding the regulation and role of chemokines in systems relevant to the kidney. Towards this end, we will endeavor to cover three specific subject areas:
- The expression and regulation of chemokine synthesis by renal cells in vitro.
- The relevance of chemokines to experimental models of renal disease in vivo, and the mechanisms by which chemokine synthesis is regulated in vivo.
- The potential relevance of chemokines to human renal disease.

In order to allow for a quick review of the literature, we have provided a table for each of the above sections which contains a condensed version of the existing data.

CHEMOKINE EXPRESSION BY RENAL CELLS IN VITRO

The expression of multiple chemokines of both the C-X-C and C-C families has been studied and characterized in cultured renal cells. The discussion following summarizes the available data on the following chemokines: cytokine-induced neutrophil chemoattractant (CINC), interleukin-8 (IL-8), macrophage inflammatory protein-2 (MIP-2) and

Chemokines in Disease, edited by Alisa E. Koch and Robert M. Strieter.
© 1996 R.G. Landes Company.

related proteins, interferon-γ induced protein (IP-10), macrophage chemotactic peptide-1 (MCP-1) and RANTES (Regulated on activation, normal T cell expressed and secreted). Recent data on the expression of the multispecific chemokine receptor are also presented. The studies reviewed are presented in concise form in Table 6.1.

CYTOKINE-INDUCED NEUTROPHIL CHEMOATTRACTANT (CINC)

To date, the most investigated chemokine with respect to renal cells is probably cytokine-induced neutrophil chemoattractant (CINC). CINC is an 8 kDa peptide originally purified from media conditioned by IL-1β-stimulated normal rat kidney epi-

Table 6.1. Chemokine synthesis by renal cells in vitro

Chemokine	Cell of Origin	Stimuli	Inhibitors	Kinetics of Expression
CINC	mesangial cells (rat)	TNF-α, IL-1β, IL-α, LPS, serum, cycloheximide	dexamethasone, genistein	rapid
	NRK-52E (tubular epithelial cell, rat)	TNF-α, IL-1β, LPS		rapid
	NRK-49F (renal fibroblast, rat)	TNF-α, IL-1β, LPS		rapid
IL-8	mesangial cells (human)	TNF-α, IL-1β, LPS	dexamethasone	rapid
	epithelial cells (human) tubular	TNF-α, IL-1β, LPS		rapid
	transitional and renal cell carcinomas (human)	TNF-α, IL-1β, cycloheximide		
MIP-2	mesangial cells (rat)	TNF-α, IL-1β, LPS	genistein	rapid
IP-10	mesangial cells (mouse)	IFN-γ, LPS, TNF-α, immune complexes		slow
MCP-1	mesangial cells (human, mouse)	IL-1β, TNF-α, IFN-γ, immune complexes, thrombin, also constitutive	free radical scavengers, forskolin, PGE2	rapid
	tubular epithelial cells (human)	IL-1β, TNF-α, IFN-γ		rapid
	renal capillary endothelial cells (rat)	LPS		
RANTES	MMC mesangial cells (mouse)	TNF-α, TNF-β, IL-1β, LPS		slow
	MCT tubular epithelial cells (mouse)	TNF-α, IL-1β, also constitutive		

For each chemokine, renal cells which have been established to synthesize each are noted along with the relevant stimuli and in vitro inhibitors. The kinetics of mRNA expression are categorized as either rapid (within minutes) or slow (within hours).

thelioid clone NRK-52E[1,2] and subsequently, from medium conditioned by a highly metastatic rat cell line, RC20, which is a spontaneously transformed variant of the normal rat kidney fibroblastic clone NRK-49F.[3] Amino acid sequence analyses have shown that CINC is 92% homologous to mouse KC, 69% homologous to human MGSA/GRO, but only 47% homologous to IL-8.[2] Consequently CINC is often referred to as the rat homologue of human GROα.

CINC appears to be the major C-X-C chemokine expressed by both NRK cell lines as well as rat mesangial cells.[2,4-6] Data are as yet unavailable on the synthesis of CINC by glomerular endothelial cells or primary lines of glomerular epithelial cells. However, the data on NRK-52E cells suggests that epithelial cells have the potential to make this cytokine.[2] Moreover, MPA (a male rat pulmonary artery endothelial cell line) expresses CINC in vitro (Dolecki GJ, unpublished observations).

Treatment of mesangial cells or the NRK cell lines with either IL-1α, IL-1β, TNF-α or LPS results in the rapid appearance of the 1.2 kb CINC mRNA on Northern transfers.[4-6] The kinetics of expression in these cells lines, however, appear to differ in subtle ways. Mesangial cells exhibit prolonged expression of the CINC mRNA in response to either IL-1β or TNF-α (peaking at 6-8 hours after cytokine stimulation, decreasing by 24 hours), but much more transient expression in response to LPS.[5,6] In contrast, in NRK-49F cells induction of CINC mRNA in response to both TNF-α and LPS is relatively transient (especially in response to TNF-α), whereas the response to IL-1β is prolonged and relatively constant for 24 hours after stimulation.[4]

The different cell lines are nonetheless similar with respect to the potency of cytokine agonists for CINC expression. For NRK-49F or mesangial cells, IL-1β is more potent than TNF-α in terms of CINC mRNA expression, and the level of CINC mRNA produced in response to IL-1β is several-fold greater than for TNF-α.[4,6]

There is also notable synergy between IL-1β and TNF-α with respect to CINC mRNA expression in mesangial cells.[6] A subthreshold concentration of IL-1β shifts the dose-response curve for CINC mRNA expression in response to TNF-α markedly to lower concentrations and appears to increase maximal levels of expression (and vice versa).

Although TGF-β has been noted to diminish expression of cytokine-induced genes,[7] such suppression is not observed with mesangial cells. TGF-β is neither an agonist for CINC mRNA expression, nor does TGF-β inhibit the expression of CINC mRNA in response to either IL-1β or TNF-α.[6]

In addition to cytokines, serum stimulates NRK-49F and mesangial cells to transiently express CINC mRNA in a manner similar to LPS.[4,5] Expression of CINC mRNA is also superinducible with cycloheximide.[4] Furthermore, in rat mesangial cells, dexamethasone partially inhibits the induction of CINC mRNA by IL-1β and cycloheximide blocks this inhibition and increases the half-life of CINC mRNA.[4] Thus, new protein synthesis is required for the glucocorticoid inhibition of induction of the CINC gene and for the relative instability of the CINC mRNA. Nuclear runoff assays indicate that dexamethasone exerts its inhibitory effect at the transcriptional level. These properties (serum stimulation of expression, superinducibility with cycloheximide, and inhibition by dexamethasone) clearly categorize CINC as an immediate-early response type gene. Expression of CINC, however, does not necessarily parallel all other immediate-early response genes in mesangial cells. A recent study examining the expression of the inducible isoform of cyclooxygenase (cyclooxygenase-2), suggests that this immediate-early response gene is turned on in mesangial cells by reactive oxygen intermediates, whereas that for CINC is not.[8]

The signal transduction pathways involved in cytokine-stimulated CINC expression in renal cells is largely unelucidated. However, the observation that

TNF-α and IL-1β are synergistic for CINC expression suggests that more than one signal transduction pathway exists. Regardless, expression of CINC in response to either cytokine is markedly decreased in response to inhibition of tyrosine kinases.[6] This tyrosine kinase dependence of CINC expression is likely due to tyrosine phosphorylation-dependent activation of NF-κB enhancer binding protein which induces GRO chemokine transcription via an NF-κB site in the GRO gene promoter region.[9]

With both mesangial cells and NRK-49F cells, additional mRNA species are seen which hybridize to the CINC cDNA but which are not other GRO family cytokines. In response to TNF-α, a second, smaller CINC transcript appears.[4,6] Through deadenylation experiments and by probing with oligonucleotides, this 0.9 kb RNA was shown to be the product of poly(A) tail removal and 3' cleavage of the larger 1.2 kb RNA.[4] Larger mRNA species hybridizing to CINC cDNA probes are also occasionally seen and likely represent nuclear transcripts.[4,6]

Synthesis of CINC protein by renal cells largely parallels expression. Renal cells (NRK-49F or -52E) produce little CINC constitutively, but synthesize nanogram levels when stimulated by LPS, TNF-α and IL-1β.[3,4,10] The small amount of CINC present in the conditioned media of unstimulated cells in the absence of any detectible CINC mRNA probably results from subtle degrees of injury to cells due to their in vitro manipulation (Dolecki GJ, unpublished observations). This constitutive level, however, may be substantial when examining isolated glomeruli in vitro.[11]

In terms of function, CINC (like human MGSA/GRO and IL-8) is a potent and selective neutrophil chemoattractant in vitro and in vivo,[12] and likely functions in vivo in glomerular inflammation as a secondary neutrophil chemoattractant (see following section on glomerulonephritis). It is also possible that CINC functions as an autocrine factor given that human MGSA/GRO (to which CINC is homologous) is an autocrine growth factor for the melanoma cell line HS294t which produces it.[13] Investigations into this possibility, however, have not produced definitive evidence for such a role for renal cells. CINC does not appear to be an autocrine mitogen or growth factor for either NRK-49F cells, or the metastatic RC-20 subline derived from these cells, although it modestly enhances adherence of these cells to tissue culture dishes.[10]

INTERLEUKIN-8 (IL-8)

IL-8 is the most studied chemokine of the C-X-C family with respect to human renal cells. IL-8, like CINC, is a selective chemoattractant for neutrophils.[14] While IL-8 is less homologous to CINC than MGSA/GRO, the evidence in vivo suggests that IL-8 functions similarly to CINC, and thus one may conceptualize these two chemokines as functional equivalents (see following discussion on glomerulonephritis). Accordingly, expression of IL-8 by human renal cells rather closely parallels that for CINC.

In human mesangial cells, the 1.8 kb IL-8 mRNA can be detected by Northern analyses of RNA from cytokine-stimulated cultures, and IL-8 protein can be detected both in the media as well as associated with the cells.[15-18] Human mesangial cells are stimulated to produce IL-8 by a set of cytokines which is similar to that which stimulates CINC by rat mesangial cells, specifically IL-1β, IL-1α and TNF-α.[15-17] Dose-response relationships and time course data are also similar to the data for CINC and rat mesangial cells. In general, IL-1β and IL-1α are more potent agonists than TNF-α. The effect of LPS on IL-8 expression by human mesangial cells appears to be variable. Interestingly, neither phorbol myristate acetate (which induces other immediate-early response genes), nor thromboxane A_2 (a prominent pro-inflammatory mediator implicated in glomerulonephritis), induce IL-8 mRNA expression.[16] As with

CINC and rat mesangial cells, dexamethasone inhibits cytokine-induced IL-8 mRNA production and IL-8 secretion.[15]

Similar to human mesangial cells, cultured human renal cortical epithelial cells respond to either IL-1β, TNF-α or LPS in both a time- and dose-dependent manner by expressing IL-8 mRNA and secreting antigenic IL-8 peptide.[19] As with human mesangial cells, IL-1β is relatively more potent an agonist than TNF-α or LPS. However, with human renal cortical epithelial cells, IL-8 mRNA expression may be more prolonged than that observed either for IL-8 with human mesangial cells or for CINC with rat mesangial cells.[19] Expression of IL-8 mRNA appears to continue through the 24 hours following cytokine expression.

Human transitional and renal cell carcinoma cells also exhibit the capacity to express IL-8 either constitutively or in response to IL-1β or TNF-α but not LPS.[20] This capacity of tumor cells to produce chemokines may be important in the inflammatory response to tumors in vivo (see following section on renal cell carcinoma). A role for IL-8 as a tumor autocrine growth factor (as for MGSA/GRO[13]) is possible.

MACROPHAGE INFLAMMATORY PROTEIN-2 (MIP-2) AND RELATED CHEMOKINES

It was recently appreciated that in addition to CINC, rat mesangial cells also express the related C-X-C chemokine MIP-2.[6] Rat MIP-2 is 67% homologous to CINC at the amino acid sequence level and is equipotent in terms of neutrophil chemoattractant activity (and equally selective).[21] RT-PCR experiments and Northern analysis show that MIP-2 mRNA (1.2 kb by Northern analysis) expression parallels CINC mRNA expression in rat mesangial cells treated with LPS, IL-1β and TNF-α in all discernible respects.[6] The only apparent difference between expression of MIP-2 and CINC is that CINC mRNA expression predominates over MIP-2 mRNA expression by several-fold.[6]

Recently, two additional cytokine-induced neutrophil chemoattractants have been identified and termed CINC-2α and CINC-2β.[21] Under this terminology, CINC is referred to as CINC-1 and MIP-2 as CINC-3. CINC-2α and -2β are virtually identical to each other except for the three C-terminal amino acids which may be coded by a possible fourth exon in the gene.[21] These two new members of the subfamily of C-X-C chemokines are equally active to CINC and MIP-2 in terms of chemotactic activity for neutrophils.[21] Rat NRK-49F cells have been observed to synthesize a form of CINC-2, tentatively identified as CINC-2α.[22] Presumably, synthesis of these newly described CINC cytokines parallels that for CINC and MIP-2, although this speculation remains to be established experimentally.

INTERFERON-γ INDUCED PROTEIN (IP-10)

IP-10 is a member of the C-X-C family of chemokines whose biologic activity remains unknown.[14] Despite this lack of understanding regarding biologic activity, its synthesis by mesangial cells has already been determined.[23] Mouse mesangial cells exhibit IP-10 mRNA in vitro in response to IFN-γ and LPS. TNF-α and immune complexes also induce IP-10 mRNA, albeit much more weakly than IFN-γ or LPS. The kinetics of expression of IP-10 mRNA are more prolonged than those of the above mentioned C-X-C chemokines. Expression of IP-10 mRNA in response to IFN-γ is evident only by 3 hours and increases through 24 hours, whereas the response to LPS is evident only at 8 hours after stimulation and is not sustained.

Although IP-10 is a member of the C-X-C chemokine family, the profile of cytokine agonists and kinetics of expression of IP-10 in mesangial cells more closely resemble those of the C-C chemokines as detailed in the following sections. Moreover, the data to date suggest that IP-10 is more likely to mediate chronic inflammation (e.g., the delayed hypersensitivity response).[14] A recent study specifically suggests that IP-10 may be a pro-inflammatory mediator acting through T cells.[24] These data all suggest that IP-10 is more similar to the C-C chemokines than the C-X-C chemokines.

MACROPHAGE CHEMOTACTIC PEPTIDE-1 (MCP-1)

MCP-1 is a member of the C-C family of chemokines and, unlike the aforementioned chemokines, is a selective chemoattractant for monocytes.[14] MCP-1, however, is produced by multiple renal cells in response to a similar set of stimuli as for the C-X-C chemokines discussed above. As with CINC and IL-8, IL-1β and TNF-α induce cultured human and mouse mesangial cells to express MCP-1 mRNA and secrete biologically active MCP-1.[16,25-27] Also, as for CINC and IL-8, IL-1β tends to be more potent than TNF-α in inducing MCP-1 mRNA.[26] In contrast to CINC and IL-8, however, MCP-1 is often expressed constitutively.[25,27]

With respect to the kinetics of expression, MCP-1 mRNA expression in response to cytokines largely parallels the kinetics of C-X-C chemokine expression.[25] This parallelism is somewhat disconcerting given that the kinetics of neutrophil migration are distinct from those of monocyte migration. The kinetics of MCP-1 expression in vivo, however, are much slower (see following section on glomerulonephritis). Apropos these comments, it is noteworthy that conditioned media from cytokine-stimulated human mesangial cells have been observed to exhibit chemotactic activity only for monocytes (and not neutrophils) despite containing biologically active amounts of IL-8.[16] Why the IL-8 in these media is inactive (i.e., whether there are inactive processed forms of IL-8 or whether there are inhibitors of IL-8) remains to be clarified.

MCP-1 mRNA is also induced, and the protein secreted, by cultured mesangial cells in response to IFN-γ and aggregated IgG.[27-29] Immune complexes cause a rapid and sustained induction of MCP-1 mRNA

(0.7 kb) expression which is not inhibited by perturbing phagocytosis, indicating that Fc receptor occupancy is sufficient for signaling (i.e., phagocytosis is not necessary).[28] Expression of MCP-1 in response to aggregated IgG (or TNF-α) is also attenuated by free radical scavengers, suggesting that reactive oxygen species mediate, at least in part, induction of MCP-1.[29] Conversely, forskolin and PGE$_2$, which elevate intracellular cAMP levels, attenuate the induction of MCP-1 in response to the aforementioned agonists by decreasing MCP-1 gene transcription.[30]

It was recently noted that the serine protease α thrombin will induce MCP-1 expression in human mesangial cells.[31] This effect depends on both receptor binding to the recently characterized thrombin receptor as well as catalytically active thrombin. This study suggests a novel role by which this coagulation factor may participate in glomerular disease, and suggests a potential avenue of future investigation.

Renal cortical epithelial cells also produce MCP-1 in a fashion which largely parallels that seen for mesangial cells.[19] Of particular note, however, is the observation that IFN-γ serves to selectively stimulate MCP-1 and not IL-8.[19] Such selectivity is not observed with IL-1β or TNF-α and may be critical to understanding the different kinetics of neutrophils and monocytes in renal inflammatory states. Renal endothelium also has the capacity to express MCP-1. If LPS is infused into the renal artery of an isolated perfused kidney, MCP-1 expression (along with IL-1β and TNF-α) is observed predominantly in the peritubular capillary endothelium.[32] Thus, the three major intrinsic cells types of the kidney (mesangial, epithelial and endothelial) all have the capacity to express this chemokine.

With respect to the mechanisms underlying the transcription of MCP-1 mRNA, two distinct regulatory elements have been identified.[33] One is a κB site located far upstream of the MCP-1 gene which appears to be necessary for agonist-stimulated induction. The second is a GC box/Sp1 binding site located closer to the 5' end of the gene which appears to be necessary for basal transcription and which may play a role in tissue specific regulation.

It is additionally noteworthy with respect to the potential biologic importance of MCP-1 that induction of MCP-1 is often accompanied by the expression of CSF-1, a cytokine required for the proliferation, maturation, activation and survival of monocytes/macrophages.[28,29] Conjecturally, the expression of CSF-1 may act as an in situ factor perpetuating the chronic phase of inflammation. Monocyte/macrophage proliferation within glomeruli may, in fact, be an important part of the chronic scarring phase of glomerular inflammation.[34-36]

RANTES (REGULATED ON ACTIVATION, NORMAL T CELL EXPRESSED AND SECRETED)

RANTES, a member of the chemokine C-C family, is chemotactic for CD4+ T lymphocytes and monocytes.[14] Murine MMC cells, a transformed mouse mesangial cell line, express RANTES mRNA (1.1 kb) constitutively and upregulate this mRNA in response to the cytokines TNF-α, TNF-β, IL-1β and LPS.[37] In contrast to the C-X-C chemokines, RANTES mRNA is more potently induced by TNF-α than IL-1β and the kinetics of expression are much slower, peaking at 24-48 hours after cytokine exposure.[37] Low level RANTES mRNA expression is also observed in glomeruli perfused with TNF-α.[37]

MCT cells, a cultured line of proximal tubule epithelial cells from the renal cortex of mice, also express the 1.1 kb RANTES mRNA and RANTES peptide constitutively.[38] RT-PCR experiments further show that IL-1α and TNF-α significantly increase the steady-state level of RANTES mRNA in these cells. RANTES expression in these cells, however, is not upregulated by TGF-β, IFN-γ or IL-6.

CHEMOKINE RECEPTORS

No information is available on the expression of chemokine receptors in renal cells specifically. However, a recent study has established that the human erythrocyte chemokine receptor (i.e., Duffy blood group antigen) is expressed in the kidney, specifically on postcapillary endothelial cells.[39] The pathophysiologic role of this chemokine receptor has yet to be determined; consequently its role in renal pathobiology is uncertain. Apropos of this issue, no definite abnormality in the inflammatory response in Duffy antigen negative individuals has been established to date.

ROLE OF CHEMOKINES IN EXPERIMENTAL MODELS OF RENAL DISEASE

To date, the role of chemokines has been most intensively investigated in experimental models of glomerulonephritis. A small number of studies, however, exist which examine the potential contribution of chemokines to tubulointerstitial disease, renal ischemia and renal carcinoma. The following discussion will cover the role of chemokines in these disease categories endeavoring, in particular, to provide an integrated view of the role chemokines play in inflammation. As in the initial section, the literature is summarized in Table 6.2 for rapid review.

GLOMERULONEPHRITIS

Although there are many different experimental models of immune complex-mediated glomerulonephritis, in general this disease state is characterized by the acute deposition (or in situ formation) of immune complexes in glomeruli, followed by complement activation, and then leukocyte emigration from the vasculature into the glomerulus.[40] The initial influx of leukocytes is comprised of neutrophils and is wholly dependent on the activation of complement.[40] Monocyte/macrophage migration follows the acute influx of neutrophils and is independent of the activation of complement as well as the prior influx of neutrophils.[41] Recent work on chemokines in glomerulonephritis has begun to cast light on the biochemical basis of the independent migration of neutrophils and

Table 6.2. Role of chemokines in experimental renal disease

Disease Model	Chemokine	Data
anti-GBM nephritis (rat)	CINC	mRNA/protein expressed in glomeruli mediates part of neutrophil influx synthesis complement/leukocyte dependent
	MIP-2	mRNA/protein expressed in glomeruli mediates part of neutrophil influx synthesis complement/leukocyte dependent
	MCP-1	mRNA/protein expressed in glomeruli
BSA/anti-BSA nephritis (rabbit)	IL-8	protein expressed in glomeruli urinary IL-8 elevated mediates part of neutrophil influx
anti-thymocyte serum nephritis (rat)	MCP-1	mRNA/protein expressed in glomeruli
autoimmune interstitial nephritis (rat)	MCP-1	mRNA expressed in kidney
hydronephrosis (rat)	MCP-1	mRNA/protein expressed by tubules
pyelonephritis (mouse)	MIP-1β	mRNA expressed in kidney
renal ischemia—	CINC, MCP-1	CINC mRNA expressed in cortex rapidly
reperfusion (rat)		MCP-1 mRNA/protein expressed in cortex following CINC
renal carcinoma (mouse)	KC, JE, IP-10	expressed by renal carcinoma in response to systemic cytokine therapy (IL-2 and IFN-α)

For each disease model, the chemokines implicated in pathogenesis are listed along with a brief summary of the existing data.

macrophages in this disease state. Additionally, these studies have clarified the relationship of C-X-C chemokines to the complement cascade.

In one recent study, a convincing role for CINC in antiglomerular basement membrane (GBM) nephritis in rats was established.[11] It was observed that glomeruli exhibit mRNA for CINC rapidly after injection of the inducing anti-GBM antibody, that the protein is elaborated by glomeruli ex vivo, that the cytokines which induce expression of CINC (TNF-α and IL-1β) are coexpressed in response to immune complex deposition, and that anti-CINC antibody attenuates (by approximately 50%) the influx of neutrophils. A commensurate reduction in acute phase proteinuria was also seen and likely reflects the diminished degree of neutrophil emigration. This role of CINC as a mediator of neutrophil influx in glomerulonephritis, however, is not specific to the kidney. Deposition of immune complexes intradermally leads to a neutrophil influx which is also blocked by administration of anti-CINC antibody to a similar degree.[11]

The incomplete efficacy of anti-CINC antibody in diminishing neutrophil influx in anti-GBM nephritis suggests that another chemokine may participate in this process. This issue was recently addressed by a second study in rats which established that MIP-2 mRNA and protein are also produced acutely after the induction of inflammation with anti-GBM antibody, and that anti-MIP-2 antibody attenuates both the influx of neutrophils and the accompanying proteinuria.[42] As for CINC, the protective effect of the antibody is partial (approximately 50%). Although the anti-MIP-2 antibody used in this study did not react with CINC (and that of the aforementioned study did not react with MIP-2), it is unclear whether the anti-MIP-2 antibody may have reacted with the recently identified CINC-2α and CINC-2β which are highly homologous to MIP-2.

These findings have been corroborated in the rabbit model of BSA/anti-BSA glomerulonephritis.[43] In this study, it was observed that IL-8 was present antigenically in inflamed glomeruli and that an anti-IL-8 antibody partially inhibited the influx of neutrophils. It should be noted that rabbits, unlike small rodents, have an IL-8 chemokine. Although the effects of the anti-IL-8 antibody on neutrophil migration were partial, the antibody completely inhibited the accompanying proteinuria. The discrepancy between neutrophil influx and activation noted in this study has been observed in other studies of glomerulonephritis and points out that neutrophil migration and activation are separable and mechanistically distinct.[44,45] Also of note in this study were observations that urinary (but not plasma) IL-8 was elevated during nephritis, suggesting that urinary IL-8 may be an indicator of acute glomerular inflammation, a hypothesis that has some support in human disease (see following section on human renal disease). Whether the IL-8 independent influx of neutrophils is due to the elaboration of the rabbit homologue of MIP-2 or a related chemokine as noted for rat remains to be proved.

It is clear from the aforementioned in vivo studies that the production of chemokines in vivo is more complex than can be appreciated from published in vitro work. In particular, the expression of CINC and MIP-2 mRNA by inflamed glomeruli in the model of anti-GBM nephritis is highly leukocyte-dependent. Abrogation of leukocyte influx using either irradiation-induced leukopenia or anti-PMN antibody completely prevents the expression of both CINC and MIP-2 mRNA.[6] Although both neutrophils and macrophages have the capacity to express both chemokines (Wu X and Lefkowith JB, unpublished observations),[42] it is not necessarily true that these cells are the exclusive source of chemokines in this model of inflammation. In situ hybridization studies, in fact, suggest that MIP-2 may be expressed by both infiltrating neutrophils and mesangial cells.[42] Additionally, chemokine expression in this model is highly complement-dependent.[6] This dependence appears to be indirect, however, and mediated through neutrophils. As noted above, irradiation-induced leukopenia or PMN depletion (which do not inhibit antibody deposition or complement activation) also prevent chemokine expression. It is further noteworthy in this regard that a similar leukocyte-dependence is observed for both TNF-α and IL-1β expression by glomeruli in anti-GBM nephritis (Wu X and Lefkowith JB, unpublished observations).[11]

The chemokine which has been implicated in the influx of monocytes/macrophages in glomerulonephritis is MCP-1. Expression of MCP-1 mRNA and protein is upregulated in glomeruli in both anti-GBM and antithymocyte serum induced glomerulonephritis.[46,47] MCP-1 mRNA expression in glomeruli during anti-GBM nephritis is delayed relative to that of CINC and MIP-2 mRNAs, peaking 24 hours after disease induction.[46] Upregulated MCP-1 is also observed during the more chronic phase of antithymocyte serum induced glomerulonephritis.[47] Although the kinetics of MCP-1 expression appear to parallel those of monocyte/macrophage migration, a causal connection between these two parameters remains to be established. Also of note, despite the apparent linked expression of MCP-1 and CSF-1 observed in mesangial cells in vitro, expression of CSF-1 by glomeruli is not altered in the course of antithymocyte serum induced nephritis.[47]

Regarding the mechanisms underlying the production of MCP-1, it was observed that complement depletion attenuates the expression of MCP-1 mRNA in antithymocyte serum induced nephritis.[47] Whether this dependence on complement activation is direct or indirect remains to be determined. It should be noted also that monocyte/macrophage migration in this model of nephritis, unlike that of anti-GBM nephritis, appears to be in part complement-dependent.[47]

The existing body of data would suggest the following scheme for the role of chemokines in immune complex-mediated glomerulonephritis (Fig. 6.1). Immune complex formation leads to complement activation and the formation of C3b, C3bi and C5a which initiates the influx of neutrophils. The opsonized immune complexes stimulate the production of cytokines (TNF-α, IL-1β) and chemokines (CINC, MIP-2) by the resident mesangial macrophages and infiltrating neutrophils. TNF-α and IL-1β further induce CINC and MIP-2 production by the resident glomerular cells (mesangial, epithelial and endothelial). Together, CINC and MIP-2 mediate the influx of neutrophils after complement activation. The immune complexes independent of complement stimulate the production of MCP-1 (or perhaps other C-C chemokines) by mesangial cells (and possibly resident macrophages) to produce an influx of monocytes/macrophages following that of neutrophils. The infiltrating monocytes/macrophages may amplify this phase by the autocrine production of MCP-1 or other C-C chemokines.

This hypothetical scheme provides a potential explanation of the biochemical basis of the selective and independent migration of neutrophils and monocytes into inflamed glomeruli. The specific neutrophil chemoattractants, CINC and MIP-2, presumably mediate the acute influx of neutrophils, whereas MCP-1 (or other C-C

chemokines), which are selective chemoattractants for monocytes/macrophages, mediate the subsequent influx of monocyte/macrophages. Complement is required to initiate the influx of neutrophils, and to stimulate neutrophils and resident macrophages both to express CINC/MIP-2 and to stimulate the production of these chemokines by endogenous glomerular cells via cytokines. MCP-1 (and possibly other C-C chemokines) are produced by mesangial cells (or possibly resident macrophages) in response to immune complexes in a manner which does not necessarily require complement. This scheme also suggests that chemokines may play an important role in amplifying the response to complement activation temporally. The kinetics of CINC and MIP-2 expression and production are slower than those for complement activation and likely serve to prolong the response to this process.[48]

TUBULOINTERSTITIAL DISEASE

Data on the role of chemokines in tubulointerstitial disease are more scant than for glomerulonephritis and largely correlative. Recent work on a model of autoimmune interstitial nephritis in rat established that IL-1β, TNF-α and MCP-1 are coexpressed during the acute phase of the disease in which the dominant leukocytes were PMNs.[49] Expression of these cytokines was downregulated as the inflammatory infiltrate became dominated by macrophages. In hydronephrosis, upregulated expression of MCP-1 mRNA and protein by renal tubules has been observed and is accompanied by an interstitial inflammatory infiltrate which is largely macrophages.[50] The expression of MIP-1β has also been observed in the kidney in a murine model of pyelonephritis.[51]

RENAL ISCHEMIA

One study has shown the sequential expression of CINC and MCP-1 mRNA in renal cortex following ischemia-reperfusion of the kidney (CINC and MCP-1 are identified in this study as rat KC and JE,

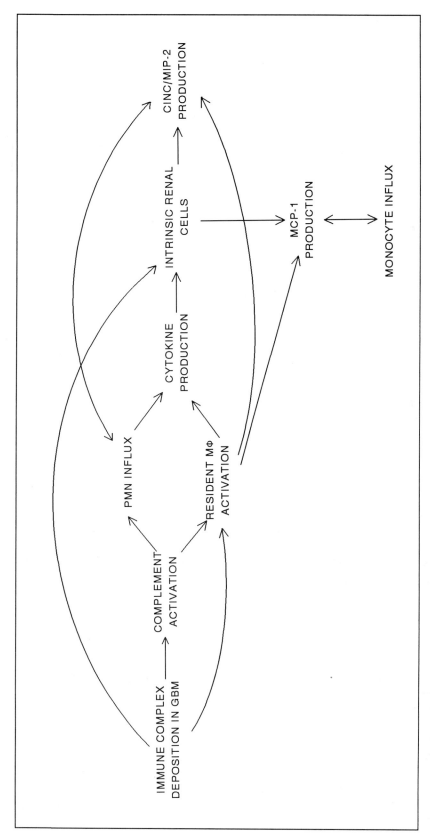

Fig. 6.1. Hypothetical scheme for the production of chemokines in immune complex-mediated glomerulonephritis.

respectively).[52] The kinetics of CINC expression were rapid (peaking at 1 hour after reperfusion), while those for MCP-1 were considerably slower (peaking at 24 hours after reperfusion). Antigen expression of MCP-1 was noted in the apical regions of the cortical and medullary thick ascending limbs and in the lumen of the distal tubule. Glomerular cells and proximal tubules did not express MCP-1.

The significance of CINC expression in renal ischemia likely relates to the potential role that neutrophils play in ischemia-reperfusion injury. There are recent studies suggesting that IL-8 is important in the ischemia-reperfusion lung injury in rabbits.[53] The tissue injury in this model appears to be mediated by neutrophils.[53] There are also data which implicate neutrophils in ischemia-reperfusion injury of the kidney.[54,55] The role of MCP-1 in renal ischemia-reperfusion injury is uncertain, but conjecturally monocytes/macrophages may be important for the reparative process. Whether chemokines play a role in the regrowth and migration of epithelial cells following ischemia-reperfusion injury has been suggested but remains to be supported experimentally.[52]

RENAL CARCINOMA

A potential role for chemokines in the inflammatory response to renal carcinoma is suggested by a recent study which showed the expression of KC (the mouse homologue of CINC), JE (the mouse homologue of MCP-1), IP-10 and TNF-α in renal carcinoma in vivo after the administration of a therapeutic cytokine regimen (IL-2 and IFN-α).[56] The expression of chemokines in vivo correlated with the infiltration of Mac-1+ (CD11bCD18) leukocytes (neutrophils, macrophages) into the tumor. Although the tumor was capable of chemokine expression in response to IL-2 and IFN-α in vitro, the TNF-α expression in these tumors in vivo appeared to be derived from infiltrating leukocytes. The induction of chemokines in tumors by invading leukocytes may be an ·important part of the host defense to tumors.

CHEMOKINES AND HUMAN RENAL DISEASE

There is currently a paucity of data on the relevance of chemokines to human renal disease; however a few studies published over the past two years have suggested that both C-X-C and C-C chemokines may contribute to a variety of pathophysiologic conditions in man. As in the previous section, the following discussion is organized according to disease state and covers glomerulonephritis, tubulointerstitial disease and allograft rejection. A summary of the available human data are provided in Table 6.3.

GLOMERULONEPHRITIS

IL-8 appears to be involved in the pathogenesis of several different inflammatory glomerulonephritides in humans. Upregulated urinary levels of IL-8 were recently observed in membranoproliferative glomerulonephritis, cryoglobulinemia, lupus nephritis, IgA nephropathy, purpura nephritis and poststreptococcal glomerulonephritis.[57] Urinary levels appeared to correlate with clinical activity and the degree of glomerular leukocyte infiltration. Although urinary IL-8 was elevated in these patients, serum IL-8 was in general not increased. IL-8 was also detected in glomeruli by immunohistochemistry in several of these patients, suggesting that production was local. In contrast to the aforementioned glomerulonephritides, urinary IL-8 was not elevated in patients with minimal change disease, focal glomerulosclerosis or membranous nephropathy.

A correlation of serum IL-8 levels and disease activity has been noted in patients with systemic lupus erythematosus.[58] Patients with renal disease particularly exhibited high levels of serum IL-8. Overall, it was noted that serum IL-8 was better correlated with clinical measures of disease activity than several more traditional markers of disease such as C4 levels or anti-dsDNA antibodies. This increase in serum IL-8 may thus reflect more a systemic inflammatory state than renal disease specifically. Elevated serum levels of IL-8 have

Table 6.3. Chemokine association with human disease

Disease State	Chemokine Association
membranoproliferative glomerulonephritis	IL-8 (elevated urinary level) MCP-1 (immunostaining of glomerulus)
acute poststreptococcal glomerulonephritis	IL-8 (elevated urinary level)
lupus nephritis	IL-8 (elevated serum and urinary levels) MCP-1 (immunostaining of glomerulus)
minimal change disease	IL-8 (elevated serum level, spontaneous production by blood monocytes)
cryoglobulinemia	IL-8 (elevated urinary level)
IgA nephropathy	IL-8 (elevated urinary level)
purpura nephritis	IL-8 (elevated urinary level)
Wegener's granulomatosis	MCP-1 (immunostaining of glomerulus)
chronic glomerulonephritis	IL-8 (elevated urinary level)
interstitial fibrosis	IL-8 (spontaneous release by fibroblasts via autocrine production of IL-1)
pyelonephritis	IL-8 (elevated urinary level)
allograft rejection	IL-8 (immunostaining of tubular epithelium) RANTES (immunostaining of tubular epithelium, endothelium, inflammatory cells)

The chemokine associations with human disease are summarized, along with the basis of the noted association.

also been noted in patients with chronic renal disease.[59] However, such elevated levels usually occur in the context of renal failure, in peritoneal dialysis patients with peritonitis, or following hemodialysis.[59]

One recent report has suggested that elevated serum IL-8 occurs in minimal change disease and nephrotic syndrome, and that such levels appear to parallel disease activity.[60] The elevated serum IL-8 in these patients was attributed to the spontaneous production of IL-8 by peripheral blood mononuclear cells. It was also observed that peripheral blood mononuclear cells were able to alter the synthesis of GBM by glomeruli in vitro, that this effect was prevented by anti-IL-8 antibodies, and that purified IL-8 could reproduce the effect of peripheral blood mononuclear cells. These data were taken to suggest that IL-8 might contribute to the renal lesion by altering the synthesis of GBM proteins,

thereby altering the permeability of the GBM. This speculation remains to be established more definitively.

MCP-1 expression has also been observed in a variety of human glomerulonephritides. Immunocytochemical evidence of local MCP-1 production has been noted in lupus nephritis, idiopathic crescentic or proliferative glomerulonephritis and Wegener's granulomatosis.[46] MCP-1 expression was absent in minimal change disease, thin basement membrane disease, membranous nephropathy or nodular glomerulosclerosis which are in general not characterized by a marked glomerular inflammatory infiltrate. Biopsies from patients with IgA nephropathy were also negative for MCP-1 expression; however, it was noted that none of the biopsies examined were from patients with a significant inflammatory infiltrate.

TUBULOINTERSTITIAL DISEASE

IL-8 has been implicated in the loss of renal function which accompanies chronic glomerulonephritis and which may be due to interstitial inflammation.[61] In a recent study, it was observed that both normal renal interstitial fibroblasts and fibroblasts derived from a kidney exhibiting both glomerulonephritis and interstitial fibrosis spontaneously produced IL-8 as well as IL-6. Both sets of fibroblasts also produced IL-8 and IL-6 in response to IL-1β and TNF-α, although fibroblasts from the fibrotic kidney exhibited greater maximal responses. A similar constitutive release by normal skin fibroblasts was not observed, although these cells could be stimulated to produce IL-8 and -6 in vitro by IL-1β and TNF-α to a degree comparable to normal renal fibroblasts. The constitutive IL-8 and IL-6 release by renal fibroblasts was partially due to the spontaneous release of IL-1 in vitro since IL-1RA inhibited the response. The differential responsiveness of normal vs. pathologic renal fibroblasts could not be attributed to differences in IL-1 receptors and was postulated to be due to a postreceptor event. The mechanism by which IL-8 contributes to the chronic inflammatory process of interstitial fibrosis remains to be established.

Studies of patients with acute pyelonephritis have demonstrated that high levels of urinary IL-8 are a ubiquitous feature of this condition, whereas IL-8 is undetectable in the urine of normal controls.[62,63] The presence of urinary IL-8 correlates with urinary leukocyte counts and likely reflects the presence of neutrophils within the kidney in the setting of acute inflammation/infection. Interestingly, only a portion (approximately 50%) of the chemotactic activity in urine from patients with pyelonephritis is inhibited by an anti-IL-8 antibody implying the presence of other chemoattractants.[63]

A recent study has suggested that a factor purified from the ultrafiltrate of chronic renal failure patients, referred to as granulocyte inhibitory protein, was able to stimulate human mesangial cells in vitro

to produce IL-6 and IL-8.[64] The nature of this cytokine, as well as the relevance of its ability to stimulate IL-6 and IL-8 production to renal disease, remain to be clarified.

ALLOGRAFT REJECTION

IL-8 expression by renal proximal and distal tubules has been observed by immunohistochemistry in the context of acute allograft rejection.[19] Presumably, expression of this cytokine is induced by the infiltrating leukocytes and their production of cytokines. The pathophysiologic role for IL-8 in the rejection response, however, remains to be addressed.

A recent report on human renal allografts has established that RANTES expression is upregulated in the context of chronic cell-mediated rejection.[65] In contrast, RANTES expression by allografts is not seen either acutely after transplantation (i.e., at 1 hour) or in the context of cyclosporin nephrotoxicity. RANTES is expressed by the infiltrating mononuclear cells, the renal tubular epithelium, and the renal vascular endothelium. Given the known chemotactic activity of RANTES for lymphocytes and monocytes, one would logically conclude that this chemokine may act as a mediator of the interstitial inflammation which characterizes allograft rejection.

SUMMARY

In sum, a substantial body of data has established that intrinsic renal cells are capable of the synthesis of a number of C-X-C and C-C chemokines, and that chemokines from both subgroups are potentially important mediators of renal inflammation in vivo. Nascent work on humans additionally suggests that the data derived from the investigation of experimental renal disease are likely to be applicable clinically.

Issues that remain to be addressed, however, are numerous. The regulation of chemokine mRNA expression and peptide synthesis in vitro remains to be further clarified, particularly how chemokines of the C-X-C and C-C subgroups are differentially expressed and how synthesis is turned off. Further studies of the in vivo contribution of chemokines to experimental models of renal disease and the in vivo regulation of chemokine synthesis also remain to be performed. In particular, more detailed investigations of the role of chemokines in both glomerulonephritis and tubulointerstitial disease are needed, particularly with respect to the role of C-C chemokines. Further investigations into renal allograft rejection and ischemic renal failure also seem warranted. Finally, additional studies of human renal disease states with respect to chemokine expression and production may help in determining which diseases can be ultimately approached by pharmacologic manipulations of chemokine synthesis or chemokine receptor blockade.

REFERENCES

1. Watanabe K, Kinoshita S, Nakagawa H. Purification and characterization of cytokine-induced neutrophil chemoattractant produced by epithelioid cell line of normal rat kidney (NRK-52E cell). Biochem Biophys Res Commun 1989; 161:1093-1099.

2. Watanabe K, Konishi K, Fujioka M, Kinoshita S, Nakagawa H. The neutrophil chemoattractant produced by the rat kidney epithelioid cell line NRK-52E is a protein related to the KC/gro protein. J Biol Chem 1989; 264:19559-19563.

3. Wittwer AJ, Carr LS, Zagorski J, Dolecki GJ, Crippes BA, De Larco JE. High-level expression of cytokine-induced neutrophil chemoattractant (CINC) by a metastatic rat cell line: purification and production of blocking antibodies. J Cell Physiol 1993; 156:421-427.

4. Dolecki GJ, DeLarco JE. Regulation of cytokine-induced neutrophil chemoattractant (CINC) mRNA production in cultured rat cells. DNA Cell Biol 1994; 13:883-889.

5. Feng L, Xia YY, Kreisberg JI, Wilson CB. Interleukin-1 alpha stimulates KC synthesis in rat mesangial cells: glucocorticoids inhibit KC induction by IL-1. Am J Physiol 1994; 266:F713-F722.

6. Wu X, Dolecki GJ, Lefkowith JB. GRO chemokines: a transduction, integration, and amplification mechanism in acute renal inflammation. Amer J Physiol 1995; 269:F248-F256.

7. Bogdan C, Paik J, Vodovotz Y, Nathan C. Contrasting mechanisms for suppression of macrophage cytokine release by transforming growth factor-beta and interleukin-10. J Biol Chem 1992; 267:23301-23308.

8. Feng L, Xia Y, Garcia GE, Hwang D, Wilson CB. Involvement of reactive oxygen intermediates in cyclooxygenase-2 expression induced by interleukin-1, tumor necrosis factor-α, and lipopolysaccharide. J Clin Invest 1995; 95:1669-1675.

9. Johsi-Barve SS, Rangnekar VV, Sells SF, Rangnekar VM. Interleukin-1-inducible expression of gro-beta via NF-κB activation is dependent upon tyrosine kinase signaling. J Biol Chem 1993; 268: 18018-18029.

10. Crippes BA, Zagorski J, Carr LS, Wittwer AJ, Dolecki GJ, De Larco JE. Investigation of possible autocrine functions for rat GRO/CINC (cytokine-induced neutrophil chemoattractant). J Cell Physiol 1993; 156: 412-420.

11. Wu X, Wittwer AJ, Carr LS, Crippes BA, De Larco JE, Lefkowith JB. Cytokine-induced neutrophil chemoattractant mediates neutrophil influx in immune complex glomerulonephritis in rat. J Clin Invest 1994; 94:337-344.

12. Suzuki H, Suematsu M, Miura S et al. Rat CINC/gro: a novel mediator for locomotive and secretagogue activation of neutrophils in vivo. J Leukocyte Biol 1994; 55:652-657.

13. Richmond A, Lawson DH, Nixon DW, Stevens JS, Chawla RK. Extraction of a melanoma growth-stimulatory activity from culture medium conditioned by the Hs294t human melanoma cell line. Cancer Res 1983; 43:2106-2112.

14. Oppenheim JJ, Zachariae CO, Mukaida N, Matsushima K. Properties of the novel proinflammatory supergene "intercrine" cytokine family. Annu Rev Immunol 1991; 9:617-648.

15. Brown Z, Strieter RM, Chensue SW et al. Cytokine-activated human mesangial cells generate the neutrophil chemoattractant, interleukin 8. Kidney Int 1991; 40:86-90.

16. Zoja C, Wang JM, Bettoni S et al. Interleukin-1 beta and tumor necrosis factor-alpha induce gene expression and production of leukocyte chemotactic factors, colony-stimulating factors, and interleukin-6 in human mesangial cells. Am J Pathol 1991; 138:991-1003.

17. Abbott F, Ryan JJ, Ceska M, Matsushima K, Sarraf CE, Rees AJ. Interleukin-1beta stimulates human mesangial cells to synthesize and release interleukin-6 and interleukin-8. Kidney Int 1991; 40: 597-605.

18. Kusner DJ, Luebbers EL, Nowinski RJ, Konieczkowski M, King CH, Sedor JR. Cytokine- and LPS-induced synthesis of interleukin-8 from human mesangial cells. Kidney Int 1991; 39:1240-1248.

19. Schmouder RL, Strieter RM, Wiggins RC, Chensue SW, Kunkel SL. In vitro and in vivo interleukin-8 production in human renal cortical epithelia. Kidney Int 1992; 41:191-198.

20. Abruzzo LV, Thornton AJ, Liebert M et al. Cytokine-induced gene expression of interleukin-8 in human transitional cell carcinomas and renal cell carcinomas. Amer J Pathol 1992; 140:365-373.

21. Nakagawa H, Komorita N, Shibata F et al. Identification of cytokine-induced neutrophil chemoattractants (CINC), rat GRO/CINC-2 alpha and CINC-2 beta, produced by granulation tissue in culture: purification, complete amino acid sequences and characterization. Biochem J 1994; 301: 545-550.

22. Nakagawa H, Ikesue A, Hatakeyama S et al. Production of an interleukin-8-like chemokine by cytokine-stimulated rat NRK-49F fibroblasts and its suppression by anti-inflammatory steroids. Biochem Pharmacol 1993; 45:1425-1430.

23. Gomez-Chiarri M, Hamilton TA, Egido J, Emancipator SN. Expression of IP-10, a lipopolysaccharide- and interferon-gamma-inducible protein, in murine mesangial cells in culture. Amer J Pathol 1993; 142: 433-439.

24. Luster AD, Leder P. IP-10, a C-X-C chemokine, elicits a potent thymus-dependent antitumor response in vivo. J Exp Med 1995; 178:1057-1065.

25. Rovin BH, Yoshiumura T, Tan L. Cytokine-induced production of monocyte chemoattractant protein-1 by cultured human mesangial cells. J Immunol 1992; 148: 2148-2153.

26. Brown Z, Strieter RM, Neild GH, Thompson RC, Kunkel SL, Westwick J. IL-1 receptor antagonist inhibits monocyte chemotactic peptide-1 generation by human mesangial cells. Kidney Int 1992; 42: 95-101.

27. Grandaliano G, Valente AJ, Rozek MM, Abboud HE. Gamma interferon stimulates monocyte chemotactic protein (MCP-1) in human mesangial cells. J Lab Clin Med 1994; 123:282-289.

28. Hora K, Satriano JA, Santiago A et al. Receptors for IgG complexes activate synthesis of monocyte chemoattractant peptide-1 and colony-stimulating factor-1. Proc Natl Acad Sci USA 1992; 89:1745-1749.

29. Satriano JA, Shuldiner M, Hora K, Xing Y, Shan Z, Schlondorff D. Oxygen radicals as second messengers for expression of the monocyte chemoattractant protein, JE/MCP-1, and the monocyte colony-stimulating factor, CSF-1, in response to tumor necrosis factor-α and immunoglobulin-G—evidence for involvement of reduced nicotinamide adenine dinucleotide phosphate (NADPH)-dependent oxidase. J Clin Invest 1993; 92:1564-1571.

30. Satriano JA, Hora K, Shan Z, Stanley ER, Mori T, Schlondorff D. Regulation of monocyte chemoattractant protein-1 and macrophage colony-stimulating factor-1 by IFN-gamma, tumor necrosis factor-alpha, IgG aggregates, and cAMP in mouse mesangial cells. J Immunol 1993; 150:1971-1978.

31. Grandaliano G, Valente AJ, Abboud HE. A novel biologic activity of thrombin—stimulation of monocyte chemotactic protein production. J Exp Med 1994; 179: 1737-1741.

32. Xia YY, Feng LL, Yoshimura T, Wilson CB. LPS-induced MCP-1, IL-1-beta, and TNF-alpha messenger RNA expression in isolated erythrocyte-perfused rat kidney. Am J Physiol 1993; 264:F774-F780.

33. Ueda A, Okuda K, Ohno S et al. NF-kappaB

and Sp1 regulate transcription of the human monocyte chemoattractant protein-1 gene. J Immunol 1994; 153:2052-2063.

34. Scandrett AL, Kissane J, Lefkowith JB. Acute inflammation is the harbinger of glomerulosclerosis in antiglomerular basement membrane nephritis. Amer J Physiol 1995; 37:F258-F265.

35. Ren KY, Brentjens J, Chen YX, Brodkin M, Noble B. Glomerular macrophage proliferation in experimental immune complex nephritis. Clin Immunol Immunopath 1991; 60:384-398.

36. Bloom RD, Florquin S, Singer GG, Brennan DC, Kelley VR. Colony stimulating factor-1 in the induction of lupus nephritis. Kidney Int 1993; 43:1000-1009.

37. Wolf G, Aberle S, Thaiss F et al. TNF-alpha induces expression of the chemoattractant cytokine RANTES in cultured mouse mesangial cells. Kidney Int 1993; 44: 795-804.

38. Heeger P, Wolf G, Meyers C et al. Isolation and characterization of cDNA from renal tubular epithelium encoding murine RANTES. Kidney Int 1992; 41:220-225.

39. Hadley TJ, Lu Z, Wasniowska K et al. Postcapillary venule endothelial cells in kidney express a multispecific chemokine receptor that is structurally and functionally identical to the erythroid isoform, which is the Duffy blood group antigen. J Clin Invest 1994; 94:985-991.

40. Couser WG. Pathogenesis of glomerulonephritis. Kidney Int 1993; 44:S19-S26.

41. Schreiner GF, Cotran RS, Pardo V, Unanue ER. A mononuclear cell component in experimental immunological glomerulonephritis. J Exp Med 1978; 147:369-384.

42. Feng LL, Xia YY, Yoshimura T, Wilson CB. Modulation of neutrophil influx in glomerulonephritis in the rat with anti-macrophage inflammatory protein-2 (MIP-2) antibody. J Clin Invest 1995; 95: 1009-1017.

43. Wada T, Tomosugi N, Naito T et al. Prevention of proteinuria by the administration of anti-interleukin 8 antibody in experimental acute immune complex-induced glomerulonephritis. J Exp Med 1994; 180:1135-1140.

44. Wu X, Helfrich MH, Horton MA, Feigen LP, Lefkowith JB. Fibrinogen mediates platelet-polymorphonuclear leukocyte cooperation during immune-complex glomerulonephritis in rats. J Clin Invest 1994; 94:928-936.

45. Wu X, Lefkowith JB. Attenuation of immune-mediated glomerulonephritis with an anti-CD11b monoclonal antibody. Amer J Physiol 1993; 264:F715-F721.

46. Rovin BH, Rumancik M, Tan L, Dickerson J. Glomerular expression of monocyte chemoattractant protein-1 in experimental and human glomerulonephritis. Lab Invest 1994; 71:536-542.

47. Stahl RAK, Thaiss F, Disser M, Helmchen U, Hora K, Schlondorff D. Increased expression of monocyte chemoattractant protein-1 in antithymocyte antibody-induced glomerulonephritis. Kidney Int 1993; 44:1036-1047.

48. Muller-Eberhard HJ. Complement: chemistry and pathways. In: Gallin JI, Goldstein IM, Snyderman R, eds. Inflammation: basic principles and clinical correlates. 2nd ed. New York: Raven Press, 1992:33-62.

49. Tang WW, Feng LL, Mathison JC, Wilson CB. Cytokine expression, upregulation of intercellular adhesion molecule-1, and leukocyte infiltration in experimental tubulointerstitial nephritis. Lab Invest 1994; 70:631-638.

50. Diamond JR, Kees-Folts D, Ding G, Frye JE, Restrepo NC. Macrophages, monocyte chemoattractant peptide-1, and TGF-β in experimental hydronephrosis. Amer J Physiol 1994; 266:F926-F933.

51. Rugo HS, O'Hanley P, Bishop AG et al. Local cytokine production in a murine model of Escherichia coli pyelonephritis. J Clin Invest 1992; 89:1032-1039.

52. Safirstein R, Megyesi J, Saggi SJ et al. Expression of cytokine-like genes JE and KC is increased during renal ischemia. Amer J Physiol 1991; 261:F1095-F1101.

53. Sekido N, Mukaida N, Harada A, Nakanishi I, Watanabe Y, Matsushima K. Prevention of lung reperfusion injury in rabbits by a monoclonal antibody against interleukin-8. Nature 1993; 365:654-657.

54. Kelly KJ, Williams WW, Colvin RB,

Bonventre JV. Antibody to intercellular adhesion molecule 1 protects the kidney against ischemic injury. Proc Natl Acad Sci USA 1994; 91:812-816.

55. Rabb H, Mendiola CC, Dietz J et al. Role of CD11a and CD11b in ischemic acute renal failure in rats. Amer J Physiol 1994; 36:F1052-F1058.

56. Sonouchi K, Hamilton TA, Tannenbaum CS, Tubbs RR, Bukowski R, Finke JH. Chemokine gene expression in the murine renal cell carcinoma, RENCA, following treatment in vivo with interferon-alpha and interleukin-2. Amer J Pathol 1994; 144: 747-755.

57. Wada T, Yokoyama H, Tomosugi N et al. Detection of urinary interleukin-8 in glomerular diseases. Kidney Int 1994; 46: 455-460.

58. Holcombe RF, Baethge BA, Wolf RE et al. Correlation of serum interleukin-8 and cell surface lysosome-associated membrane protein expression with clinical disease activity in systemic lupus erythematosus. Lupus 1994; 3:97-102.

59. Nakanishi I, Moutabarrik A, Okada N et al. Interleukin-8 in chronic renal failure and dialysis patients. Nephrology, Dialysis, Transplantation 1994; 9:1435-1442.

60. Garin EH, Blanchard K, Matsushima K, Djeu JY. IL-8 production by peripheral blood mononuclear cells in nephrotic patients. Kidney Int 1994; 45:1311-1317.

61. Lonnemann G, Englerblum G, Muller GA, Koch KM, Dinarello CA. Cytokines in human renal interstitial fibrosis. II. intrinsic interleukin (TL)-1 synthesis and IL-1-dependent production of IL-6 and IL-8 by cultured kidney fibroblasts. Kidney Int 1995; 47:845-854.

62. Tullus K, Fituri O, Burman LG, Wretlind B, Brauner A. Interleukin-6 and interleukin-8 in the urine of children with acute pyelonephritis. Pediatr Nephrol 1994; 8:280-284.

63. Ko YC, Mukaida N, Ishiyama S et al. Elevated interleukin-8 levels in the urine of patients with urinary tract infections. Infect Immun 1993; 61:1307-1314.

64. Ziesche R, Roth M, Papakonstantinou E et al. A granulocyte inhibitory protein overexpressed in chronic renal disease regulates expression of interleukin-6 and interleukin-8. Proc Natl Acad Sci USA 1994; 91:301-305.

65. Pattison J, Nelson PJ, Hule P et al. RANTES chemokine expression in cell-mediated transplant rejection of the kidney. Lancet 1994; 343:209-211.

CHAPTER 7

NEUTROPHIL RECRUITMENT IN ACUTE LUNG INJURY:
THE INTERPLAY OF EARLY RESPONSE CYTOKINES, ADHESION MOLECULES, AND C-X-C CHEMOKINES

Robert M. Strieter, Theodore J. Standiford,
Lisa M. Colletti and Steven L. Kunkel

INTRODUCTION

Acute lung injury is a consequence of the host response to a variety of direct or indirect stimuli leading to pulmonary inflammation. Many clinical entities, including trauma, pneumonia/sepsis, ischemia-reperfusion injury, as well as the adult respiratory distress syndrome (ARDS), are characterized by varying degrees of pulmonary insult and the resulting functional impairment of normal gas exchange of the lung. These inflammatory responses are specifically initiated, maintained, and resolved, depending upon a complex yet coordinated interaction between immune and nonimmune cells. For example, the capacity of the lung to generate an acute inflammatory response is necessary to assure adequate clearance of an offending agent. The host response to a bacterial pneumonitis is characterized by an acute inflammatory reaction. The histopathology of bacterial pneumonia is composed of proteinaceous exudate and massive neutrophil extravasation leading to consolidation of the lung. Once the inciting agent is cleared, the inflammatory reaction resolves and normal repair and tissue remodeling occurs. This reestablishes normal lung function without the sequela of chronic pulmonary fibrosis. In contrast, the acute inflammatory response associated with ARDS may culminate in severe lung injury, ultimately impacting on host survival. The basic

Chemokines in Disease, edited by Alisa E. Koch and Robert M. Strieter.
© 1996 R.G. Landes Company.

mechanisms and mediators that induce acute pulmonary inflammation remain to be fully elucidated. However, it is known that the participation of a variety of mediators, produced by both immune and nonimmune cells, are involved in the co-ordination of these activities, including reactive oxygen metabolites, carbohydrates, lipids and protein mediators, of which a group has been classified as cytokines.

The fidelity of pulmonary inflammation is dependent upon cellular communication. While this is often accomplished through direct cell-to-cell adhesive inter-action via specific cellular adhesion molecules, cells also signal each other through soluble mediators, such as cytokines. These polypeptide molecules often have pleiotropic effects on a number of biological functions including proliferation, differentiation, recognition and cellular recruitment. Their actions are mediated through paracrine and autocrine signaling through receptor-ligand interactions on specific cell population targets. However, under certain conditions, these molecules may behave as hormones. Cytokines display concentration-dependent effects, being expressed in low concentrations during normal homeostasis, with modest increases exerting local effects, and still greater elevations resulting in systemic effects. Cytokine research investigating the biology of these proteins is rapidly expanding, and currently over 40 specific cytokines have been isolated and characterized. Individual subpopulations of immune cells possess different capacities to elaborate and secrete specific cytokines in response to particular stimuli. Nonimmune cells, including endothelial cells, fibroblasts and epithelial cells also demonstrate particular responses to specific signals resulting in the production of other cytokines. Furthermore, cell populations vary in their expression of receptors for individual cytokines, and, as a result, differ in their capacity to respond to specific cytokine signals.

Investigations into the interactions between various cell populations have lead to the concept of cytokine networking. Simply stated, one population of cells may respond directly to specific stimuli by the elaboration of a particular cytokine to exert distinct effects upon another population of cells. The targets respond by producing cytokines which may serve as feedback signals to the primary cell, or alternatively, initiate a cascade of events by affecting yet another array of target cells. Still other inflammatory effector cells, such as monocytes and neutrophils, may be recruited locally in response to specific chemotactic signals. As many of the complexities of the inflammatory cytokine cascade have been elucidated, an increasing amount of evidence now suggests that nonimmune cells play crucial roles in the generation, maintenance, and resolution of both local and systemic inflammatory responses.

The lungs comprise a unique interface between the body and the environment, presenting a tremendous alveolar surface area of 75 square meters and only a minimal barrier of 4-8 µm between the alveolar space and the extensive microvasculature. While this configuration is ideal for gas exchange, it also increases vulnerability to noxious stimuli and pathogens. Consequently, the pulmonary tissue must possess the capacity to generate brisk inflammatory responses to both inhaled and hematogenous challenges, in order to provide prompt clearance of the offending agent and avoid compromise of essential gas exchange function. This acute inflammatory response typically results in local increases in vascular permeability and a predominantly neutrophilic influx. Once successful containment of the noxious agent has occurred, inflammation should then resolve with normal repair, tissue remodeling and return to homeostasis. However, because of the great capacity to initiate potent inflammatory responses, the lung may also be predisposed to tissue injury by excessive reactions generated by both local or distant precipitants. In conditions such as ARDS, the over-exuberant tissue inflammation may result in severe irreversible lung injury mediated primarily by elicited and activated neutrophils. In this chapter, we will focus on recent advances in inflammation research that address the interplay of early response cytokines, adhesion molecules and C-X-C chemokine-induced neutrophil recruitment into the lung during the pathogenesis of acute pulmonary inflammation.

ELICITATION OF NEUTROPHILS INTO THE LUNG: THE ROLE OF ADHESION MOLECULES

The extravasation and sequestration of neutrophils during acute lung injury is dependent upon a complex series of events that include: generation of early response cytokines that lead to endothelial cell activation and surface expression of endothelial cell-derived neutrophil adhesion molecules, production of C-X-C chemokines for the elicitation of neutrophils, neutrophil-endothelial cell adhesion, neutrophil activation and expression of neutrophil-derived adhesion molecules, neutrophil diapedesis and migration beyond the vascular barrier in response to continued adhesion molecule expression and established tissue chemotactic gradients.

Neutrophil adhesion to the endothelium is a prerequisite event for successful neutrophil extravasation. In the last decade, significant progress has been made in the study of the basic mechanisms of neutrophil-endothelial cell interaction. The development of monoclonal antibody technology, together with the discovery of the genetic disorder leukocyte adhesion deficiency (LAD), have provided tremendous insight into the molecular mechanisms of neutrophil-endothelial cell adhesion events. Patients suffering with LAD are clinically characterized as having leukocytosis and recurrent episodes of sepsis, which are characterized by the failure to form "pus" at sites of infection. The molecular basis for their disease is due to genetic mutations of the common β_2 subunit of the leukocyte β_2 integrin adhesion molecule family and is usually fatal in childhood.[1,2]

NEUTROPHIL-DERIVED ADHESION MOLECULES

The β_2 integrin family consists of heterodimeric glycoproteins that are expressed on the surface of leukocytes. The three members of this family display a variable α- and a constant β-chain with the following cluster designations: CD11a/CD18, CD11b/CD18 and CD11c/CD18.[2-6] While CD11a/CD18 complex is expressed on all leukocytes, only CD11b/CD18 appears to be significantly expressed on neutrophils.[2-6] Neutrophils have a substantial pool of CD11b/CD18 present within secondary and tertiary granules, and when activated by chemotaxins this β_2 integrin is rapidly translocated and expressed on the cell surface.[5-7] The ligand/receptor for CD11b/CD18 is either a split product of complement (iC3b) or the intercellular adhesion molecule-1 (ICAM-1) found on the surface of both immune and nonimmune cells.[6] The role of leukocyte β_2 integrins during the pathogenesis of acute lung injury has been studied using specific neutralizing monoclonal antibodies against either the variable α- or constant β-chain of the CD11b/CD18 complex. These investigations demonstrated that neutralizing either CD11b or CD18 resulted in attenuation of neutrophil-dependent pulmonary vascular permeability, hemorrhage and neutrophil extravasation in the lung.[8-11]

An additional group of adhesion molecules that function independently of β_2 integrin ligand/receptor interaction with ICAM-1 have been identified and are referred to as selectins or LEC-CAMs (Lectin, Epidermal Growth Factor, Complement, Cellular Adhesion Molecules).[7,12,13] The Selectin family is also important in mediating neutrophil-endothelial cell adhesion and includes the following members: L-selectin (leukocyte-endothelial cell adhesion molecule-1; LECAM-1), E-selectin (endothelial-leukocyte adhesion molecule-1; ELAM-1) and P-selectin (granule membrane protein-140; GMP-140 or platelet activation-dependent granule to external membrane; PADGEM). While L-selectin is constitutively expressed on leukocytes, E-selectin gene expression and functional presence on endothelium requires endothelial cell activation by either endotoxin, or the early response cytokines, tumor necrosis factor-α (TNF) and interleukin-1 (IL-1).[12,13] In contrast, P-selectin is rapidly expressed on the surface of platelets and endothelial cells after release from either the α-granules or Weibal-Palade bodies, respectively.[14] While the specific adhesion of neutrophils to endothelium appears to be related to either β₂ integrin or selectin molecules, recent studies have demonstrated the importance of the combination of these adhesion molecules in neutrophil-endothelial cell adhesion and transendothelial migration. Neutrophil (L-selectin) interaction with activated endothelium (E- and P-selectin) is an early event leading to margination or "rolling" under conditions of heighten shear force,[13,15,16] while neutrophil β₂ integrin interaction with endothelial cell ICAM-1 appears to be essential in promoting stable intravascular adhesion and transendothelial cell migration.[6,7,16]

ENDOTHELIAL CELL-DERIVED ADHESION MOLECULES

ICAM-1, a member of the immunoglobulin supergene family, is an important ligand/receptor for CD11b/CD18 expressed on neutrophils. While ICAM-1 can be found constitutively expressed on endothelial cells, this adhesion molecule can be induced in response to endotoxin, TNF or IL-1.[5,6] In addition, ICAM-1 can be detected on the surface of mononuclear phagocytes as well as nonimmune cells (e.g., fibroblasts and epithelial cells).[6] ICAM-1 has been demonstrated in the lung to play an important role in the mediation of neutrophil-dependent inflammation, as passive immunization with neutralizing ICAM-1 antibodies has been shown to attenuate pulmonary injury in an animal model of inflammation.[6,9]

In addition to ICAM-1, E-selectin is also expressed on the surface of endothelial cells in response to endotoxin, TNF or IL-1.[12,13,15-18] E-selectin expression on endothelium appears to be more rapid than the expression of ICAM-1.[6] In contrast, P-selectin is rapidly mobilized to the surface of endothelial cells following exposure to either split products of complement, thrombin or histamine.[12-14] Endothelial cell expression of E-selectin and P-selectin is important for the promotion of neutrophil adhesion, and this interaction is dependent upon the recognition of sialylated derivatives of the Lewis x oligosaccharide (sLe^x) on the neutrophil.[12-15,19] These findings support the notion that adhesive interaction between neutrophils and the endothelium is an important event leading to neutrophil-dependent lung injury.

ELICITATION OF NEUTROPHILS INTO THE LUNG: THE ROLE OF CYTOKINES

Cytokines represent a diverse group of biologically active proteins that, in addition to many other activities, are instrumental in the evolution of acute lung injury. In order to illustrate potentially important cytokine networks operative in pulmonary inflammation which mediate neutrophil recruitment, we will focus our discussion on the early response cytokines (IL-1 and TNF) and the C-X-C chemokine family.

TNF AND IL-1

Although biochemically unrelated, TNF and IL-1 demonstrate similar pleiotropic and overlapping effects on a variety of cellular functions.[20-25] These cytokines are primarily produced by mononuclear phagocytes and, because of their role for initiating further inflammatory responses, have been termed "early response cytokines". At sites of local inflammation, modest concentrations are essential, and serve to closely regulate cellular function. These early response cytokines dictate the events leading to initiation, maintenance and repair of tissue injury in a cascade of cytokine activity. In marked contrast to the controlled events of local production of TNF and IL-1, the exaggerated systemic release of these cytokines can result in a syndrome of multiorgan injury with increased host morbidity and mortality. Thus, TNF and IL-1 have a broad spectrum of biologic activity that can influence the outcome of an inflammatory response on both the local and the systemic levels.

Although the pathogenesis of septic shock and the development of acute lung injury are multifactorial, the role of TNF and IL-1 in mediating septic shock and ARDS has been clearly demonstrated in a number of studies. Waage and colleagues[26] examined sera from patients suffering from meningococcal septicemia with acute lung injury. They found a significant correlation between serum TNF levels and mortality. In a similar study of 55 patients with a clinical diagnosis of sepsis and purpura fulminans due to meningococcemia, serum levels of both TNF and IL-1 correlated with mortality.[27] In another study, patients were prospectively randomized to assess the efficacy of methylprednisolone administered in septic shock.[28] Serum levels of TNF were detected in 33% of the patients with septic shock. TNF levels were elevated with equal frequency in patients with shock due to either gram-positive or negative bacteria. The magnitude of TNF measured also correlated with a higher incidence and severity of ARDS and mortality.

In several animal studies, systemically administered TNF induced similar pathophysiological effects as compared to either endotoxin or infusion of live gram-negative bacteria. Animals demonstrated metabolic acidosis, elevated body temperature and circulating levels of catecholamines, consumptive coagulopathy-DIC, multiorgan dysfunction (renal, hepatic, gastrointestinal and pulmonary), alterations in circulating leukocytes and hypotension leading to shock.[29] In other studies the concomitant administration of both TNF and IL-1 have been found to be synergistic in mediating similar pathophysiological effects.[30] Interestingly, when in vivo protein synthesis was inhibited by actinomycin D and sublethal TNF or IL-1 administered to mice, a 100% mortality occurred within 8 to 12 hours, as compared to the absence of lethality without actinomycin D.[31] These findings suggest that de novo protein synthesis is required to protect against the lethal effects of either TNF or IL-1. Inhibition of endogenously produced TNF during bacteria-induced septic shock has been shown in animal models to significantly attenuate the pathogenesis of multiorgan injury and mortality. Tracey and associates,[29] using a baboon model of septic shock, administered a monoclonal antihuman TNF antibody both prior to and after the injection of a LD100 dose of live E. coli. Only the monoclonal antibody administration prior to the lethal dose of E. coli decreased mortality. In contrast, Hinshaw and colleagues,[32] employing a similar model of E. coli-induced lethal septicemia in a baboon model, could delay the addition of monoclonal anti-TNF antibodies for up to 30 minutes after E. coli challenge and all animals survived. Interestingly, our laboratory[33] has studied the endogenous expression and regulation of TNF from a murine model of endotoxemia and have shown that TNF is rapidly produced after a LD_{100} infusion of endotoxin. Peak levels of TNF were seen at one hour, with a rapid decline to relatively undetectable levels by 8 hours. Similar findings have been seen in human volunteer subjects injected with low doses of endotoxin.[34] These results suggest that TNF is under strict regulation. However, the expression of TNF and IL-1, in the context of septic shock, are potent mediators that trigger a cascade of events that lead to acute lung injury and multiorgan failure.

The host response to infection or injury in the lung is associated with the generation of early response cytokines, IL-1 and TNF. When endotoxin, IL-1 or TNF are intratracheally injected, these inflammatory mediators induce an intra-alveolar inflammatory response composed of a neutrophilic exudate that peaks at 6 to 12 hours, followed by a monocytic and lymphocytic infiltrate peaking at 24 and 48 hours, respectively.[35] However, IL-1 on a molar basis has been shown to be more potent than TNF. In addition, these same investigators found that endotoxin was capable of inducing both TNF and IL-1 gene expression from whole lung homogenates. Recently, reports of an IL-1 inhibitor have led to the isolation, purification, cloning and expression of an IL-1 receptor antagonist (IRAP).[36-41] IRAP is a 22 kDa polypeptide that has 40% homology with IL-1-β and has been shown to be produced from PBM or monocytic tumor cell lines in response to either endotoxin or adherent IgG.[36,40,41] The inhibitory activity of IRAP appears to be at the level of competitive occupation of the IL-1 receptor without agonist activity.[36,40,41] Immunologic effects of IRAP have been shown in vitro to inhibit IL-1-induced dermal fibroblast-derived PGE_2 production and neutrophil adherence to endothelial cells.[36,40,41] IRAP has been shown in vivo to be a potent inhibitor of *E. coli*-induced septic shock and lung injury in rabbits.[42] In addition, IRAP was found to have a protective role in the lungs of rats receiving either intratracheal endotoxin or IL-1.[43] These findings suggest that IRAP has an important immunomodulating influence on IL-1, and its production by mononuclear phagocytes in the lung may impact on the pathogenesis of acute lung injury mediated by IL-1.

TNF and IL-1 have a number of effects on endothelial cell function including the expression of cell surface adhesion molecules for leukocytes (ICAM-1 and E-selectin),[6,17,18] production of a neutrophil chemotactic/activating factor IL-8,[44] induction of a procoagulant surface with the generation of tissue factor,[45] plasminogen activator inhibitor,[46,47] and a reduction in the cell surface expression of thrombomodulin leading to a decline in thrombomodulin-dependent activation of protein C.[48-50] These cytokines may prime neutrophils in response to specific activating factors with enhanced respiratory burst and release of reactive oxygen metabolites, phagocytosis and degranulation of specific and azurophilic granules containing a number of proteolytic enzymes.[20-25] Thus, these two cytokines act as initiators and promoters,

setting into motion an intricate cascade of events leading to microvascular inflammation. The neutrophil-endothelial cell interaction is dynamic, resulting in endothelial injury and migration of neutrophils into the extravascular space.

C-X-C CHEMOKINE FAMILY

The primary feature of both TNF- and IL-1-dependent acute inflammation in the lung is the sequestration of neutrophils and subsequent neutrophil-dependent lung injury. Although TNF and IL-1 were initially reported to be chemotactic for neutrophils,[51] more recent studies have definitively demonstrated that neither IL-1 nor TNF have direct chemotactic activity in vitro for neutrophils.[52] These findings suggest that cytokine networks are operative in vivo which are dependent upon the initial expression of early response cytokines (TNF and IL-1), followed by the generation of more specific distal mediators which directly influence neutrophil activation and recruitment.

Recently, the C-X-C chemokine family of cytokines have been identified that appear to have proinflammatory and reparative activities.[53-60] These cytokines in their monomeric forms are all less than 10 kDa and are characteristically basic heparin-binding proteins. This family displays four highly conserved cysteine amino acid residues, with the first two cysteines separated by one nonconserved amino acid residue. In general, these cytokines appear to have specific chemotactic activity for neutrophils. Because of their chemotactic properties and the presence of the C-X-C cysteine motif, these cytokines have been designated the C-X-C chemokine family. Interestingly, these chemokines are all clustered on human chromosome 4, and exhibit between 20% to 50% homology on the amino acid level.[53-63] Over the last decade, 13 different human C-X-C chemokines have been identified and include platelet factor-4 (PF4), NH_2-terminal truncated forms of platelet basic protein [PBP; connective tissue activating protein-III (CTAP-III), β-thromboglobulin (β–TG) and neutrophil activating protein-2 (NAP-2)], IL-8, growth-related oncogene (GROα), GROβ, GROγ, interferon-γ-inducible protein (IP-10), monokine induced by interferon-γ (MIG), epithelial neutrophil activating protein-78 (ENA-78) and granulocyte chemotactic protein-2 (GCP-2).[53-63] The murine homologues to the human C-X-C chemokine family include KC, macrophage inflammatory protein-2 (MIP-2), crg-2 and MIG, and are structurally homologous to human GROα, GROβ and GROγ, IP-10 and MIG, respectively.[53-63] No murine or rat structural homologue exists for human IL-8.[53-63] IL-8, ENA-78 and GCP-2 were all initially identified on the basis of their ability to induce neutrophil activation and chemotaxis.[53-63] C-X-C chemokines have been found to be produced by an array of cells including monocytes, alveolar macrophages, neutrophils, platelets, eosinophils, mast cells, T lymphocytes, natural killer cells (NK cells), keratinocytes, mesangial cells, epithelial cells, hepatocytes, fibroblasts, smooth muscle cells, mesothelial cells and endothelial cells.[53-78] The production of C-X-C chemokines by both immune and nonimmune cells within the lung supports the contention that these cytokines may play a pivotal role in orchestrating pulmonary inflammation.

ACUTE PULMONARY INFLAMMATION: THE INTERPLAY OF EARLY RESPONSE CYTOKINES, ADHESION MOLECULES AND C-X-C CHEMOKINES

The common histopathologic feature of acute inflammation and injury in the lung is the presence of intrapulmonary neutrophils. During the initiation phase of acute inflammation the movement of neutrophils from the pulmonary vascular compartment to interstitium and alveolar space is an early event in the propagation of further lung inflammation. Inflammatory stimuli from either side of the alveolar-capillary membrane may result in pulmonary microvascular alterations which lead to local increases in neutrophil adhesion. These adhered neutrophils, under the influence of adhesion molecules and chemokines, then undergo directed migration along chemotactic gradients to the inflamed area. During recruitment, these neutrophils also become activated, releasing various proteases, reactive oxygen metabolites and cytokines, which result in acute lung injury. As the acute inflammatory process changes from the initiation to maintenance and resolution stages, the cellular composition of the inflammatory lesions change to a predominately mononuclear cell population. Thus, leukocyte elicitation is dynamic, with specific chemoattractants expressed at specific temporal windows of the inflammatory response. In bacterial infection and other clinical conditions, the recruitment of neutrophils is mediated by a number of biologically active agents, including C-X-C chemokines.

The importance of cytokine networks between immune and nonimmune cells of the alveolar-capillary membrane or airway of the lung is necessary for cellular communication during inflammation. The subsequent events of these cellular/cytokine interactions are crucial to initiating and propagating the inflammatory response which leads to pulmonary injury. Both TNF and IL-1 are early response cytokines that are necessary not only for the initiation of acute inflammation, but also are required for persistence of the inflammatory response, leading to chronic inflammation. The production of C-X-C chemokines by the major cellular components of the alveolar-capillary membrane or airway of the lung, and their participation in the inflammatory response, may be critical for the orchestration of the directed migration of leukocytes into the lung (Fig. 7.1). The alveolar-capillary membrane has traditionally been viewed only as a structure for gas exchange, but an understanding of a more complex role has emerged with advances in molecular biological techniques and investigations of individual cell components. The alveolar-capillary membrane can now be viewed as a dynamic assembly of immune and nonimmune cells that,

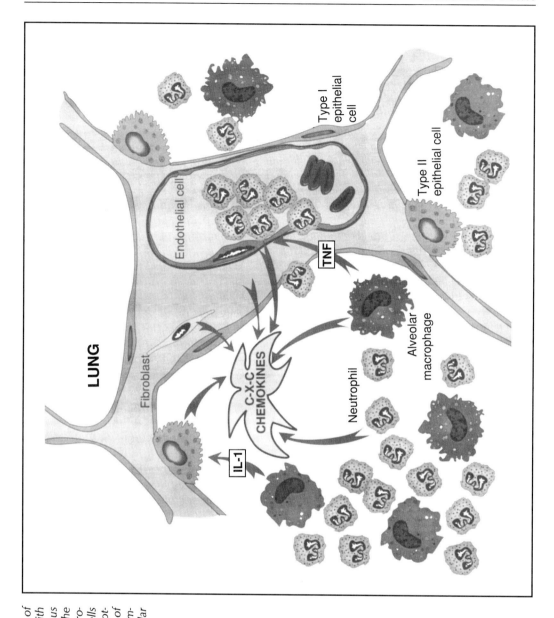

Fig. 7.1. The alveolar-capillary membrane of the lung is a dynamic assembly of cells with the capability to respond to both exogenous and endogenous agonists resulting in the generation of C-x-C chemokines. The production of C-x-C chemokines by these cells establishes an effective neutrophil chemotactic gradient that leads to the elicitation of neutrophils from the microvascular compartment into the interstitium and alveolar space of the lung.

through cytokine networking, can generate significant quantities of C-X-C chemokines. Importantly, the expression of C-X-C chemokines by the major cellular constituents of the lung is stimulus specific. Neutrophils, mononuclear phagocytes and endothelial cells produce C-X-C chemokines in response to either LPS, TNF or IL-1, but not to IL-6. Pulmonary fibroblasts and epithelial cells express C-X-C chemokines in response to specific host-derived signals, such as TNF or IL-1. These findings are significant since cells once thought of as "targets" of the inflammatory response, can actively participate as effector cells in the production of potent neutrophil chemoattractants. Thus, during acute inflammation, the production of TNF and IL-1 can act in either an autocrine or paracrine fashion to stimulate contiguous cells, both immune and nonimmune, to express C-X-C chemokines.

Cytokine networks between immune and nonimmune cells of the alveolar-capillary membrane are necessary for cellular communication during pulmonary inflammation. The subsequent events of these cellular/humoral interactions are pivotal to the initiation and propagation of the inflammatory response leading to pulmonary injury. The interrelationship of early response cytokines, adhesion molecules and the C-X-C chemokines orchestrates the recruitment of neutrophils into the lung. The paradigm for neutrophil extravasation is likely operative in the microvasculature of the lung, and consists of four or more steps (Fig. 7.2). First, lung injury results in the activation of microvascular endothelium in response to the local generation of TNF or IL-1, leading to expression of endothelial cell-derived E-and P-selectins and ICAM-1. The constitutive presence of neutrophil-derived L-selectin and other lectin moieties allows for the initial adhesive interaction of these cells with endothelial cell selectins, leading to the "rolling" effect. Second, generation of C-X-C chemokines leads to the activation of neutrophils in the vascular compartment and expression of β_2 integrins,

while L-selectin is concomitantly shed. Third, the interaction of the neutrophil β_2 integrins with their receptor/ligand, ICAM-1, results in the rapid arrest of neutrophils on the endothelium. Fourth, the subsequent events leading to neutrophil extravasation beyond the vascular compartment are dependent upon a combination of haptotaxis, migration in response to an insoluble gradient (the continued expression of β_2 integrins on neutrophils and ICAM-1 on nonimmune cells), and the maintenance of a C-X-C chemokine specific neutrophil chemotactic gradient. The participation of C-X-C chemokines in the inflammatory response appears to be critical for the orchestration of the directed migration of neutrophils into the lung. After arriving in the lung, these activated leukocytes can further respond to noxious or antigenic stimuli and induce pulmonary injury through the release of reactive oxygen metabolites, proteolytic enzymes and additional cytokines.

THE ROLE OF C-X-C CHEMOKINES IN PULMONARY INFLAMMATION

Clinical studies examining elevations in pulmonary IL-8 levels and the development and mortality of the adult respiratory distress syndrome have conflicted; however most have suggested a strong correlation.[79-83] Of particular interest is the recent findings of Donnelly and colleagues,[84] that correlated early increases in bronchoalveolar lavage fluid IL-8 content of patients at risk for subsequent development of ARDS and, importantly, also demonstrated the alveolar macrophage as an important cellular source of IL-8 prior to neutrophil influx. High concentrations of IL-8 were found in the bronchoalveolar lavage fluid from trauma patients, some within 1 hour of injury and prior to any evidence of significant neutrophil influx. Patients who progressed to ARDS had significantly greater bronchoalveolar lavage fluid levels of IL-8 than those patients who failed to develop ARDS. Interestingly, plasma levels

Fig. 7.2. Neutrophil elicitation is dependent upon the orchestrated events of the generation of early response cytokines, the expression of neutrophil- and endothelial cell-derived adhesion molecules, and the production of C-X-C chemokines to establish an extravascular neutrophil chemotactic gradient. Panel A, the microvasculature under conditions of normal homeostasis. Panel B represents the microvasculature immediately after an injury; the early response cytokines, TNF and IL-1, are produced leading to an autocrine and paracrine activation of contiguous cells. L-selectin on neutrophils interacts with its receptor/ligand (E- and P-selectin) on endothelium, leading to the "rolling effect". Panel C, ICAM-1 expression is induced on the surface of the endothelium and C-X-C chemokines are produced by both immune and nonimmune cells of the vascular wall in response to both the initiating event and host-derived early response cytokines. C-X-C chemokine activation of neutrophils in the microvascular compartment results in the concomitant shedding and expression of L-selectin and CD11b/CD18 on the surface of the neutrophil, respectively, leading to firm ICAM-1-dependent intravascular adhesion of neutrophils to the endothelium. Panels D and E, the extravasation of neutrophils from the vascular to extravascular compartment is dependent upon the combination of haptotaxis [migration in response to an insoluble gradient (the continued polar expression of β_2 integrins on neutrophils and ICAM-1 on nonimmune cells)] and the maintenance of a neutrophil specific (C-X-C chemokine) chemotactic gradient.

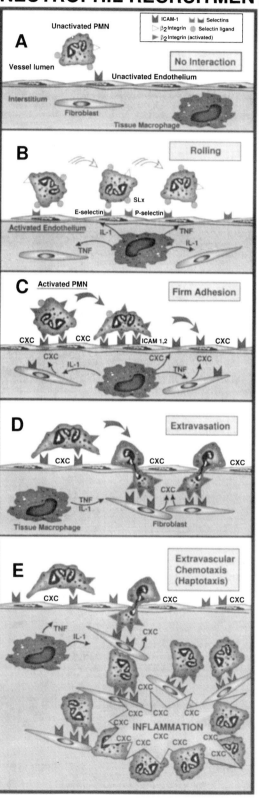

of IL-8 from these patients were not found to be significantly different from patients who developed ARDS as compared to those that did not develop ARDS.

Recent investigations have also shown that anoxia/hyperoxia simulating ischemia-reperfusion can lead to an induction of IL-8 gene expression with a significant increase in IL-8 production by mononuclear cells and endothelial cells.[85,86] IL-8 gene induction was associated with the presence of increased binding activity in nuclear extracts from hypoxic endothelial cells for the NF-κB site.[86] Of further clinical significance, endotoxin was found to further potentiate this hyperoxic response (see ref. 85 and unpublished observations). While these in vitro studies suggested that IL-8 may be a major neutrophil chemotaxin produced in the context of simulated ischemia-reperfusion, Sekido and associates[87] demonstrated that IL-8 significantly contributed to reperfusion lung injury using a rabbit model of lung ischemia-reperfusion injury. Reperfusion of the ischemic lung resulted in the production of IL-8 that correlated with maximal pulmonary neutrophil infiltration. Passive immunization of the animals with neutralizing antibodies to IL-8, prior to reperfusion of the ischemic lung, prevented neutrophil extravasation and tissue injury, suggesting a causal role for IL-8 in this model. In another model of ischemia-reperfusion injury demonstrating the importance of cytokine cascades between the liver and lung, Colletti and colleagues[88] demonstrated that hepatic ischemia-reperfusion injury and the generation of TNF can result in pulmonary-derived ENA-78. The production of ENA-78 in the lung was correlated with the presence of neutrophil-dependent lung injury, and passive immunization with neutralizing ENA-78 antibodies resulted in significant attenuation of lung injury in this model.

C-X-C chemokines have also been found to play a significant role in mediating neutrophil infiltration in the lung parenchyma and pleural space in response to endotoxin and bacterial challenge. Frevert and associates[89] found that passive immunization of rats with neutralizing GROα antibodies prior to intratracheal LPS resulted in 71% reduction in neutrophil accumulation within the lung. Broaddus and associates[90] found that passive immunization with neutralizing IL-8 antibodies blocked 77% of endotoxin-induced neutrophil influx in the pleura. Greenberger and colleagues,[91] using a murine model of *Klebsiella* pneumonia, demonstrated that neutralization of MIP-2 results in both a reduction in the recruitment of neutrophils to the lung and pulmonary clearance of bacteria. The depletion of MIP-2 in this model during bacterial pneumonia was associated with a higher early mortality. These studies support the notion that C-X-C chemokines are important in the elicitation of neutrophils in the lung under conditions of acute inflammation.

The above studies underscore the interrelationship of early response cytokines, adhesion molecules and C-X-C chemokines in the orchestration of the recruitment of neutrophils into the lung. The discovery of the C-X-C chemokine supergene families has greatly enhanced our understanding of the biology of leukocyte recruitment. These protein mediators of inflammation play an important role during the initiation and maintenance of pulmonary diseases associated with inflammation. They are responsible for the induction of leukocyte-derived adhesion molecules resulting in enhanced leukocyte-endothelial cell interaction, leukocyte activation and chemotaxis, and subsequent transendothelial extravasation at the site of lung inflammation.

ACKNOWLEDGMENTS

This research was supported in part by the National Institutes of Health grants HL50057, CA66180 and 1P50HL46487 (RMS), HL58200 and AA10571 (TJS), HL02401 (LMC) and HL31693 and HL35276 (SLK). We would like to acknowledge Robin G. Kunkel for her outstanding artwork.

REFERENCES

1. Anderson DC, Springer TA. Leukocyte adhesion deficiency: An inherited defect in the Mac-1, LFA-1, and p150, 95 glycoproteins. Annu Rev Med 1987; 38:175-94.

2. Kishimoto TK, Larson RS, Corbi AL, Dustin AL, Staunton AL, Springer TA. The leukocyte integrins: LFA-1, Mac-1, and p150,95. Adv Immunol 1989; 46:149-82.

3. Hogg N. The leukocyte integrins. Immunology Today 1989; 10:111-14.

4. Kishimoto TK, Larson RS, Corbi AL, Dustin ML, Staunton ML, Springer TA. Leukocyte integrins. In: Leukocyte adhesion molecules: Structure, function, and regulation. Springer TA, Anderson DC, Rosenthal AS et al, eds. New York: Springer-Verlag, 1990:7-43.

5. Arnaout MA. Structure and function of the leukocyte adhesion molecules CD11/CD18. BLOOD 1990; 75:1037-50.

6. Springer TA. Adhesion receptors of the immune system. Nature 1990; 346:425-34.

7. Springer TA. The sensation and regulation of interactions with the extracellular environment: The cell biology of lymphocyte adhesion receptors. Annu Rev Cell Biol 1990; 6:359-402.

8. Vedder NB, Winn RK, Rice CL, Chi EY, Arfors KE, Harlan JM. A monoclonal antibody to the adherence-promoting leukocyte glycoprotein CD18, reduces organ injury and improves survival from hemorrhagic shock and resuscitation in rabbits. J Clin Invest 1988; 81:939-44.

9. Barton RW, Rothlein R, Ksiazek J, Kennedy C. Role of anti-adhesion monoclonal antibodies in rabbit lung inflammation. In: Leukocyte adhesion molecules: Structure, function, and regulation. Springer TA, Anderson DC, Rosenthal AS et al, eds. New York: Springer-Verlag, 1990:149-55.

10. Mulligan MS, Varani J, Warren JS, Till GO, Smith CW, Anderson DC, Todd RF III, Ward PA. Roles of $\beta 2$ integrins of rat neutrophils in complement- and oxygen radical-mediated acute inflammatory injury. In: Leukocyte emigration and its sequelae. Movat HZ, ed. Basle: Karger, 1987:79.

11. Mulligan MS, Warren JS, Smith CW, Anderson DC, Yeh CG, Rudolph AR, Ward PA. Lung injury after deposition of IgA immune complexes: Requirements for CD18 and L-arginine. J Immunol 1992; 148: 3086-92.

12. Lasky LA. Lectin cell adhesion molecules (LEC-CAMs): A new family of cell adhesion proteins involved with inflammation. J Cell Biochem 1991; 45:139-46.

13. Stoolman LM. Selectins (LEC-CAMs): Lectin-like receptors involved in lymphocyte recirculation and leukocyte recruitment. In: Fukuda M, ed. Cell surface carbohydrates and cell development. Boca Raton: CRC Press, 1992:71-98.

14. McEver RP, Beckstead JH, Moore KL, Marshall-Carlson L, Bainton DF. GMP-140, a platelet alpha-granule membrane protein, is also synthesized by vascular endothelial cells and is localized in Weibel-Palade bodies. J Clin Invest 1989; 84:92-97.

15. Stoolman LM. Adhesion molecules controlling lymphocyte migration. Cell 1989; 56:907-10.

16. Butcher EC. Leukocyte-endothelial cell recognition: Three (or more) steps to specificity and diversity. Cell 1991; 67:1033-36.

17. Bevilacqua MP, Stengelin S, Gimbrone MA, Seed B. Endothelial leukocyte adhesion molecule 1: An inducible receptor for neutrophils releated to complement regulatory proteins and lectins. Science 1989; 243: 1160-65.

18. Miller EJ, Cohen AB, Najao S, Griffith D, Maunder RJ, Martin TR, Weiner-Kronish JP, Sticherling M, Christopher E, Matthay MA. Elevated levels of NAP-1/Interleukin-8 are present in the airspaces of patients with the adult respiratory distress syndrome and are associated with increased mortality. Am Rev Respir Dis 1992; 146:427-32.

19. Picker LJ, Warnock RA, Burns A, Doerschuk CM, Berg EL, Butcher EC. The neutrophil selectin LECAM-1 presents carbohydrate ligands to the vascular selectins ELAM-1 and GMP-140. Cell 1991; 66: 921-33.

20. Larrick JW, Kunkel SL. The role of tumor necrosis factor and interleukin-1 in the immunoinflammatory response. Pharm Res . 1988; 5:129-39.

21. Kunkel SL, Remick DG, Strieter RM, Larrick JW. Mechanisms that regulate the

production and effects of tumor necrosis factor-α. Crit Rev of Immunol 1989; 9:93-117.

22. Le J, Vilcek J. TNF and IL-1: Cytokines with multiple overlapping biological activities. Lab Invest 1987; 56:234-82.

23. Sherry B, Cerami A. Cachectin/tumor necrosis factor exerts endocrine, paracrine, and autocrine control of the inflammatory responses. J Cell Biol 1988; 107:1269-77.

24. Dinarello CA. Interleukin-1 and its biologically related cytokines. Adv Immunol 1989; 44:153-205.

25. Cerami A. Inflammatory cytokines. Clin Immunol Immunopathol 1992; 62:S3-S10.

26. Waage A, Halstensen A, Espevik T. Association between tumour necrosis factor in serum and fatal outcome in patients with meningococcal disease. Lancet 1987; 1:355-57.

27. Girardin E, Grau GE, Dayer JM, Roux-Lombard P. The J5 Study Group, Lambert PH. Tumor necrosis factor and interleukin-1 in the serum of children with severe infectious purpura. N Engl J Med 1988; 319:397-400.

28. Marks JD, Marks CB, Luce JM, Montgomery AB, Turner J, Metz CA, Murray JF. Plasma tumor necrosis factor in patients with septic shock: Mortality rate, incidence of adult respiratory distress syndrome. Am Rev Respir Dis 1990; 141:94-97.

29. Tracey KJ, Fong Y, Hesse DG, Manogue KR, Lee AT, Kuo GC, Lowry SF, Cerami A. Anti-cachectin/TNF monoclonal antibodies prevent septic shock during lethal bacteraemia. Nature 1987; 330:662-64.

30. Sipe JD. The molecular biology of interleukin 1 and the acute phase response. Adv Intern Med 1989; 34:1-20.

31. Shalaby MR, Halgunset J, Haugen OA, Aarset H, Aarden L, Waage A, Matsushima K, Kvithyll H, Boraschi D, Lamvil L, Espevik T. Cytokine-associated tissue injury and lethality in mice: A comparative study. Clin Immunol Immunopath 1991; 61:69-82.

32. Hinshaw LB, Tekamp-Olson P, Chang ACK, Lee PA, Taylor FB, Murray CK, Peer GT, Emergon TE, Poassey RB, Juo GC. Survival of primates in LD100 septic shock following therapy with antibody to tumor necrosis factor (TNF-alpha). Circ Shock 1990; 30:279-92.

33. Remick DG, Strieter RM, Lynch JP, III, Nguyen D, Eskandari M, Kunkel SL. In vivo dynamics of murine tumor necrosis factor-α gene expression: Kinetic of dexamethasone-induced suppression. Lab Invest 1989; 60:766-71.

34. Michie HR, Mangue KR, Spriggs DR, Revhaug A, O'Dwyer S, Dinarello CA, Ceram A, Wolff SM, Wilmore DW. Detection of circulating tumor necrosis factor after endotoxin administration. N Engl J Med 1988; 318:1481-86.

35. Ulich TR, Watson LR. Songmei Y, Guo K, Wang P, Thang H, Castillo JD. The intratracheal administration of endotoxin and cytokines: I. Characterization of LPS-induced IL-1 and TNF mRNA expression and LPS-, IL-1-, and TNF-induced inflammatory infiltrate. Am J Pathol 1991; 138:1485-96.

36. Dinarello CA. Interleukin-1 and interleukin-1 antagonism. BLOOD 1991; 77:1627-52.

37. Eisenberg SP, Evans RJ, Arend WP, Verderber E, Brewer MT, Hannum CH, Thompson RC. Primary structure and functional expression from complementary DNA of a human interleukin-1 receptor antagonist. Nature 1990; 343:343-46.

38. Mazzei GJ, Seckinger PL, Dayer JM, Shaw AR. Purification and characterization of a 26-kDa competitive inhibitor of interleukin 1. Eur J Immunol 1990; 20:683-89.

39. Hannum CH, Wilcox CJ, Arend WP, Joslin FG, Dripps DJ, Heimdal PL, Armes LJ, Sommer A, Einsenberg SP, Thompson RC. Interleukin-1 receptor antagonist activity of a human interleukin-1 inhibitor. Nature 1990; 343:336-40.

40. Carter DB, Deibel MR, Dunn CJ et al. Purification, cloning, expression, and biological characterization of an interleukin-1 receptor antagonist protein. Nature 1990; 334:633-38.

41. Arend WP. Interleukin 1 receptor antagonist a new member of the interleukin 1 family. J Clin Invest 1991; 88:1445-51.

42. Ohlsson K, Bjork P, Bergenfeldt M, Hageman R, Thompson RC. IL-1ra reduces mortality from endotoxin shock. Nature

1990; 348:550-52.

43. Ulich TR, Yin S, Guo K, Castillo JD, Eisenberg SP, Thompson RC. The intracheal administration of endotoxin and cytokines: III. The interleukin-1 (IL-1) receptor antagonist inhibits endotoxin- and IL-1-induced acute inflammation. Am J Pathol 1991; 138:521-24.

44. Strieter RM, Kunkel SL, Showell HJ, Remick DG, Phan SH, Ward PA, Marks RM. Endothelial cell gene expression of a neutrophil chemotactic factor by TNF-alpha, LPS, and IL-1-beta. Science 1989; 243:1467-69.

45. Bevilacqua MP, Pober JS, Majeau GR, Fiers W, Cotran RS, Gimbrone MA. Recombinant tumor necrosis factor induces procoagulant activity in cultured human vascular endothelium: Characterization and comparison with the actions of interleukin 1. Proc Natl Acad Sci USA 1986; 83:4533-37.

46. Stern DM, Kaiser E, Nawroth PP. Regulation of the coagulation system by vascular endothelial cells. Haemostasis 1988; 18:202-14.

47. Crutchley DJ, Conanan LB. Endotoxin induction of an inhibitor of plasminogen activator in bovine pulmonary artery endothelial cells. J Biol Chem 1986; 261:154-59.

48. Esmon CT. The regulation of natural anticoagulation pathways. Science 1987; 235:1348-52.

49. Clouse LH, Comp PC. The regulation of hemostasis: The protein C system. N Engl J Med 1986; 314:1298-1304.

50. Moore KL, Andreoli SP, Esmon NL, Esmon CT, Bang NU. Endotoxin enhances tissue factor and suppresses thrombomodulin expression of human vascular endothelium in vitro. J Clin Invest 1987; 79:124-30.

51. Sauder DN, Mounessa NL, Katy SI, Dinarello CA, Gallin JI. Chemotactic cytokines: The role of leukocyte pyrogen and epidermal cell thymocyte-activating factor in neutrophil chemotaxis. J Immunol 1984; 132:828-37.

52. Yoshimura T, Matsushima K, Oppenheim JJ, Leonard EJ. Neutrophil chemotactic factor produced by LPS-stimulated human blood mononuclear leukocytes: Partial characterization and separation from interleukin-1. J Immunol 1987; 139:788-94.

53. Baggiolini M, Dewald B, Walz A. Interleukin-8 and related chemotactic cytokines. In: Gallin JI, Goldstein IM, Snyderman R, eds. Inflammation: Basic Principles and Clinical Correlates. New York: Raven Press Ltd, 1992.

54. Baggiolini M, Walz A, Kunkel SL. Neutrophil-activating peptide-1/interleukin 8, a novel cytokine that activates neutrophils. J Clin Invest 1989; 84:1045-49.

55. Matsushima K, Oppenheim JJ. Interleukin 8 and MCAF: Novel inflammatory cytokines inducible by IL-1 and TNF. Cytokine 1989; 1:2-13.

56. Oppenheim JJ, Zachariae OC, Mukaida N, Matsushima K. Properties of the novel proinflammatory supergene "intercrine" cytokine family. Annu Rev Immunol 1991; 9:617-48.

57. Miller MD, Krangel MS. Biology and biochemistry of the chemokines: a family of chemotactic and inflammatory cytokines. Crit Rev Immunol 1992 12:17-46.

58. Baggiolini M, Dewald B, Walz A. Interleukin-8 and related chemotactic cytokines. In: Gallin JI, Goldstein IM, Snyderman R, eds. Inflammation: Basic Principles and Clinical Correlates. New York: Raven Press Ltd, 1992.

59. Baggiolini M, Dewald B, Moser B. Interleukin-8 and related chemotactic cytokines-C-X-C and C-C chemokines. Adv Immunol 1994; 55:97-179.

60. Taub DD, Oppenheim JJ. Chemokines, inflammation and immune system. Therapeutic Immunol 1994; 1:229-46.

61. Farber JM. HuMIG: a new member of the chemokine family of cytokines. Biochem Biophys Res Comm 1993; 192:223-30.

62. Proost P, DeWolf-Peeters C, Conings R, Opdenakker G, Billiau A, Van Damme J. Identification of a novel granulocyte chemotactic protein (GCP-1) from human tumor cells: in vitro and in vivo comparison with natural forms of GROa, IP-10, and IL-8. J Immunol 1993; 150:1000-10.

63. Walz A, Burgener R, Car B, Baggiolini M, Kunkel SL, Strieter RM. Structure and neutrophil-activating properties of a novel inflammatory peptide (ENA-78) with homol-

ogy to interleukin-8. J Exp Med 1991; 174:1355-62.

64. Walz A, Baggiolini M. Generation of the neutrophil-activating peptide NAP-2 from platelet basic protein or connective tissue-activating peptide III through monocyte proteases. J Exp Med 1990; 171:449-54.

65. Yoshimura T, Matsushima K, Oppenheim JJ, Leonard EJ. Neutrophil chemotactic factor produced by LPS-stimulated human blood mononuclear leukocytes: Partial characterization and separation from interleukin-1. J Immunol 1987; 139:788-94.

66. Matsushima K, Morishita K, Yoshimura T, Lavu S, Obayashi Y, Lew W, Appella E, Kung HF, Leonard EJ, Oppenheim JJ. Molecular cloning of a human monocyte-derived neutrophil chemotactic factor (MDNCF) and the induction of MDNCF mRNA by interleukin-1 and tumor necrosis factor. J Exp Med 1988; 167:1883-93.

67. Strieter RM, Kunkel SL, Showell HJ, Marks RM. Monokine-induced gene expression of human endothelial cell-derived neutrophil chemotactic factor. Biochem Biophys Res Commun 1988; 156:1340-45.

68. Strieter RM, Kunkel SL, Showell HJ, Remick DG, Phan SH, Ward PA, Marks RM. Endothelial cell gene expression of a neutrophil chemotactic factor by TNF-α, LPS, and IL-1β. Science 1989; 243:1467-69.

69. Strieter RM, Phan SH, Showell HJ, Remick DG, Lynch JP, Genard M, Raiford C, Eskandari M, Marks RM, Kunkel SL. Monokine-induced neutrophil chemotactic factor gene expression in human fibroblasts. J Biol Chem 1989 264:10621-26.

70. Thornton AJ, Strieter RM, Lindley I, Baggiolini M, Kunkel SL. Cytokine-induced gene expression of a neutrophil chemotactic factor/interleukin-8 by human hepatocytes. J Immunol 1990; 144:2609-13.

71. Elner VM, Strieter RM, Elner SG, Baggiolini M, Lindley I, Kunkel SL. Neutrophil chemotactic factor (IL-8) gene expression by cytokine-treated retinal pigment epithelial cells. Am J Path 1990; 136: 745-50.

72. Strieter RM, Chensue SW, Basha MA, Standiford TJ, Lynch JP, Kunkel SL. Human alveolar macrophage gene expression

of interleukin-8 by TNF-α, LPS and IL-1β. Am J Respir Cell Mol Biol 1990; 2:321-26.

73. Standiford TJ, Kunkel SL, Basha MA, Chensue SW, Lynch JP, Toews GB, Strieter RM. Interleukin-8 gene expression by a pulmonary epithelial cell line: A model for cytokine networks in the lung. J Clin Invest 1990; 86:1945-53.

74. Strieter RM, Kasahar K, Allen R, Showell HJ, Standiford TJ, Kunkel SL. Human neutrophils exhibit disparate chemotactic factor gene expression. Biochem Biophys Res Comm 1990; 173:725-30.

75. Brown Z, Strieter RM, Chensue SW, Ceska P, Lindley I, Nield GH, Kunkel SL, Westwick J. Cytokine activated human mesangial cells generate the neutrophil chemoattractant—interleukin 8. Kidney International 1991; 40:86-90.

76. Rolfe MW, Kunkel SL, Standiford TJ, Chensue SW, Allen RM, Evanoff HL, Phan SH, Strieter RM. Pulmonary fibroblast expression of interleukin-8: a model for alveolar macrophage-derived cytokine networking. Am J Respir Cell Mol Biol 1991; 5:493-501.

77. Nickoloff BJ, Karabin GD, Barker JNWN, Giffiths CEM, Sarma V, Mitra RS, Elder JT, Kunkel SL, Dixit VM. Cellular localization of interleukin-8 and its inducer, tumor necrosis factor-alpha in psoriasis. Am J Pathol 1991; 138:129-40.

78. Strieter RM, Kasahara K, Allen RM, Standiford TJ, Rolfe MW, Becker FS, Chensue SW, Kunkel SL. Cytokine-induced neutrophil-derived interleukin-8. Am J Pathol 1992; 141:397-407.

79. Jorens PG, VanDamme J, DeBecker W, Bossaert L, DeJongh RF, Herman AG, Rampart M. Interleukin-8 in the broncho-alveolar lavage fluid from patients with the adult respiratory distress syndrome (ARDS) and patients at risk for ARDS. Cytokine 1992; 4:592-97.

80. Miller EJ, Cohen AB, Nago S, Griffith D, Maunder RJ, Martin TR, Weiner-Kronish JP, Sticherling M, Christophers E, Matthay MA. Elevated acute inflammatory injury. J Immunol 1992; 148:1847-57.

81. Hack CE, Hart M, VanSchijndel RJMS, Eerenberg AJM, Nuijens JH, Thijs LG,

Aarden LA. Interleukin-8 in sepsis: Relation to shock and inflammatory mediators. Infect Immun 1992; 60:2835-42.

82. Chollet-Martin S, Montravers P, Gilbert C, Elbim C, Desmonts JM, Fagon JY, Gougerot-Pocidalo MA. High levels of interleukin-8 in the blood and alveolar spaces of patients with pneumonia and Adult Respiratory Distress Syndrome. Infect Immun 1993; 61:4553-59.

83. Donnelly TJ, Meade P, Jagels M, Cryer HG, Law MM, Hugli TE, Shoemaker WC, Abraham E. Cytokine, complement, and endotoxin profiles associated with the development of the adult respiratory distress syndrome after severe injury. Crit Care Med 1994; 22:768-76.

84. Donnelly SC, Strieter RM, Kunkel SL, Walz A, Robertson CR, Carter DC, Grant IS, Pollock AJ, Haslett C. Interleukin-8 and development of adult respiratory distress syndrome in at-risk patient groups. Lancet 1993; 341:643-47.

85. Metinko AP, Kunkel SL, Standiford TJ, Strieter RM. Anoxia-hyperoxia induces monocyte derived interleukin-8. J Clin Invest 1992; 90:791-98.

86. Karakurum M, Shreeniwas R, Chen J, Pinsky D, Yan SD, Anderson M, Sunouchi K, Major J, Hamilton T, Kuwabara K, Rot A, Nowygrod R, Stern D. Hypoxic induction of interleukin-8 gene expression in human endothelial cells. J Clin Invest 1994; 93:1564-70.

87. Sekido N, Mukaida N, Harada A, Nakanishi I, Watanabe Y, Matsushima K. Prevention of lung reperfusion injury in rabbits by a monoclonal antibody against interleukin-8. Nature 1993; 365:654-57.

88. Colletti LM, Kunkel SL, Walz A, Burdick MD, Kunkel RG, Wilke CA, Strieter RM. Chemokine expression during hepatic ischemia/reperfusion induced lung injury in the rat: the role of epithelial neutrophil activating protein. J Clin Invest 1995; 95:134-141.

89. Frevert CW, Huang S, Danaee H, Paulauskis JD, Kobzik L. Functional characterization of the rat chemokine KC and its importance in neutrophil recruitment in a rat model of pulmonary inflammation. J Immunol 1995; 154:335-44.

90. Broaddus VC, Boylan AM, Hoeffel JM, Kim KJ, Sadick M, Chutharapal A, Hebert CA. Neutralization of IL-8 inhibits neutrophil influx in a rabbit model of endotoxin-induced pleurisy. J Immunol 1994; 152:2960-67.

91. Greenberger MJ, Strieter RM, Kunkel SL, Danforth JM, Laichalk LL, McGillicuddy DC, Standiford TJ. Neutralization of MIP-2 attenuates neutrophil recruitment and bacterial clearance in murine Klebsiella pneumonia. Infect Immunity (in press).

========== CHAPTER 8 ==========

THE ROLE OF CHEMOKINES IN PNEUMONIA

Gary B. Huffnagle, Robert M. Strieter, Steven L. Kunkel,
Galen B. Toews and Theodore J. Standiford

INTRODUCTION

The lung represents one of the most complex and multifunctional organ systems. Not only is the lung involved in the critical process of gas exchange, but this organ is also an active and important participant in a variety of immunologic responses. Through its continuous contact with ambient air and its enormous vascular bed, the lung is exposed to a large and quite varied burden of foreign antigens, including infectious agents. The lung utilizes multiple systems of host defense, which include mechanical, phagocytic, and immunologic components, to rid itself of injurious substances.[1] The initial barriers to entrance of infectious agents into the lung include specific mechanical defenses, such as the glottis, the cough reflex, airway secretions, and an intact mucociliary system that lines the entire surface of the large conducting airways. When defense mechanisms of the conducting airways are breached, the phagocytic system of the terminal airspaces then becomes critical to effectively eliminating injurious agents from the lung.

Innate, or natural immunity, is the principal pathway for effective elimination of bacterial organisms from the alveolus.[1,2] The three phagocytic cells that constitute innate immunity in the lung include alveolar macrophages, neutrophils (PMN), and recruited mononuclear phagocytes.[1-3] The alveolar macrophage represents the primary resident phagocytic cell of the alveolus. In the setting of a low bacterial burden, or exposure to less virulent gram-positive organisms, the alveolar macrophage can effectively phagocytize and kill invading organisms. However, when the bacterial burden is large, or when more virulent encapsulated gram-negative organisms, such as *Pseudomonas aeruginosa* or *Klebsiella*

Chemokines in Disease, edited by Alisa E. Koch and Robert M. Strieter.
© 1996 R.G. Landes Company.

pneumoniae, gain access to the lower air-spaces, the recruitment of neutrophils (PMN) is essential for effective containment and clearance of bacteria. In addition, specific bacterial infections, including *K. pneumoniae*, are associated with an appreciable influx of blood mononuclear phagocytes, although the contribution of these cells to the clearance of *K. pneumoniae* in vivo is not known.[3] While phagocytosis of bacteria can occur in the presence of natural opsonins (i.e., complement, surfactant) alone, this process is greatly enhanced by acquired immunity, in particular the presence of specific opsonizing antibody secreted by sensitized B lymphocytes.[4]

In contrast to bacterial infection, host responses to viruses, fungi and mycobacteria are more complex and require also the phagocytic system, as well as antibody-mediated and cell-mediated immunity.[5,6] While PMN play a role in host defense against fungal and mycobacterial pathogens, the recruitment and activation of macrophages and T cells are essential to the effective clearance of these organisms from the lung. Macrophages engulf, process and present antigen to reactive CD4+ T cells. These macrophages are then activated by T cell-derived cytokines resulting in enhanced phagocytic, microbicidal and cytotoxic activities. CD4+ T cells also stimulate the differentiation of B cells into antibody-producing plasma cells, further facilitating microbial phagocytosis. CD8+ T cells also participate in cell-mediated immune responses in the lung, as these cells mediate cellular cytotoxicity that is crucial to effective host defense against viral agents.

CYTOKINES INVOLVED IN NATURAL AND IMMUNE HOST DEFENSE

The generation of inflammation in the setting of bacterial challenge is a complex and dynamic process which involves the coordinated expression of both pro- and anti-inflammatory cytokines. Several cytokine mediators, including tumor necrosis factor-alpha (TNF-α), interferon-gamma (IFN-γ) and granulocyte-colony stimulating factor (G-CSF), have been shown to play important roles in host defense against bacteria, mycobacteria and fungi.[7-9] Recently, two closely related families of chemotactic cytokines, referred to as chemokines, have been characterized. The C-X-C chemokine family, which includes IL-8, MIP-2, GRO, ENA-78 and NAP-2, has predominant PMN stimulatory and chemotactic activities, while the C-C family, which includes MCP-1, MCP-2, MCP-3, RANTES, MIP-1α and MIP-1β, exerts predominant chemotactic and/or activating effects on macrophages, lymphocytes and eosinophils.[10] As discussed in other chapters of this text, specific members of the C-X-C and C-C chemokine families have been linked to the pathogenesis of a variety of inflammatory disease states.[10] However, several lines of evidence would suggest that C-X-C and C-C represent integral components of host defense, particularly against infection. The well-characterized in vitro leukocyte activating and chemotactic activities would predict that these chemokines may enhance the recruitment and effector functions of PMN and macrophages in infection. In addition, a number of infectious agents, or cellular components of these agents, have been shown to induce the production of C-X-C or C-C chemokines from mononuclear phagocytes and stromal cells. Lastly, chemokines have been detected in increased amounts within the lungs of patients with a variety of pulmonary infections.

THE ROLE OF CHEMOKINES IN BACTERIAL INFECTION

BACTERIAL INFECTION AND CHEMOKINE INDUCTION

A number of studies have demonstrated that bacteria or bacterial cellular constituents are potent inducers of chemokines both in vitro and in vivo. Lipopolysaccharide and lipoteichoic acid, cell wall components of gram-negative and gram-positive organisms, respectively, have been shown to be inducers of IL-8 and MIP-1α from mononuclear phagocytes.[10-12] Similarly, capsular and membrane polysaccharides from *S. aureus* and *K. pneumoniae*, respectively, can stimulate the production of both C-X-C and C-C chemokines.[13,14] Moreover, the entry of invasive bacterial species (*Listeria monocytogenes* and *Salmonella* spp.) into epithelial cell monolayers has been shown to trigger IL-8 release, whereas coincubation of these cells with noninvasive bacteria (*Eschericia coli* and *Enterococcus faecium*) failed to induce IL-8 secretion.[15] Finally, the phagocytosis of bacterial and fungal organisms can serve as a signal for the secretion of chemokines, including IL-8 and MCP-1.[16-18]

Additional indirect evidence supporting a role of chemokines in bacterial pneumonia stems from the observation that chemokines, in particular IL-8, have been detected in increased amounts within the sputum, bronchoalveolar lavage fluid (BALF) or pleural fluid obtained from patients with acute pulmonary or pleural bacterial infection. Rodriguez and colleagues found an increased incidence and severity of bacterial pneumonia in trauma patients who had IL-8 present in bronchial secretions.[19] Our laboratory has detected increased IL-8 in the sputum and bronchoalveolar lavage fluid of patients with cystic fibrosis in exacerbation (unpublished observations). In this study, IL-8 accounted for approximately 40-50% of the increased PMN chemotactic activity found in the BALF obtained from these patients during exacerbation of disease, and IL-8 levels were closely correlated with numbers of PMN in BALF and disease activity. Interestingly, a dramatic decline in the expression of IL-8 mRNA from BALF cells occurred after treatment with antibiotics with or without corticosteroids. Finally, increased levels of IL-8 have been detected in the pleural fluid of patients with bacterial empyema, with the levels of IL-8 correlating with pleural fluid neutrophilia.[20] While finding increased expression of chemokines during pleuro-pulmonary bacterial infection does not establish a role for these mediators in infection, it does suggest that specific chemokines may serve as potentially useful diagnostic and prognostic indicators in these patients.

THE EFFECT OF CHEMOKINES ON LEUKOCYTE PHAGOCYTIC AND BACTERICIDAL ACTIVITY IN VITRO

Effective clearance of microbes by leukocytes (both PMN and mononuclear phagocytes) is dependent upon initial attachment, phagocytosis, and eventual intracellular killing.[4,21] The efficacy of phagocytosis is chiefly determined by the presence of specific (immunoglobulin) and/or nonspecific (complement) opsonins on the surface of microbes, as well as the expression of specific complement (CR3) or immunoglobulin (FcγR) receptors on the surface of leukocytes.[4] Direct evidence demonstrating that chemokines regulate leukocyte phagocytic activity has been lacking. Since PMN are of critical importance in host defense against bacterial infection, and these cells are regulated by C-X-C rather than C-C chemokines, most studies have examined the effect of specific C-X-C chemokines on PMN phagocytic and antibacterial activities. Hostoffer and colleagues observed that IL-8 did not alter IgA-mediated phagocytosis of *P. aeruginosa* by PMN, although IL-8 did increase the cell surface expression of CR3 on PMN.[22] In contrast, studies in our laboratory indicate that treatment of human PMN with either human recombinant (hr) IL-8 or murine recombinant (mr) MIP-2 (the functional murine homologue of IL-8) for 1 hour in the presence of 10% human serum resulted in an approximately 1.6- and 2.1-fold increase in phagocytosis of *E. coli*, respectively, as compared to PMN incubated in serum alone (data not shown). These effects could not be completely explained by changes in leukocyte CR3 or FcγR expression, as incubation of PMN with either IL-8 or MIP-2 resulted in only modest increases in PMN FcγRII and CR3 expression, with no significant change in FcγRIII expression.

The effect of chemokines on leukocyte bactericidal activity has been studied in somewhat more detail. Interleukin-8 has been shown to enhance the killing of _E. coli_ by PMN isolated from patients with myelodysplastic syndrome.[23] Similarly, we have observed that both hrIL-8 and mrMIP-2 enhanced the ability of PMN to kill intracellular _E. coli_ in a dose-dependent fashion, resulting in a maximal 4- and 5.6-fold increase in killing, respectively, as compared to untreated PMN (Table 8.1). The mechanism of chemokine-induced PMN bacterial killing has not yet been fully elucidated; however, nonoxidative events are more likely involved than oxidative events. In PMN, C-X-C chemokines such as IL-8 and MIP-2 are more potent inducers of degranulation than of respiratory burst activation [10,24,25]. IL-8-induced PMN microbicidal activity also has been shown previously to be unaffected by coincubation with antioxidants.[26] Furthermore, IL-8 and MIP-2 failed to induce the secretion of nitric oxide from PMN, indicating that chemokine effects on PMN bactericidal activity occur by nitric-oxide independent mechanisms.

Just as C-X-C chemokines regulate PMN phagocytic and bactericidal activities, C-C chemokines can enhance the antibacterial effects of mononuclear phagocytes. Nakano and associates have demonstrated that hrMCP-1 greatly augmented the phagocytosis and killing of _P. aeruginosa_ and _Salmonella typhimurium_ by murine peritoneal macrophages.[27] Similarly, we have observed that treatment of murine alveolar macrophages with mrMIP-1α resulted in both an increase in phagocytosis (data not shown) and an approximately 2-fold increase in _E. coli_ killing, as compared to unstimulated alveolar macrophages. Collectively, the above studies indicate that members of both the C-X-C and C-C chemokine families can significantly enhance the ability of the primary phagocytic cells of the lung (PMN and alveolar macrophages) to phagocytize and kill bacterial pathogens.

THE ROLE OF CHEMOKINES IN A MURINE MODEL OF BACTERIAL PNEUMONIA

The relative contribution of chemokines to effective containment and eventual clearance of bacterial pathogens from the lung in vivo has not previously been defined. Some evidence obtained in murine

Table 8.1. Bacterial killing of phagocytosed E. coli by resting and stimulated human PMN

Treatment	Leukocyte Bactericidal Activity	
	E. coli CFU	Killing Index
Control	$21.8 \pm 0.12 \times 10^3$	22.5×10^3
fMLP (10^{-7}M)	$12.2 \pm 0.24 \times 10^3$	7.36×10^3
mrMIP-2		
1 ng/ml	$17.7 \pm 0.34 \times 10^3$	18.2×10^3
10 ng/ml	$4.26 \pm 0.11 \times 10^{3*}$	2.47×10^3
50 ng/ml	$3.88 \pm 0.27 \times 10^{3*}$	1.87×10^3
hrIL-8		
1 ng/ml	$17.8 \pm 0.14 \times 10^3$	18.2×10^3
10 ng/ml	$5.44 \pm 0.13 \times 10^{3*}$	4.35×10^3
50 ng/ml	$7.16 \pm 0.47 \times 10^{3*}$	6.90×10^3

Resting or cytokine-stimulated PMN (1×10^6) were incubated with 10% human serum and _E. coli_ (1×10^7) in HBSS x 1 hour, then cell-lysate CFU determined. Values represent mean ± SEM of 12 separate experiments. *p < 0.01 as compared to unstimulated control. Killing index is calculated by dividing mean number of CFU by the phagocytic index (the lower the killing index, the greater the killing). The phagocytic index is the product of mean number of intracellular bacteria per PMN x mean percent of PMN containing intracellular bacteria.

models of bacterial peritonitis suggest that specific C-X-C and C-C chemokines represent biologically relevant mediators of bacterial clearance in vivo. For example, the administration of hrIL-8 to nonneutropenic mice challenged with *K. pneumoniae* i.p. was protective, whereas IL-8 treatment in neutropenic mice administered *K. pneumoniae*, or mice (neutropenic and nonneutropenic) challenged with *P. aeruginosa* resulted in no change in mortality or, in some instances, increased mortality.[28] In other murine models of *P. aeruginosa* or *S. typhimurium* peritonitis, the i.p. administration of hrMCP-1 (2.5 mg/animal) resulted in complete protection from lethality.[27]

To begin to address the role of specific chemokines in lung antibacterial host defense, we have developed a murine model of *Klebsiella* pneumonia. *Klebsiella pneumoniae* is an encapsulated gram-negative organism that is one of the most common causes of both community-acquired and nosocomial gram-negative pneumonia. In this model, CD-1 or CBA/J mice were intratracheally inoculated with 10^3 CFU of *K. pneumoniae,* strain 43816, serotype 2 (ATCC, Rockville, MD). This strain was used in our experiments, as this organism is a heavily-encapsulated species that is particularly virulent in mice.[29,30] Histologic examination of the lungs 48 hours after the i.t. inoculation with *K. pneumoniae* revealed substantial accumulation of PMN and moderate numbers of macrophages within the lung airspace and interstitium.[30] Temporally correlating with the development of pulmonary inflammation was the production of TNF-α, MIP-2 and MIP-1α.[30,31] A significant time-dependent increase in the levels of these cytokines was noted in lung homogenates after the i.t. administration of *K. pneumoniae* at 48 hours, with a maximal 13-, 14- and 8-fold increase in lung homogenate TNF-α, MIP-2 and MIP-1α levels observed, respectively, as compared to saline-treated control (Fig. 8.1). Immunohistochemical analysis indicated that the alveolar macrophage was the major cellular source of these cytokines. However, recruited PMN also appear to express cell-associated TNF-α and MIP-2, indicating that PMN not only function as effector cells in the phagocytosis and killing

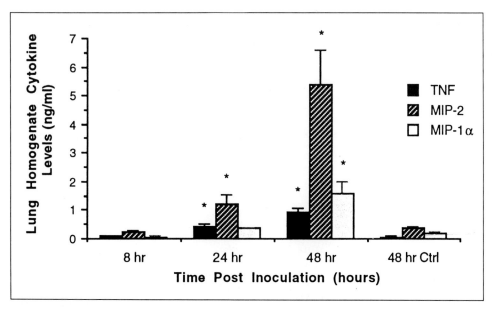

Fig. 8.1. Time-dependent production of TNF-α, MIP-2 and MIP-1α protein in lung homogenates after the i.t. administration of saline or K. pneumoniae (10³ CFU). *p < 0.05 as compared to 48 hour control. Experimental n = 5 per group.

of bacteria, but these cells can also amplify the inflammatory response by expressing chemotactic and activating cytokines.

To determine the biologic relevance of MIP-2 to PMN influx in *Klebsiella* pneumonia, animals were passively immunized with either rabbit pre-immune serum or rabbit antimurine MIP-2 antibody i.p. 2 hours prior to the i.t. administration of *K. pneumoniae* (or saline control), then lungs removed 48 hours later and assayed for myeloperoxidase (MPO) activity as a measure of PMN influx.[31] Lung MPO activity in anti-MIP-2-treated animals inoculated with *Klebsiella* was decreased by 60% at 48 hours, as compared to animals receiving pre-immune serum (p < 0.05). In addition, treatment with anti-MIP-2 antibodies resulted in a 4.4- and 1.6-fold increase in viable *K. pneumoniae* in the lungs at 24 and 48 hours postinoculation, respectively, as compared to animals receiving pre-immune serum (Table 8.2). Furthermore, inhibition of MIP-2 bioactivity in vivo resulted in early dissemination of *K. pneumoniae* to both blood and liver (Table 8.2). Finally, as compared to animals receiving pre-immune serum, passive immunization with anti-MIP-2 serum resulted in a 40-50% increase in early (24-48 hours), but not late (>72 hours) mortality. These studies indicate that MIP-2 is an important mediator of PMN influx and of effective bacterial clearance in murine *Klebsiella* pneumonia. The contribution of MIP-1α to lung antibacterial host defense in *Klebsiella* pneumonia is the focus of ongoing studies. However, preliminary studies suggest that neutralization of MIP-1α in vivo does not substantially alter mortality in animals inoculated with either 10^2 CFU (LD50 dose) or 10^3 CFU (LD100 dose) of *K. pneumoniae*.

THE ROLE OF CHEMOKINES IN MYCOBACTERIA INFECTION

INTRODUCTION

Mycobacterium tuberculosis infections in the lungs elicit an acute or chronic inflammatory cellular infiltrate.[5] Chronic *M. tuberculosis* infections result in the formation of well-defined granulomas. Granulomas are comprised of cells of the monocyte lineage together with mycobacteria-specific T lymphocytes. To date, IL-8 and MCP-1 have been the most extensively studied chemokines in mycobacterial infections owing to the spectrum of their chemotactic activity (neutrophils/T cells and monocytes/T cells, respectively) and the cellular sources of these chemokines (macrophages and parenchymal cells).

CHEMOKINE INDUCTION BY MYCOBACTERIA

Phagocytosis of *M. tuberculosis* by human monocytic cell lines (THP-1 and Mono Mac 6) and peripheral blood monocytes stimulates the production of IL-8 and MCP-1 by these cells.[17,18,32,33] The kinetics

---

Table 8.2. K. pneumoniae CFU in plasma and liver 24 hours post inoculation

Site	Treatment	K. pneumoniae CFU
Plasma	pre-immune	$1.17 \pm 0.21 \times 10^1$
	anti-MIP-2	$2.82 \pm 0.45 \times 10^1$
Liver	pre-immune	$3.47 \pm 0.35 \times 10^1$
	anti-MIP-2	$11.2 \pm 0.18 \times 10^{1*}$
Lung	pre-immune	$1.74 \pm 0.10 \times 10^3$
	anti-MIP-2	$10.1 \pm 0.40 \times 10^{3*}$

Effect of anti-MIP-2 serum on *K. pneumoniae* CFU in plasma, liver, and lung at 24 hour postinoculation. Animals were pretreated with either 0.5 ml rabbit anti-MIP-2 antibody or rabbit pre-immune serum i.p. 2 hours prior to i.t. inoculation. *p < .05 as compared to animals receiving pre-immune serum.

of MCP-1 expression is rapid with MCP-1 mRNA detectable as early as 4 hours postingestion.[33] IL-8 but not MCP-1 expression is stimulus specific, e.g., phagocytosis of latex beads or zymosan results in the expression and secretion of MCP-1 but not IL-8.[32,33] Stimulation of human monocytes or blood mononuclear cells with purified protein derivative of *M. tuberculosis* (PPD) induces both IL-8 and MCP-1.[17,34] Purified recombinant mycobacterial 65 kDa heat shock protein, a major immunogenic protein in the activation of both α-β and γ-δ T cells, also stimulates THP-1 cells to secrete IL-8.[35] Lipoarabinomannan (LAM), a major cell wall associated glycolipid of *M. tuberculosis* and *M. leprae*, can induce the expression of both MCP-1 and MIP-2 by murine bone marrow-derived macrophages (MBMM).[36,37] LAM and other cell wall components (lipomannan and phosphoinositolmannoside) also stimulate IL-8 expression and secretion by human alveolar macrophages in vitro but deacylated-LAM does not.[38] Thus, phagocytosis by monocytic cells of particulates, mycobacteria or mycobacterial components stimulates MCP-1 production whereas phagocytosis specifically of mycobacteria-derived proteins or bacilli is required for stimulation of IL-8 production.

Mycobacterial virulence factors are a determining factor in the production of chemokines by phagocytes. The avirulent H37Ra strain and virulent Erdman strain of *M. tuberculosis* differ in the structure of their LAM. Incubation of MBMM with H37Ra LAM induces increased levels of mRNA for both MCP-1 and MIP-2 while Erdman LAM, even at high concentrations, is unable to stimulate MCP-1 or MIP-2 expression.[36,37] Addition of IFN-γ will stimulate a small amount of MCP-1 production by MBMM cocultured with Erdman LAM.[36] In contrast, IL-8 production by human monocytic cell lines is unaffected by the virulence of the *M. tuberculosis* strain.[17] Genetic differences in host resistance to mycobacterial infection (bcg^r vs. bcg^s strains of mice) appear to play only a minor role in the capacity of MBMM to express MIP-2 or MCP-1 following stimulation with mycobacterial cell wall components from the H37Ra or Erdman strains.[37] Thus, the ability to avoid stimulating chemokine production by phagocytes may be a mechanism by which mycobacteria evade elimination by host defenses.

Cytokines such as TNF, IL-1 and IFN-γ play an important modulatory role in chemokine production following stimulation by *M. tuberculosis* or mycobacterial components. Neutralizing antibodies to TNF or IL-1 block IL-8 production by alveolar macrophages following incubation with mycobacterial cell wall components or phagocytosis of whole organisms.[37] In contrast, IL-8 production by human monocytic cell lines following phagocytosis of *M. tuberculosis* is independent of TNF production.[17] MCP-1 gene expression by human monocytic cell lines under similar conditions is also unaffected by anti-TNF pretreatment or HIV infection.[33] However, IFN-γ augments LAM-induced MCP-1 expression but inhibits LAM-induced MIP-2 expression in MBMM.[36,37] Incubation of these cells with the nitric oxide inhibitor NG-monomethyl-L-arginine blocks MIP-2 expression.[37] Taken together, these observations demonstrate that both cytokines and phagocytic stimuli determine chemokine production by phagocytes in mycobacterial defenses.

CHEMOKINE ACTIVITY AGAINST MYCOBACTERIA IN VITRO AND IN VIVO

IL-8 also may enhance mycobactericidal activity in neutrophils. Intracellular killing of *Mycobacteria fortuitum* by human PMN is augmented by IL-8 via an oxygen-independent mechanism.[26] While IL-8 alone does not stimulate hydrogen peroxide production or phagocytosis, it does prime PMN for enhanced hydrogen peroxide production upon stimulation with opsonized *M. fortuitum*.[26] These observations suggest that IL-8 may play a role in both the recruitment and activation of PMN in mycobacterial infections.

Few studies have addressed the role of chemokines in mycobacterial infections in vivo. In one study, antibodies to purified, nonrecombinant MIP-1 and MIP-2 were effective in reducing neutrophilia in mice during a peritoneal infection with *M. bovis* BCG or *M. avium*.[39] These antibodies were effective even when administered late in the infection, an observation consistent with an in vivo chemotactic activity for these chemokines. In another study, IL-8 levels were significantly elevated in the lavage fluid obtained from patients with pulmonary tuberculosis compared to normal controls.[38] In addition, there was an upregulation of IL-8 mRNA and protein in macrophages obtained by bronchoalveolar lavage of these patients. Overall, these two studies and the previously described in vitro data implicate a significant role for chemokines in the pathogenesis of mycobacterial infections.

ROLE OF CHEMOKINES IN FUNGAL INFECTION

INTRODUCTION

Protection against fungal infection relies predominantly on cell-mediated defenses.[6] This includes innate and acquired immune defenses. While lymphocytes and eosinophils can have direct fungicidal activity, neutrophils and macrophages are the major effector cells in host defense against fungal infection. In addition, antifungal effector cells may be enhanced by or require antigen-specific T cell help. Since cell-mediated defenses depend upon the recruitment and activation of inflammatory cells, chemokines likely play an important role in this process.

However, little is known about the role of chemokines in fungal infections. IL-8, MIP-1α and MCP-1 have been demonstrated in vitro to stimulate a number of cellular events associated with phagocyte activation including production of hydrogen peroxide and release of lysozomal enzymes.[26,40,41] IL-8 also increases neutrophil fungistatic activity against *Candida albicans* in vitro.[42] Although chemokines have received significant attention as mediators of pathologic processes, chemokines are critical mediators of protective inflammatory responses such as seen in infection by the opportunistic fungus *Cryptococcus neoformans*.

CRYPTOCOCCOSIS

C. neoformans is a ubiquitous, encapsulated yeast that is the leading cause of fatal mycosis in AIDS patients.[43] *C. neoformans* is acquired via the respiratory tract and cleared via a T cell-mediated inflammatory response.[44] In the absence of an effective T cell response, a cryptococcal infection will disseminate to the central nervous system resulting in meningitis. Effective clearance of the infection from the alveoli requires both CD4+ and CD8+ T cells. Significant numbers of these lymphocytes are recruited into the lungs, and while the exact function of CD8+ T cells in pulmonary cryptococcosis is unknown, CD4+ T cells are critical for inflammatory cell recruitment and activation.[45] Activated macrophages, neutrophils, NK cells and some T cells have all been demonstrated to kill or growth-inhibit *C. neoformans* in vitro.[43] These leukocytes all play a role in eliminating *C. neoformans* in vivo; however, macrophages (recruited and resident) are generally held to be the major effector cell in the alveoli. Taken together, the recruitment of monocyte/macrophages and CD4+ T cells is crucial for effective pulmonary defense against *C. neoformans* infection.

Strain variation in virulence of *C. neoformans* in mice can serve as a powerful tool in dissecting host-microbe interactions including the mechanism(s) of inflammatory cell recruitment. *C. neoformans* strain 52 and strain 145 differ significantly in virulence.[46,47] Strain 52 is a moderately virulent or "opportunistic" strain while strain 145 is highly virulent. The difference in virulence between these two strains of *C. neoformans* lies in their ability to evade inducing an inflammatory response in the lungs.[46,47] The moderately virulent strain 52 induces a vigorous immune-mediated inflammatory response that progressively clears the infection (Fig. 8.2A). In contrast,

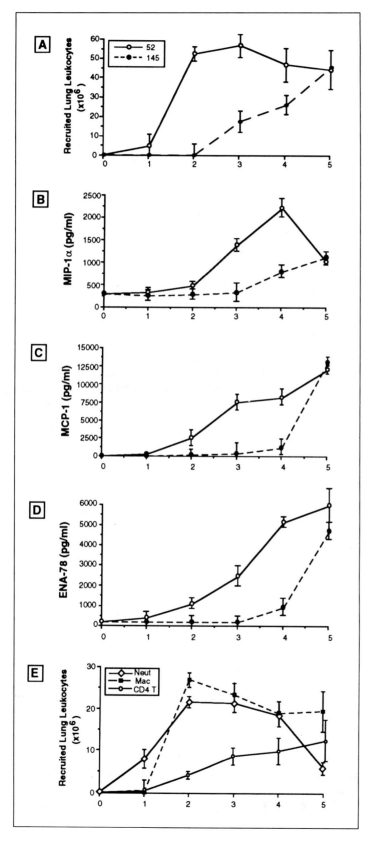

Fig. 8.2. Chemokine production and inflammatory cell recruitment during a pulmonary cryptococcosis infection. (A) Recruitment of leukocytes into the lungs following intratracheal infection with either C. neoformans 52 or C. neoformans 145. leukocytes were isolated and counted following enzymatic digestion of lungs. [Recruited Lung Leukocytes] = [Lung Leukocytes in Infected Lungs]-[Lung Leukocytes in Uninfected Lungs]. (B-D) MIP-1α, MCP-1, and ENA-78 levels in the bronchoalveolar lavage fluid of C. neoformans 52 and C. neoformans 145 infected CBA/J mice. (E) Leukocyte subset (neutrophil, macrophage, and CD4+ T cell) recruitment into the lungs of C. neoformans 52 infected mice. (Adapted from ref. 47.)

the pulmonary inflammatory response to strain 145 is delayed in onset, slower to develop and ineffective in eliminating the infection (Fig. 8.2A). Thus, these two strains of *C. neoformans* provide an opportunity to dissect the events critical for the development of a protective inflammatory response in the lungs.

CHEMOKINE INDUCTION AND LEUKOCYTE RECRUITMENT IN PULMONARY CRYPTOCOCCOSIS

Experimental evidence suggests that one of the major differences in the host response to infection by these two strains of *C. neoformans* is in the production of chemokines. A strain 52 infection induces significant levels of MIP-1α in the alveoli while strain 145 fails to elicit the production of MIP-1α (Fig. 8.2B). Similarly, strain 52 induces significant amounts of MCP-1 while strain 145 does not (Fig. 8.2C). The same is also true for ENA-78 (Fig. 8.2D). Overall, the production of MCP-1, MIP-1α and ENA-78 in the alveoli correlates with inflammatory cell recruitment following pulmonary *C. neoformans* infection.

Analysis and quantification of the different leukocyte subsets in the inflammatory infiltrate of strain 52 infected mice suggests some interesting correlations (Fig. 8.2E). First, the production of the C-C chemokines MCP-1 and MIP-1α correlates with the recruitment of mononuclear but not granulocytic cells into the lungs (Figs. 8.2B and 8.2E). Second, the kinetics of MCP-1 production is most similar to the kinetics of CD4+ T cell recruitment into the lungs (Figs. 8.2C and 8.2E). Finally, the levels of ENA-78 in the bronchoalveolar lavage fluid of strain 52 infected mice do not parallel the recruitment of neutrophils into the lungs of these mice (Figs. 8.2D and 8.2E). Rather, as ENA-78 levels increase, neutrophil recruitment decreases. Although the significance of this observation is unknown, it suggests that ENA-78 plays a role other than as a neutrophil chemotactic factor in this infection. Currently, no such activity has been

described for ENA-78. Taken together, the data in Figure 8.2 demonstrate that strain differences in *C. neoformans*, resulting from differences in the production of virulence factors, are important determinants in the induction of chemokines. These analyses also provide evidence, albeit circumstantial, that chemokines are important mediators of pulmonary inflammatory cell recruitment during a *C. neoformans* infection.

To directly test whether MCP-1 and MIP-1α mediate inflammatory cell recruitment during a *C. neoformans* infection, mice can be treated with neutralizing anti-MCP-1 or anti-MIP-1α specific antisera. This protocol is effective in reducing the bronchoalveolar lavage fluid levels of these two chemokines (Fig. 8.4). Treatment of *C. neoformans* 52 infected mice with anti-MIP-1α antisera significantly decreases the total number of inflammatory cells in the lungs (Fig. 8.3). Anti-MCP-1 serum also significantly reduces the number of inflammatory cells (Fig. 8.3). However, neither antichemokine treatment achieves the same degree of inhibition of leukocyte recruitment as can be achieved by treatment with anti-T cell antibodies (Fig. 8.3). MCP-1 and MIP-1α appear to share overlapping roles in total leukocyte recruitment since either antichemokine alone can decrease inflammation by >50%. While it is not known what effect the combination of anti-MIP-1α plus anti-MCP-1 serum would have on total inflammatory cell numbers, the observation that anti-T cell antibodies completely ablated inflammation suggests that other chemokines are involved in this process and that T cell help is a proximal event in the induction of MIP-1α and MCP-1 production. Both of these antisera also have the predicted effect of increasing the pulmonary burden of *C. neoformans* by 2- to 4-fold as a result of decreasing inflammation (data not shown). In summary, the production of MIP-1α and MCP-1 is critical for the recruitment of inflammatory cells into the lungs following *C. neoformans* infection.

Both anti-MCP-1 or anti-MIP-1α sera appear to be equally efficacious in block-

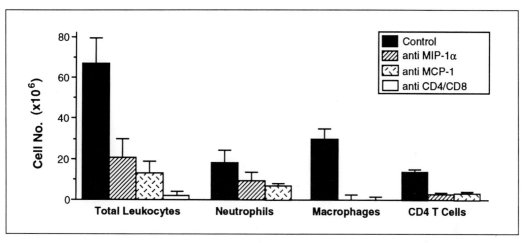

Fig. 8.3. Effect of anti-MCP-1, anti-MIP-1α or anti-CD4/CD8 antibodies on leukocyte recruitment into the lungs of C. neoformans 52 infected mice at 2 weeks postinfection. Leukocytes were isolated and counted following enzymatic digestion of lungs. [Recruited Lung Leukocytes] = [Lung Leukocytes in Infected Lungs]-[Lung Leukocytes in Uninfected Lungs].

ing the recruitment of monocyte/macrophages, neutrophils and CD4⁺ T cells (Fig. 8.3). Both of these antisera completely ablate the recruitment of macrophages into the lungs. In addition, the number of CD4⁺ T cells is reduced by 60-70%. Somewhat surprisingly, neutrophil recruitment is also decreased by 60%. Since MIP-1α has only chemokinetic activity for neutrophils and MCP-1 has no activity for neutrophils, [48,49] the reduction in the number of neutrophils by these antisera is an indirect effect of reducing the number of macrophages and CD4⁺ T cells in the lungs (cellular sources of neutrophil chemotactic factors). Thus, MIP-1α and MCP-1 mediate leukocyte recruitment directly and indirectly during a pulmonary C. neoformans infection.

INFLAMMATORY CYTOKINE CASCADE AND PROXIMAL SIGNALS FOR CHEMOKINE PRODUCTION IN CRYPTOCOCCOSIS

What are the proximal signals for chemokine induction in the lungs during pulmonary cryptococcosis? The first event that happens in the alveoli following intratracheal instillation of C. neoformans is the interaction of the organism with the alveolar macrophage. Preliminary results suggest that coculture of cryptococci with alveolar macrophages in vitro does not yield detectable amounts of MCP-1, MIP-1α or ENA-78 (data not shown). Thus, the phagocytosis of C. neoformans alone is insufficient to elicit chemokine production, suggesting that there must be an event proximal to the induction of chemokines. Alveolar macrophages do produce TNF upon coculture with cryptococci,[47] suggesting that TNF may be a proximal mediator of chemokine induction.

Several lines of evidence support the idea that TNF production is a proximal signal for chemokine expression in pulmonary cryptococcal infection. Due to differences in virulence factor production, a strain 52 infection elicits TNF production in the alveoli while a strain 145 infection does not.[47] Treatment of C. neoformans 52 infected mice with anti-TNF at the onset of infection results in a significant reduction in pulmonary inflammation, the ablation of pulmonary clearance and the dissemination of the infection to the central nervous system (Huffnagle et al, submitted). Thus, the pathogenesis of a strain 52 infection becomes similar to that of a strain 145 infection. More importantly for this discussion, treatment with anti-TNF serum significantly reduces the levels of MCP-1,

Fig. 8.4. Effect of (A) anti-TNF, (B) anti-MIP-1α or (C) anti-MCP-1 neutralizing antibodies on TNF, MIP-1α, and MCP-1 levels in the bronchoalveolar lavage fluid of C. neoformans 52 infected mice at 2 weeks postinfection.

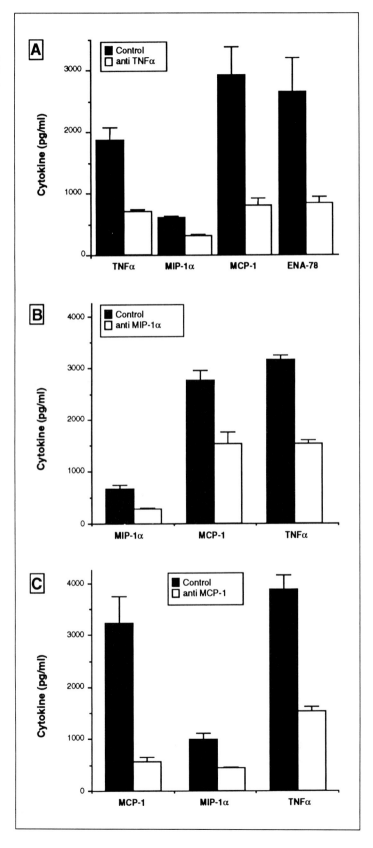

MIP-1α and ENA-78 in the bronchoalveolar lavage fluid of *C. neoformans* strain 52 infected mice (Fig. 8.4A). Anti-TNF treatment also prevents the development of protective T cell mediated immunity, again linking T cell immunity to chemokine production (Huffnagle et al, submitted). These observations suggest that TNF is a crucial proximal signal for chemokine expression in the lungs during a *C. neoformans* infection.

The inflammatory cascade is not a linear progression of events. As illustrated in Figures 8.4B and 8.4C, treatment of *C. neoformans* infected mice with anti-MCP-1 decreases MIP-1α levels in the lungs and treatment with anti-MIP-1α decreases MCP-1 levels (while chemokines all share a high degree of homology, these two antisera have no crossreactivity towards the other chemokine). These results suggest that MCP-1 is required for maximal induction of MIP-1α and MIP-1α for MCP-1 induction. Antichemokine treatment also reduces the level of the "proximal mediating cytokine" TNF. Thus, there are two phases of chemokine induction in the inflammatory response to *C. neoformans*. The first is production of chemokines by resident leukocytes or parenchymal cells. As inflammatory cells begin to accumulate in the lungs, the second phase begins as these cells also serve as rich sources of additional chemokines and proinflammatory cytokines such as TNF. Therefore, chemokine induction during an inflammatory response does not occur in a linear fashion, rather it occurs as a "feedback loop" whereby inflammatory cell recruitment and activation are amplified during the response.

THE ROLE OF IL-10 IN BACTERIAL, MYCOBACTERIAL AND FUNGAL PNEUMONIA

Other chapters in this book discuss some of the events which occur when chemokine production is not regulated in a controlled, orderly fashion. However, in a protective, nonpathologic inflammatory response, little is known about the signals that downregulate chemokine production

allowing inflammation to resolve. Preliminary evidence from cryptococcal and *Klebsiella* pneumonia models suggest that IL-10 may be a major downregulatory signal for chemokine production. Interleukin-10 (IL-10) is a cytokine that was initially identified as an important mediator of Th2-driven immune responses.[50] More recently, this cytokine has been shown to exert anti-inflammatory properties, in part by downregulating the expression of TNF, IL-1 and members of both the C-X-C and C-C chemokine families.[51,52] We have recently shown that endogenously-produced IL-10 plays an important role in dampening the overzealous production of cytokines in endotoxemia, as the passive immunization of mice with anti-IL-10 followed by challenge with sublethal doses of lipopolysaccharide (100 μg) i.p. resulted in a marked increase in the magnitude of TNF-α and MIP-2 expression, enhanced lung injury and substantial increases in mortality.[53] Furthermore, the administration of IL-10 to mice has been shown by others to markedly attenuate endotoxin-induced lethality.[54] However, IL-10-mediated suppression of activating and chemotactic cytokines may be detrimental to the host in the setting of infectious pneumonia, where a vigorous inflammatory response is essential for effective microbial clearance. In support of this premise, IL-10 inhibits macrophage antimicrobial activity in vitro.[55] In addition, the exaggerated expression of IL-10 in patients with leprosy has been associated with persistent and chronic infection,[56] and the inhibition of IL-10 bioactivity in vivo promotes effective clearance of *M. avium-intracellulare* in mice.[57]

To test the hypothesis that IL-10 may have detrimental effects on lung antimicrobial host defense, we first assessed the effect of mrIL-10 on PMN phagocytic activity. Treatment of PMN with IL-10 resulted in a 33% reduction in phagocytosis of *E. coli*, and a maximal 3.9-fold decrease in killing of intracellular *E. coli*, as compared to unstimulated PMN. We next assessed the contribution of IL-10 to effective clearance of bacteria in vivo.[30] Interestingly, inoculation of animals with *K. pneumoniae* resulted in the time-dependent production of both IL-10 mRNA and protein, with maximal expression occurring at 48 hours postinoculation (data not shown). To further define the biologic role of endogenously-produced IL-10 in *Klebsiella* pneumonia, animals were pretreated with rabbit antimurine IL-10 serum 2 hours prior to inoculation with *K. pneumoniae*. Treatment with anti-IL-10 antibodies resulted in a 3.6-, 2.5- and 1.8-fold increase in TNF-α, MIP-2 and MIP-1α protein levels in lung homogenates at 24 hours, as compared to animals receiving pre-immune serum (Fig. 8.5), indicating the expression of activating and chemotactic cytokines in the lung is regulated by endogenous IL-10. Furthermore, passive immunization with anti-IL-10 antibodies resulted in an 3.3-fold reduction in lung *K. pneumoniae* CFU, and a greater than 100-fold decrease in numbers of *K. pneumoniae* cultured from blood at 48 hours. Importantly, survival in anti-IL-10-treated animals inoculated with *K.*

pneumoniae was 40% at 5 days, with 20% of animals surviving past 14 days, whereas no animals in the control group survived to 5 days (data not shown). Collectively, these observations indicate that while the endogenous expression of IL-10 plays an important role in controlling the inappriate secretion of activating and chemotactic cytokines in endotoxemia, IL-10 production appears to be detrimental to the host in the setting of acute bacterial infection.

Additional observations made in murine pulmonary cryptococcosis suggests that endogenously produced IL-10 may impair host anticryptococcal activity in vivo. In a *C. neoformans* strain 145 infection, there is a marked increase in the expression of IL-10 in the lungs within days post-infection (K. McAllister, personal communication). IL-10 expression remains high during the course of a strain 145 infection but does not during a strain 52 infection. Since IL-10 can downregulate TNF production, IL-10 may indirectly (or directly)

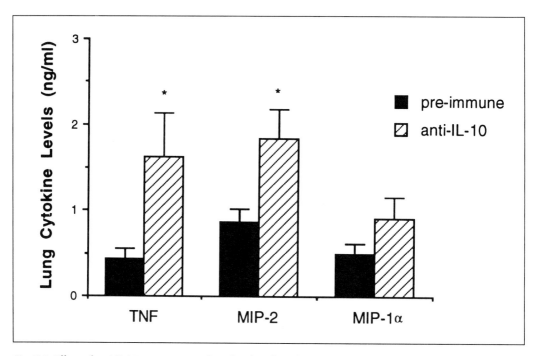

Fig. 8.5. Effect of anti-IL-10 serum on cytokine levels in lung homogenates 24 hours after inoculation with K. pneumoniae. CD-1 mice were passively immunized with 0.5 ml rabbit pre-immune or rabbit antimurine IL-10 serum 2 hours prior to inoculation with K. pneumoniae (10³ CFU).

downregulate chemokine production during a *C. neoformans* strain 145 infection. Further studies to define the role of IL-10 in pulmonary cryptococcosis are ongoing.

CONCLUSIONS

Chemokines are crucial mediators of host defense against bacterial, mycobacterial and fungal infections of the lung. The studies reviewed in this chapter have focused on selected members of the C-X-C and C-C chemokine families. However, the role of other members of the chemokine families in lung host defense against infection has been largely ignored. When one considers the tremendous overlap of biologic activity between members of each chemokine family, it is not at all difficult to speculate that these other chemokines may also participate in host defense against infection. A better understanding of the role of chemokines in lung infection may allow for the immunologic manipulation of pro- and/or anti-inflammatory cytokine expression in vivo, which may serve as an important adjuvant therapy in the treatment of immunocompromised and/or immunocompetent patients with severe bacterial, mycobacterial or fungal pneumonia.

ACKNOWLEDGMENT

This research was supported in part by National Institutes of Health grants 1P50HL46487, HL50057, HL02401, HL31693, HL35276, HL52800, HL51082, AA10571, a Department of Veterans Affairs Merit Research Award and a Parker B. Francis Award from the Francis Families Foundation, Kansas City, MO.

REFERENCES

1. Nelson S, Mason CM, Knolls J et al. Pathophysiology of pneumonia. Clin Chest Med 1995; 16:1-12.
2. Onofrio JM, Toews GB, Lipscomb MF. Granulocyte-alveolar macrophage interaction in the pulmonary clearance of *Staphylococcus aureus*. Am Rev Respir Dis 1983; 127: 335-342.
3. Toews GB, Gross GN, Pierce AK. The relationship of inoculum size to lung bacterial clearance and phagocytic cell response in mice. Am Rev Respir Dis 1979; 120:559-566.
4. Horwitz MA. Phagocytosis of microorganisms. Rev Infect Dis 1982; 4:104-123.
5. DesPrez RM, Heim CR. *Mycobacterium tuberculosis*. In: Mandell GL, Douglas RG, Bennett JE, eds. Principles and Practice of Infectious Diseases. 3rd ed. New York: Churchill Livingstone, 1990:877-1905.
6. Cox RA, ed. Immunology of the Fungal Diseases. Boca Raton: CRC Press, 1989.
7. Nakano Y, Onozuka K, Yerada Y et al. Protective effect of recombinant tumor necrosis factor-α in murine salmonellosis. J Immunol 1990; 144:1935-1941.
8. Kolls JK, Nelson S, Summer WR. Recombinant cytokines and pulmonary host defense. Am J Med Sci 1993; 306:330-335.
9. Nelson S. Overview of granulocyte colony-stimulating factor in bacterial infections in the nonneutropenic host. Clin Infect Dis 1991; 143S:398-410.
10. Oppenheim JJ, Zachariae COC, Mukaida N et al. Properties of the novel proinflammatory supergene intercrine cytokine family. Annu Rev Immunol 1991; 9:617-647.
11. Standiford TJ, Arenberg DA, Danforth JM et al. Lipotheichoic acid induces the secretion of interleukin-8 from human blood monocytes: A cellular and molecular analysis. Inf Immun 1994; 62:119-125.
12. Danforth JM, Strieter RM, Arenberg DA et al. Induction of MIP-1α in-vitro and in-vivo: The role of lipoteichoic acid. J Clin Immunol Immunopath 1995; 74:77-83.
13. Luini W, Rossi, M N, Licciardello L et al. Chemotactic cytokine gene expression and production induced in human monocytes by membrane proteoglycans from klebsiella pneumoniae. J Immunopharmac 1991; 13(6):631-637.
14. Soell M, Diab M, Haan-Archipoff G et al. Capsular polysaccharide types 5 and 8 of *Staphylococcus aureus* bind specifically to human epithelial (KB) cells, endothelial cells, and monocytes and induces release of cytokines. Infect Immun 1995; 63:1380-1386.
15. Eckmann L, Kagnoff MF, Fierer J. Epithelial cells secrete the chemokine interleukin-8 in response to bacterial entry. Infect

Immun 1993; 61:4569-4574.

16. Bazzoni F, Cassatella MA, Rossi F et al. Phagocytosing neutrophils produce and release high amounts of the neutrophil-activating peptide 1/interleukin 8. J Exp Med 1991; 173:771-774.

17. Friedland JS, Shattock RJ, Griffin GE. Phagocytosis of *mycobacterium tuberculosis* or particulate stimuli by human monocytic cells induces equivalent monocyte chemotactic protein-1 gene expression. Cytokine 1993; 5:150-156.

18. Kasahara K, Tobe T, Tomita M et al. Selective expression of monocyte chemotactic and activating factor/monocyte chemoattractant protein 1 in human blood monocytes by Mycobacterium tuberculosis. J Infect Dis 1994; 170:1238-1247.

19. Rodriguez JL, Miller CG, DeForge E et al. Local production of interleukin-8 is associated with nosocomial pneumonia. J Trauma 1992; 33:74-81.

20. Antony V, Godbey SW, Kunkel SL et al. Recruitment of inflammatory cells to the pleural space. Chemotactic cytokines, IL-8, and monocyte chemotactic peptide-1 in human pleural fluids. J Immun 1993; 151(12):7216-7223.

21. Lehrer RI, Ganz T. Antimicrobial polypeptides of human neutrophils. Blood 1990; 76:2169-2181.

22. Hostoffer RW, Krukovets I, Berger M. Enhancement by tumor necrosis factor-α of Fcα receptor expression and IgA-mediated superoxide generation and killing of peudomonas aeruginosa by polymorphonuclear leukocytes. J Infect Dis 1994; 170:82-87.

23. Zwierzina H, Holzinger I, Gaggl S et al. Recombinant human interleukin-8 restores function in neutrophils from patients with myelodysplastic syndromes without stimulating myeloid progenitor cells. Scand J Immunol 1993; 37(3):322-328.

24. Wolpe SD, Sherry B, Juers D et al. Identification and characterization of macrophage inflammatory protein 2. Proc Natl Acad Sci 1989; 86:612-616.

25. Wolpe SD, Cerami A. Macrophage inflammatory proteins 1 and 2: Members of a novel superfamily of cytokines. FASEB J 1989;

3:2565-2573.

26. Nibbering PH, Pos O, Stevenhagen A et al. Interleukin-8 enhances nonoxidative intracellular killing of *mycobacterium fortuitum* by human granulocytes. Infect Immun 1993; 6:3111-3116.

27. Nakano Y, Kasahara T, Mukaida N et al. Protection against lethal bacterial infection in mice by monocyte-chemotactic and -activating factor. Infect Immun 1994; 62:377-383.

28. Vogels MTE, Lindley IJD, Curfs JHAJ et al. Effects of interleukin-8 on nonspecific resistance to infection in neutropenic and normal mice. Antimicrob Agents Chem 1993; 37:276-280.

29. Bakker Woudenberg IAJM, Lokerse AF, ten Kate MT et al. Liposomes with prolonged blood circulation and selective localization in *Klebsiella pneumoniae*-infected lung tissue. J Infect Dis 1993; 168:164-171.

30. Greenberger MG, Strieter RM, Kunkel SL et al. Anti-interleukin-10 antibodies increase survival in a murine model of Klebsiella pneumonia. J Immunol 1995; 155:722-729.

31. Greenberger MG, Strieter RM, Kunkel SL et al. Neutralization of macrophage inflammatory protein-2 attenuates neutrophil influx and bacterial clearance in murine Klebsiella pneumonia. J Infect Dis (in press).

32. Friedland JS, Shattock RJ, Johnson JD et al. Differential cytokine gene expression and secretion after phagocytosis by a human monocytic cell line of Toxoplasma gondii compared with Mycobacterium tuberculosis. Clin Exp Immunol 1993 91:282-286.

33. Friedland JS, Shattock RJ, Griffin GE. Phagocytosis of Mycobacterium tuberculosis or particulate stimuli by human monocytic cells induces equivalent monocyte chemotactic protein-1 gene expression. Cytokine 1993; 5:150-156.

34. Wilkinson PC, Newman I. Identification of IL-8 as a locomotor attractant for activated human lymphocytes in mononuclear cell cultures with anti-CD3 or purified protein derivative of Mycobacterium tuberculosis. J Immunol 1992; 149:2689-2694.

35. Friedland JS, Shattock R, Remick DG et al. Mycobacterial 65-kDa heat shock protein induces release of proinflammatory

cytokines from human monocytic cells. Clin Exp Immunol 1993; 91:58-62.

36. Roach TI, Barton CH, Chatterjee D et al. Macrophage activation: lipoarabinomannan from avirulent and virulent strains of Mycobacterium tuberculosis differentially induces the early genes c-fos, KC, JE, and tumor necrosis factor-alpha. J Immunol 1993; 150:1886-1896.

37. Roach TI, Chatterjee D, Blackwell JM. Induction of early-response genes KC and JE by mycobacterial lipoarabinomannans: regulation of KC expression in murine macrophages by Lsh/Ity/Bcg (candidate Nramp). Infect Immun 1994; 62: 1176-1184.

38. Zhang Y, Broser M, Cohen H et al. Enhanced interleukin-8 release and gene expression in macrophages after exposure to Mycobacterium tuberculosis and its components. J Clin Invest 1995; 95:586-592.

39. Appelberg R. Interferon-gamma (IFN-γ) and macrophage inflammatory proteins (MIP)-1 and -2 are involved in the regulation of the T cell-dependent chronic peritoneal neutrophilia of mice infected with mycobacteria. Clin Exp Immunol 1992; 89:269-273.

40. Rollins BJ, Walz A, Baggiolini M. Recombinant human MCP-1/JE induces chemotaxis, calcium flux, and the respiratory burst in human monocytes. Blood 1991; 78: 1112-1116.

41. Fahey T, Tracey K, Tekamp-Olson P et al. Macrophage inflammatory protein 1 modulates macrophage function. J Immunol 1992; 148:2764-2769.

42. Djeu JY, Matsushima K, Oppenheim JJ et al. Functional activation of human neutrophils by recombinant monocyte-derived neutrophil chemotactic factor/IL-8. J Immunol 1990; 144:2205-2210.

43. Murphy JW. Cryptococcosis. In: Cox RA, ed. Immunology of the Fungal Diseases. Boca Raton: CRC Press, 1989:93-138.

44. Huffnagle GB, Lipscomb MF. Animal model of human disease: Pulmonary cryptococcosis. Am J Pathol 1992; 141: 1517-1520.

45. Huffnagle GB, Lipscomb MF, Lovchik JA et al. The role of CD4+ and CD8+ T cells in the protective inflammatory response to a pulmonary cryptococcal infection. J Leuko Biol 1994; 55:35-42.

46. Curtis JL, Huffnagle GB, Chen GH et al. Experimental murine pulmonary cryptococcosis: Differences in pulmonary inflammation and lymphocyte recruitment induced by two encapsulated strains of *Cryptococcus neoformans*. Lab Invest 1994; 71:113-126.

47. Huffnagle GB, Chen GH, Curtis JL et al. Downregulation of the afferent phase of T cell-mediated pulmonary inflammation and immunity by a high melanin-producing strain of *Cryptococcus neoformans*. J Immunol 1995; 155(in press).

48. Beall CJ, Mahajan S, Kolattukudy PE. Conversion of monocyte chemoattractant protein-1 into a neutrophil attractant by substitution of two amino acids. J Biol Chem 1992; 267:3455-3459.

49. VanOtteren GM, Standiford TJ, Kunkel SL et al. Expression and regulation of macrophage inflammatory protein-1 alpha by murine alveolar and peritoneal macrophages. Am J Respir Cell Mol Biol 1994; 10:8-15.

50. Howard M, O'Garra A, Ishida H et al. Biological properties of interleukin 10. J Clin Immunol 1992; 12:239-247.

51. Fiorentino DF, Zlotnik A, Mosmann TR et al. IL-10 inhibits cytokine production by activated macrophages. J Immunol 1991; 147:3815-3822.

52. Kasama T, Strieter RM, Lukacs NW et al. Regulation of neutrophil-derived chemokine expression by IL-10. J Immunol 1994; 152:3559-3569.

53. Standiford TJ, Strieter RM, Lukacs NW et al. Neutralization of IL-10 increases lethality in endotoxemia: Cooperative effects of macrophage inflammatory protein-2 and tumor necrosis factor. J Immunol 1995; 155:2222-2229.

54. Howard M, Muchamuel T, Andrade S et al. Interleukin 10 protects mice from lethal endotoxemia. J Exp Med 1993; 177: 1205-1208.

55. Oswald IP, Wynn TA, Sher A et al. Interleukin 10 inhibits macrophage microbicidal activity by blocking endogenous production of tumor necrosis factor α required as a costimulatory factor for interferon γ-induced activation. Proc Natl Acad

Sci USA 1992; 89:8676-8680.

56. Sieling PA, Abrams JS, Yamamura M et al. Immunosuppressive roles for IL-10 and IL-4 in human infection: In vitro modulation of T cell responses in leprosy. J Immunol 1993; 150:5501-5510.

57. Bermudez L, Champsi J. Infection with *Mycobaterium avium* induces production of interleukin-10 (IL-10), and administration of anti-IL-10 antibody is associated with enhanced resistance to infection in mice. Infect Immun 1993; 61:3093-3097.

================= CHAPTER 9 =================

THE ROLE OF CHEMOKINES IN GRANULOMATOUS DISEASES

Nicholas W. Lukacs and Stephen W. Chensue

INTRODUCTION

Granulomatous inflammation is characterized by an intense accumulation of leukocytes around an inciting agent, which can be either infectious or noninfectious in nature.[1,2] The cellular constituents of granulomas include both immune and nonimmune cell populations including macrophages, lymphocytes, mast cells, epithelioid cells and fibroblasts. In addition, multinucleated giant cells are characteristic in delayed type hypersensitivity granulomas, as are eosinophils in chronic parasitic induced granulomas (Table 9.1). All of these cell populations likely contribute to the overall pathology and local tissue damage associated with granulomatous reactions. The residual fibrosis which accompanies the resolution phase of the granuloma results in irreversible tissue damage and possible organ dysfunction. Noninfectious foreign body type granulomas can be induced by environmental or industrial agents such as talc, silica or beryllium, while infectious granulomas are induced by bacterial (tubercle bacilli), fungal, viral or parasitic (*Leishmania/Schistosoma*) infestation. In addition, other classes of granulomatous inflammation, such as sarcoid and Wegener's, have been classified as nonspecific immune type reactions (Table 9.1). These latter responses have unknown etiology but have, however, classical immune-associated characteristics, i.e., high rate of cellular turnover and cytokine producing lymphoid cells. The treatment strategies for infectious lesions have been aimed at the elimination of the infectious agent, while the vast majority of noninfectious granuloma formations have been treated with glucocorticoids to nonspecifically downregulate the inflammatory response. The use of glucocorticoids for long periods of time can immunocompromise the patient and impair the ability of the immune system to resist opportunistic infections. The limited options for treatment largely reflect the paucity of information concerning

Chemokines in Disease, edited by Alisa E. Koch and Robert M. Strieter.
© 1996 R.G. Landes Company.

Table 9.1. Granuloma formation around infectious and nonoinfectious agents

Class of Granuloma	Leukocyte Infiltrate
Foriegn Body	
Talc	Mononuclear cells
Silica	Syncytial Giant Cells
Berylium	
Infectious (DTH)	
Bacterial (Tuberculoid)	Monocytes, Lymphocytes
Parasitic (Schistosome)	Eosinophils, Mast Cells
Fungal	Langerhan's Giant Cell
Viral	
Undefined Immune	
Sarcoid	Monocytes, Lymphocytes
Wegener	Langerhan's Giant Cell

the mechanisms which are operative during the formation of granulomas.

One of the key issues in inflammation has been the determination of mechanisms which are involved in leukocyte recruitment and activation at the site of the lesion. Historically, leukocyte recruitment induced by the release of chemotactic mediators such as C5a, PAF, LTB4, etc. was a widely accepted explanation. However, these mediators demonstrated little specificity for the cells recruited and could not explain the presence of selected leukocyte populations in particular diseases. In contrast to these relatively nonspecific leukocyte recruiters, there is a recently described class of chemotactic proteins that appear to have specificity for particular subsets of leukocytes which enter inflamed tissues. The C-X-C family of chemokines, typified by IL-8, appears to be most prominently involved in acute inflammation and neutrophil recruitment, while the C-C family of chemokines, typified by MCP-1, appears to be involved in chronic inflammation and the recruitment of monocytes, lymphocytes, eosinophils and basophil/mast cell populations.[3,4] As reviewed in other chapters of this book, chemokines are now known to be involved in multiple areas of acute and chronic inflammation. In fact, chemokines appear to be central molecules which me-

diate the specificity of the leukocyte infiltrates. Given that chronic inflammation (monocytes, lymphocytes, basophils and eosinophils) is involved in the formation of granulomas, the focus has been on the role of the C-C chemokine family in granuloma formation. The following sections will discuss the production, regulation, cellular source and specific contribution of C-C family chemokines in selected types of granulomas.

CYTOKINE REGULATION OF GRANULOMA FORMATION

Granuloma formation occurs during many disease states; however, the intensity and the cellular constituency of granulomas can vary considerably. For example, foreign body type granulomas are predominantly composed of mononuclear phagocytic cells and large syncytial giant cells, whereas granulomas of an infectious nature may contain large numbers of lymphocytes, eosinophils and mast cells as well as compact Langerhan's-type multinucleated giant cells (Table 9.1). The soluble signals, or cytokines, which are produced during the development of these various lesions likely determine the cell populations which are recruited to the site of the lesion as well as the development of pathological fibrosis (Table 9.2). The differential cellular

Table 9.2. Cytokine regulation of granuloma formation

Granuloma Type	Activating Cytokines	Fibrotic Responses
Foriegn Body	IL-1, TNF	Mild
Bacterial (Th1 Type)	IL-1, TNF, IL-12, IFN-γ	Moderate
Parasitic (Th2 Type)	IL-1, TNF, IL-4, IL-5, IL-10	Severe

makeup of these lesions may be suggestive of distinct patterns of cytokine and chemokine production.

Some of the most potent classes of inflammatory cytokines have been identified as the early response cytokines IL-1 and TNF. These pleuripotent cytokines have the ability to regulate physiological parameters such as fever, malaise and appetite during inflammation, as well as to enhance production of a number of additional inflammatory cytokines and chemokines and to promote the expression of adhesion molecules necessary for cellular extravasation into tissue.[5] Studies of TNF production during schistosome egg and tuberculoid granuloma formation indicates that the production of this potent inflammatory cytokine may have a significant role during the development of the lesion.[6,7] Most convincingly, in vivo TNF depletion inhibits mycobacterial granulomas,[8] while exogenous administration of TNF into nonresponsive SCID mice reconstituted the ability of these mice to mount a circumovum schistosome egg granulomatous response.[9] This latter response in SCID mice appeared to be similar to a foreign body type reaction, consisting primarily of mononuclear cells.

The role of IL-1 in granulomatous lesions has also been investigated. Increased mRNA expression and production of IL-1 protein has been associated with the development and severity of several types of granulomatous diseases, including sarcoidosis,[10] schistosomiasis[11] and leishmaniasis,[12] as well as with foreign body reactions. The regulation of IL-1 during granuloma formation is crucial for controlling the severity of the lesion. The exogenous administration of IL-1[11] or the neutralization of endogenous IL-1 receptor antagonist[13] both accelerated lesion development and increased lesion severity.

Other cytokines appear to also regulate the development and resolution of granuloma formation. Immune-associated cytokines/lymphokines, such as interferon-γ (IFN-γ), IL-4, IL-10 and IL-12, have a striking ability to regulate the granuloma formation, leukocyte subset infiltration, chemokine production and possibly endstage fibrosis of the developing lesions. These lymphokines can be classified as Th1 (type 1) or Th2 (type 2) associated cytokines.[14] The type 1 cytokines IL-12 and IFN-γ appear to be associated primarily with intracellular infectious agents, such as *Mycobacterium*, which depend upon intracellular killing by phagocytic cells to clear the infection. In intracellular infections the ability to produce type 1 cytokines dictates the success of clearance of the agent and granuloma resolution.[15] The type 2 cytokines IL-4 and IL-10 are associated most closely with parasite-elicited responses, such as that observed in schistosomiasis[16] and leishmaniasis.[17] The production of Th2 type cytokines during intracellular infections may promote prolonged granuloma formation and increased lesion size, leading to exacerbated fibrotic responses. Utilizing a functional analysis of granuloma formation, laboratories have begun to classify granulomatous diseases by the pattern of cytokines produced during the response. This chapter will attempt to outline the role of particular chemokines in granuloma formation and the differential regulation within various types of lesions and foreign body, Th1 and Th2 type responses.

CHEMOKINE PRODUCTION WITHIN FOREIGN BODY GRANULOMAS

The initiation of foreign body granulomas is a response which lacks antigen specific lymphocyte participation. These lesions are primarily observed in the lungs and induced by inhaled or injected substances such as talc or silica. Foreign body granulomas are usually self-limited and have little tissue damage associated with them. However, some forms of foreign body lesions, such as silica-induced granulomas, have considerable associated tissue injury, with accompanying leukocyte recruitment and fibrosis. The leukocyte population which primarily infiltrates these lesions has been identified as mononuclear phagocytes. The characterization of these lesions, and of the cytokines and chemokines which initiate and maintain the limited cellular influx, have been studied using animal models.

In a yeast wall glucan rat model of foreign body granulomatous inflammation, a significant mononuclear cell infiltrate has been demonstrated to be associated with the expression and production of MCP-1.[18,19] Neutralization of MCP-1 in the glucan-challenged, treated animals significantly decreased the size of the lesion and the intensity of the mononuclear cell infiltrate into the lung.[19] The regulation of MCP-1 and mononuclear cell recruitment to the lesions appears to be via IL-1β and TNF-α production.[20] A significant attenuation of the glucan-induced lesion was mediated by passive immunization of animals with anti-IL-1 or anti-TNF-α. The expression and production of MCP-1 was also significantly attenuated when the IL-1 and TNF were neutralized in vivo, suggesting the presence of cytokine cascades leading to the accumulation of mononuclear cell populations.

In a second model of foreign body granuloma, the growth and chemokine profile of an inert sepharose bead embolized to the lungs was characterized. The induced lesion was short lived, peaking at 2-3 days, and composed of primarily mononuclear phagocytes. The resolution of the lesion appears to be complete, with little or no tissue damage. The production of chemokines during the development of this lesion was very modest. Increases in MIP-1α were observed at day 4 and day 8, while MCP-1 production was elevated at days 2 through 8 and appeared to correspond to the early accumulation of monocytes around the foreign body (unpublished data). These results were consistent with the data reported above for the more active yeast wall glucan granuloma formation.

DELAYED TYPE HYPERSENSITIVITY GRANULOMA FORMATION

The formation of delayed-type hypersensitivity granulomas occurs during several disease states, and is initiated by antigen-specific mechanisms which mediate chronic infiltration of leukocyte populations within tissues. The resulting lesion often resolves, leaving behind a fibrosed, dysfunctional region within the organ. The mechanisms of leukocyte recruitment and the role of chemokines in these chronic DTH granulomas likely dictate the severity of the end-stage fibrotic response. In recent studies, the presence of elevated levels of chemokines IL-8 and MCP-1 in the BAL fluid of patients with pulmonary sarcoidosis suggested a possible role for chemokines in human disease progression.[21] In addition, corresponding chemotaxis assays demonstrated that levels of IL-8 and MCP-1 correlated directly with the ability of the BAL samples to induce neutrophil and monocyte chemotaxis, respectively. Both chemokines have been implicated in T lymphocyte chemotaxis, suggesting that they may have a role in directing the recruitment of both T cell and monocyte components to the lesion. The interaction of monocytic and lymphocytic cell populations within the lesion likely lend to the chronicity of the response. Clinical studies examining the presence of chemokines during disease suggest that they may have a role in the inflammation and recruitment of leukocytes. However, longitudinal studies in patient populations have been very difficult due to the complications of characterizing, controlling and sampling experimental populations.

The role of chemokines in DTH granulomatous responses has been more clearly defined using animal models. A mouse model of pulmonary granuloma formation using schistosome parasite eggs has been informative for defining mechanisms of leukocyte recruitment and chemokine regulation. In this model noninfectious *S. mansoni* parasite eggs are embolized into the lungs of naive or sensitized mice.[1] The pulmonary deposited eggs secrete soluble antigen (SEA) which induces a T cell-mediated circumovum response, characterized by intense cellular recruitment, mononuclear cell accumulation and development of fibrosing granulomatous lesions. In the primary response in naive mice, granulomas develop which appear to be initially mediated by a Th1, IFN-γ response and which peak in size 16 days postembolization.[22,23] In secondary granuloma development in SEA-sensitized mice, the inflammation is mediated by a Th2, IL-4 type response.[16,24] The secondary lesion is accelerated, peaking at 4-8 days and resolving by 16 days postembolization.[24] The primary granuloma is characterized by mononuclear cell accumulation, whereas the secondary granuloma formation has an additional intense eosinophil infiltration (>50%). These two distinct phases of granuloma formation provided the unique opportunity to examine the differential role of chemokines during the progression of inflammation in lesions with distinct cytokine profiles.

Since the chronic schistosome egg granulomas primarily induce mononuclear and eosinophilic cell accumulation, the principal thrust of our research has been examining the role of C-C chemokines. MIP-1α has been shown to be chemotactic for monocytes, T lymphocytes and eosinophils, which can be found within the primary and/or secondary granuloma. Our initial observations demonstrated significant induction of MIP-1α mRNA in the primary and secondary lesions which corresponded to the growth patterns of granuloma formation.[25] The production of MIP-1α protein from isolated granulomas demonstrated a progressive increase in primary lesions until 16 days, while isolated secondary lesions had accelerated production of MIP-1α following egg deposition and initial granuloma formation. In vivo neutralization of MIP-1α during primary and secondary granuloma formation demonstrated differential results. During primary granuloma formation the size of the lesion was reduced by over 60%, whereas secondary granuloma formation was reduced by only 15-20%. Immunohistochemical localization of MIP-1α identified mononuclear phagocytes as the primary source of MIP-1α. However, granuloma fibroblasts can also produce C-C chemokines in response to multiple stimuli,[26] indicating that nonimmune cells may substantially contribute to the chronic recruitment of leukocytes to the granuloma. Interestingly, the production of MIP-1α can be induced by ICAM-1-mediated adhesion during monocyte-stromal cell interactions.[27] Correspondingly, primary granuloma formation was shown to be mediated by TNF-induced ICAM-1 expression.[28] These latter studies suggest a strong interrelationship between adhesion molecules and chemokine production, which together promote the initiation and growth of the granuloma. Altogether, these results suggest that MIP-1α plays a greater role in leukocyte recruitment during primary, type 1 cytokine-mediated, than in the secondary, type 2 cytokine-mediated granuloma.

The role of another C-C chemokine, MCP-1, in granuloma formation was also examined. Murine MCP-1 (JE) was first described as an immediate early gene in fibroblast activation.[29] MCP-1 is chemotactic for monocytes, lymphocytes and basophils and can be upregulated in a number of immune and nonimmune cell populations by IL-1 and TNF. Interestingly,

IL-4, a Th2 type cytokine, can stimulate MCP-1 production from endothelial and smooth muscle cells.[30] When the expression of MCP-1 mRNA was examined in *S. mansoni*-induced lung granulomas, a much stronger expression was observed in lungs with secondary, versus those with primary, granulomas.[31] The production of MCP-1 in isolated egg granulomas demonstrated very high constitutive levels of MCP-1 in secondary lesions, which correlated with the size of the Th2 cytokine-mediated lesion. Interestingly, when MCP-1 was neutralized in vivo, there was no evidence of diminished formation of primary lesions, but a significant decrease was observed in secondary lesions. When paraffin lung tissue sections were immunostained for MCP-1, the predominant expression of MCP-1 appeared to be within mononuclear phagocytes and vascular smooth muscle cells within the secondary lesions. The MCP-1 and MIP-1α neutralization results were novel observations, which suggested that specific chemokines were operative at certain stages of the immune response, possibly dependent upon the cytokine profile expressed (Th1 vs. Th2 type cytokines). In addition, the immunolocalization of chemokines in specific cell populations, leukocyte or stromal cell, suggests that certain cell types contribute at different phases of granuloma formation. In recent studies in our laboratory, IL-10, a Th2 cytokine with immunosuppressive activity, had potent suppressive activity on leukocyte-derived chemokines, but no effect on stromal cell-derived chemokine production (unpublished data). The latter results suggest a prominent role for stromal-derived chemokines within chronic lesions, leading to sustained leukocyte recruitment. These observations may extend to other diseases with distinct phases or cytokine profile associations, and indicate a differential role of chemokines during disease development and granuloma formation.

In another model of granuloma inflammation, mice were immunized with live *Mycobacteria* and then challenged with mycobacterial antigen (PPD) coated beads by embolization to the lungs.[32] The resulting granulomas had a Th1 cytokine phenotype, characterized by IFN-γ but no detectable IL-4. Interestingly, unlike the Th2 type cytokine-mediated schistosome egg granulomas, these lesions do not have a significant amount of fibrosis related with their development and resolution. The production of MIP-1α and MCP-1 has also been monitored within these lesions. Both of these cytokines were demonstrably upregulated during the development of the lesion, beginning at day 2 and gradually rising through day 8 of granuloma development. However, in vivo depletion studies using antibodies specific for either MIP-1α or MCP-1 demonstrated that neither chemokine had a significant role in granuloma development. The fact that specific neutralization of MIP-1α and MCP-1 did not reduce the size of the Th1 type PPD lesion suggests that other chemoattractants, perhaps for instance RANTES, may play a much larger role in tuberculoid-like granulomatous inflammation.

Other chemokines may also be differentially regulated during different types of granulomatous inflammation. RANTES, a C-C chemokine, can induce the migration of mononuclear cells and eosinophils into a site of inflammation.[33,34] The production of RANTES by epithelial cell populations can be inhibited by IL-4 and IL-10 (Th2 type cytokines), whereas IL-1, TNF and IFN-γ promote the expression of RANTES.[35] This pattern of regulation is consistent with a Th1 type response and may relegate RANTES to a role in endotoxin and Th1 cytokine-mediated inflammation. In contrast, another C-C chemokine, C10, was not induced by IL-1 or TNF, but was induced by IL-4 in macrophages, suggesting a Th2 cytokine correlation.[36] These classifications, however, must be considered carefully, as most disease states have rarely been described as strict Th1 or Th2 type inflammations. In fact, type 1 and type 2 cytokines likely collaborate in responses by dictating different aspects of cellular recruitment and activation.

The Role of Chemokines in Granuloma Activation

Chemokines produced during granulomatous inflammation may also have activational effects on the development of DTH reactions. MIP-1α has been shown to induce a prostaglandin-independent fever when injected in vivo and can induce the production of early response cytokines IL-1 and TNF in macrophage cultures.[37] As previously discussed in this chapter, both IL-1 and TNF have been shown to potentially contribute to granuloma formation. In addition, recent data has demonstrated that MIP-1α can induce ICAM-1 expression on vascular endothelial cells (Standiford et al, unpublished data), strongly linking chemokines and adhesion molecule expression. These latter studies suggest that the inflammatory activities of MIP-1α by themselves may constitute a potent cytokine contributing to the initiation and maintenance of the granulomatous reaction. MCP-1 also appears to have activational properties associated with inflammation. MCP-1 can directly activate monocytes and induce the expression of leukocyte integrins CD11b and CD11c on their surface and additionally induce the production of IL-1 and IL-6.[38] In the schistosome egg granuloma lesions discussed above, significant levels of both MCP-1 and MIP-1α were detected during the development of the lesions. Other chemokines may also have the ability to induce cytokine production as well as adhesion molecule expression. C-X-C chemokines may contribute to the development of the granulomatous lesions through novel mechanisms of activation. Recent observations indicate that the C-X-C cytokine family has strong angiogenic properties which may be critical to the development of the large fibrosing lesions observed in many diseases[39] (see chapter by Koch and Strieter). The alternative functions of chemokines during disease have only begun to be explored. Future investigations should reveal new and interesting roles for chemokines and their activational properties during disease development and physiologic homeostasis.

Table 9.3. Chemokine production and participation during experimental granuloma

Granuloma Induction	Chemokine Production	Depletion Success
Yeast Wall	MCP-1	yes
Sepharose Bead	MIP-1α	
	MCP-1	?
Schistosome egg		
Primary (Th1)	MIP-1	yes
	MCP-1	no
Secondary (Th2)	MIP-1	Modest
	MCP-1	yes
Tuberculoid (Th1)	MIP-1	no
	MCP-1	no
	RANTES	??

SUMMARY

Chemokines can induce the recruitment of specific leukocyte populations as well as activation of inflammatory cytokines and expression of adhesion molecules. Whether specific chemokines have preferential expression patterns and specific roles during various granulomatous diseases should be considered. The results from experimental models discussed in this chapter suggest that there may be particular chemokines which participate in specific lesions (Table 9.3). The targeting of chemokine molecules for therapeutic intervention during inflammation may be ideal for controlling chronic responses. However, the production patterns and function of the various chemokines during specific disease states must be analyzed and identified to fully understand their functions.

References

1. Boros DL. Immunopathology of *Schistosoma mansoni* infection. Clin Microbiol Rev 1989; 2:250-269.
2. Kunkel SL, Strieter RM, Lukacs NW, Chensue SW. Molecular aspects of granulomatous inflammation. EOS J Immunol Immunophar 1994;14:71-77.

3. Oppenheim JJ, Zachariae COC, Mukaida N, Matsushima K. Properties of the novel proinflammatory "intercrine" cytokine family. Annu Rev Immunol 1991; 9:617-634.

4. Schall TJ, Bacon K, Bacon KJ, Toy KJ, Goeddel DV. Selective attraction of monocytes and T lymphocytes of the memory phenotype by cytokine RANTES. Nature 1990; 347:669-671.

5. Beutler B, Cerami A. Tumor necrosis factor, cachexia, shock and inflammation: a common mediator. Annu Rev Biochem 1988; 57:505-545.

6. Kindler V, Sappino AP, Grau GE, Piguet PF, Vassalli P. The inducing role of tumor necrosis factor in the development of bactericidal granulomas during BCG infection. Cell 1989; 56:731-740.

7. Joseph AL, Boros DL. TNF plays a role in Schistosoma mansoni egg-induced granulomatous inflammation. J Immunol 1993; 151:5461-5468.

8. Tumang MC, Keogh C, Moldawer LL, Helfgott DC, Teitelbaum R, Hariprashad J, Murray HW. Role and effect of TNF-alpha in experimental visceral leishmaniasis. J Immunol 1994; 153:768-775.

9. Amiri P, Locksley RM, Parslow TG, Sadick M, Rector E, Ritter D, McKerrow JH. Tumor Necrosis Factor-α restores granulomas and induces parasite egg laying in schistosome-infected SCID mice. Nature 1992; 356:604-610.

10. Rolfe MW, Standiford TJ, Kunkel SL, Burdick MD, Gilbert AR, Lynch JP, Strieter RM. Interleukin-1 receptor antagonist expression in sarcoidosis. Am Rev Respir Dis 1993; 148:1378-1384.

11. Chensue SW, Otterness IG, Higashi GI, Forsh CS, Kunkel SL. Monokine production by hypersensitivity (Schistosoma mansoni egg) and foreign body (Sephadex bead)-type granuloma macrophages: evidence for sequential production of IL-1 and tumor necrosis factor. J Immunol 1992; 142:1281-1287.

12. Curry AJ, Kaye PM. Recombinant interleukin 1 alpha augments granuloma formation and cytokine production but not parasite clearence in mice infected with Leishmania donavani. Infect Immun 1992;

60:4422-4426.

13. Chensue SW, Bienkowski M, Eessalu TE, Warmington KS, Hersey SD, Lukacs NW, Kunkel SL. Endogenous interleukin 1 receptor antagonist protein (IRAP) regulates schistosome egg granuloma formation and the regional lymphoid response. J Immunol 151:3654-3662.

14. Mossmann TR, Moore KW. The role of IL-10 in crossregulation of Th1 and Th2 response. Immunol Today 1989; 12: A49-A58.

15. Huygen K, Abramowicz D, Vanderbussche P, Jacobs F, De Bruyn J, Kentos A, Drowart A, Van Vooren JP, Goldman M. Spleen cell cytokine secretion in Mycobacterium bovis SCG-infecter mice. Infect Immun 1992; 60:2880-2886.

16. Grzych JM, Pearce E, Cheever A, Caulada ZA, Caspar P, Henry S, Lewis F, Sher A. Egg deposition is the major stimulus for the production of Th2 cytokines in murine schistosomiasis mansoni. J Immunol 1991; 146:1322-1329.

17. Chakkalath HR, Titus RG. Leishmania major-parasitized macrophages augment Th2-type T cell activation. J Immunol 1994; 153:4378-4387.

18. Jones ML, Warren JS. Monocyte chemoattractant protein 1 in a rat model of pulmonary granulomatosis. Lab Invest 1992; 66:498-503.

19. Flory CM, Jones ML, Warren JS. Pulmonary granuloma formation in the rat is partially dependent on monocyte chemoattractant protein 1. Lab Invest 1993; 69:396-404.

20. Flory CM, Jones ML, Miller BF, Warren JS. Regulatory roles of tumor necrosis factor-alpha and interleukin-1 beta in monocyte chemoattractant protein-1-mediated pulmonary granuloma formation in the rat. Am J Pathol 1995; 146:450-462.

21. Car BD, Meloni F, Luisetti M et al. Elevated IL-8 and MCP-1 in the bronchoalveolar lavage fluid of patients with idiopathic pulmonary fibrosis and pulmonary sarcoidosis. Am J Respir Crit Care Med 1994; 149:655-659.

22. Lukacs NW, Boros DL. Utilization of fractionated soluble egg antigens reveals se-

lectively modulated granulomatous and lymphokine responses during murine schistomiasis mansoni. Infect Immun 60: 3209-3216.

23. Lukacs NW, Boros DL. Lymphokine regulation of granuloma formation in murine schistosomiasis mansoni. Clin Immunol Immunopath 1993; 68:57-63.

24. Chensue SW, Terebuh PD, Warmington KS et al. Role of IL-4 and IFN-gamma in *Schistosoma mansoni* egg-induced hypersensitivity granuloma formation. Orchestration, relative contribution and relationship to macrophage function. J Immunol 1992; 148:900-911.

25. Lukacs NW, Kunkel SL, Strieter RM et al. The role of macrophage inflammatory protein-1 alpha in *Schistosoma mansoni* egg-induced granulomatous inflammation. J Exp Med 1993; 177:1551-1559.

26. Lukacs NW, Chensue SW, Smith RE et al. Production of monocyte chemoattractant protein-1 and macrophage inflammatory protein-1 alpha by inflammatory granuloma fibroblasts. Am J Pathol 1993; 144: 711-718.

27. Lukacs NW, Strieter RM, Elner VM et al. Intercellular adhesion molecule-1 mediates the expression of monocyte-derived MIP-1α during monocyte-endothelial cell interactions. Blood 1994; 83:1174-1178.

28. Lukacs NW, Chensue SW, Strieter RM et al. Inflammatory granuloma formation is mediated by TNF-α inducible ICAM-1. J Immunol 152:5883-5889.

29. Rollins BJ, Morriso ED, Stiles CD. Cloning and expression of JE, a gene inducible by platelet-derived growth factor and whose product has cytokine-like properties. PNAS USA 1988; 85:3738-3742.

30. Rollins BJ, Pober JS. Interleukine 4 induces the synthesis and secretion of MCP-1/JEby human endothelial cells. Am J Pathol 138:1315-1319.

31. Chensue SW, Warmington KS, Lukacs NW et al. Monocyte chemotactic protein expression during schistosome egg granuloma formation: Sequence of production, localization, contribution and regulation. Am J Pathol 1995; 146:130-138.

32. Chensue SW, Warmington KS, Ruth JH et al. Cytokine function during mycobacterial and schistosomal antigen-induced pulmonary granuloma formation: local and regional participation of IFN-γ, IL-10 and TNF. J Immunol 1995; 154:5969-5976.

33. Meurer R, Van Riper G, Feeney W et al. Formation of eosinophilic and monocytic intradermal inflammatory sites in the dog by injection of human RANTES but not monocyte chemoattractant protein 1, human macrophage inflammatory protein 1 alpha, or human interleukin 8. J Exp Med 178:1913-1921.

34. Alam R, Stafford S, Forsythe P et al. RANTES is a chemotactic and activating factor for human eosinophils. J Immunol 1993; 150:3442-3448.

35. Heeger P, Wolf G, Meyers C et al. Isolation and characterization of cDNA from renal tubular epithelium encoding murine RANTES. Kidney Int 1992; 41:220-224.

36. Orlofsky A, Lin EY, Prystowsky MB Selective induction of the β chemokine C10 by IL-4 in mouse macrophages. J Immunol 1994; 152:5084-5091.

37. Fahey TJ, Tracey KJ, Tekamp-Olson P et al. Macrophage inflammatory protein 1 modulates macrophage function. J Immunol 148:2764.

38. Jiang Y, Beller DI, Frendl G et al. Monocyte chemoattractant protein-1 regulates adhesion molecule expression and cytokine production in human monocytes. J Immunol 1992; 145:2423-2428.

39. Koch AE, Polverini PJ, Kunkel SL et al. Interleukin-8 (IL-8) as a macrophage-derived mediator of angiogenesis. Science 1992; 258:1798-1801.

CHAPTER 10

THE ROLE OF CHEMOKINES IN ISCHEMIA AND REPERFUSION INJURY

Akihisa Harada, Naofumi Mukaida and Kouji Matsushima

INTRODUCTION

Tissue ischemia is a clinically serious event that evokes various bio-chemical, morphological and pathological changes, thereby causing cellular damage and dysfunction. Ischemia-induced tissue damage is associated with the accumulation of toxic metabolites and depletion of cellular energy. Re-establishment of blood flow is vital for the restoration of cellular metabolism and the removal of toxic metabolites in ischemic tissue. Paradoxically, severe tissue injury, often known as ischemia-reperfusion injury, occurs during reperfusion rather than during ischemia. Specifically, reperfusion of ischemic tissue causes more severe intracellular enzyme release, influx of Ca^{2+}, breakdown of phospholipids and damage of cell membrane than the injury induced by ischemia per se.[1] The idea of reperfusion injury was first formulated by cardiologists, as they had noticed that arrhythmias or stunning was induced by reperfusion of ischemic myocardium in several experimental models.[2] Later, researchers began to realize that reperfusion injury was observed in any tissue or cell undergoing ischemia, and thereafter the concept of this injury was widely acknowledged. Ischemia-reperfusion injury is involved in the pathophysiology of various types of clinical disorders including myocardial infarction, cerebral infarction, vascular disease, organ transplantation and multiple organ failure. Current evidence reveals that reperfusion injury is characterized by increased microvascular permeability, protein leakage and neutrophil sequestration. Moreover, ischemia-reperfusion models involving multiple organs can cause characteristic injury in multiple organs similar to that in a single organ, suggesting that the pathophysiological mechanism of reperfusion injury is common.

Chemokines in Disease, edited by Alisa E. Koch and Robert M. Strieter.
© 1996 R.G. Landes Company.

During the past decade, extensive efforts have been made to clarify the mechanism of the ischemia-reperfusion injury. At first, the neutrophils infiltrating injured tissue had been presumed to be beneficial for recovering from, and healing of the damaged tissue in ischemia-reperfusion injury. However, it was observed that the size of an injured area was markedly reduced by depleting neutrophils using antineutrophil antibodies in animals,[3] suggesting that neutrophils were the primary mediator of the reperfusion injury. These observations have provided critical and definitive evidence that neutrophil-mediated inflammatory processes occur in the reperfused area and contribute to tissue damage.

The potential pathogenic role of inflammation in reperfusion injury has been further examined using anti-inflammatory agents that can reduce neutrophil function or interfere with the generation of chemotactic factors or oxygen free radical scavengers in vivo.[3,4] These various agents could diminish injury size, supporting the idea that neutrophil-mediated acute inflammation is an essential factor for reperfusion injury.

Leukocyte migration into the injured site is induced not only by potent chemotactic factors such as C5a, N-formyl peptides derived from bacteria and leukotriene B4, but also by low molecular weight leukocyte chemotactic cytokines (chemokines) which exhibit cell-type specific leukocyte chemoattraction. Several chemokines have been isolated, cloned and expressed in large quantities in the past decade. These chemokines demonstrate significantly high homology with each other, having four characteristic cysteine amino acid residues, and are classified into two subgroups, C-X-C and C-C, depending on whether the first two cysteines are separated by one amino acid or are adjacent. The C-X-C chemokines generally exhibit chemotactic activities against neutrophils and lymphocytes but not against monocytes, whereas C-C chemokines exhibit chemotactic activities against monocytes and T lymphocytes

but not against neutrophils.[5] Thus, chemokines produced by the cells in ischemic tissue may govern the directed migration of activated neutrophils into the reperfused tissue.

In this review, we will discuss the biochemical, cellular and molecular basis of ischemia-reperfusion injury and the chemotactic cytokines involved in the pathogenesis of this injury.

BIOCHEMISTRY OF REPERFUSION INJURY

Reperfusion of blood flow results in reoxygenation of ischemic tissue, leading to the generation of reactive oxygen metabolites such as superoxide anion, hypochlorous acid ($HOCl$) and hydrogen peroxide (H_2O_2). Reperfusion injury is mediated at least in part by the formation of these reactive oxygen metabolites since oxygen radicals can cause damage to every component in tissue, including nucleic acids, membrane lipids, enzymes and receptors. Evidence for the involvement of reactive oxygen metabolites in reperfusion injury was initially provided by Granger et al in the cat small intestine in vivo.[6,7] In their experiments, administration of superoxide dismutase (SOD) before reperfusion significantly attenuated the capillary permeability change and the necrosis of the microvasculature. Moreover, oxidant formation was directly demonstrated in reperfused ischemic bowel by chemiluminescence.[8] These results demonstrated that reactive oxygen intermediates were generated in reperfused ischemic tissue and could mediate the injury.

The oxygen radical-producing enzyme xanthine oxidase was postulated to be important for the generation of oxygen radicals. Xanthine oxidase inhibitors such as allopurinol, pterin aldehyde and tungsten dramatically reduced reperfusion injury in animal models, suggesting that xanthine oxidase is an important source of the oxidants produced after reperfusion.[7,9,10] More than 90% of xanthine oxidase (XO) normally exists in healthy tissue in the form of xanthine dehydrogenase (XDH), which converts hypoxanthine to xanthine with NAD^+ as its electron acceptor, thus generating NADH without producing $O_2\cdot$ and H_2O_2. However, in ischemic tissue, XDH does not exist as such and is changed, probably by proteolysis, to XO, which uses oxygen as its substrate instead of NAD. Thus, the conversion of XDH to XO in hypoxic stress is the initial important step in the oxygen radical-mediated reperfusion injury. The next important event in reperfusion injury is accumulation of hypoxanthine due to catabolism of ATP in the ischemic tissue. Furthermore, since XO converts hypoxanthine to xanthine only in the presence of oxygen, XO cannot catalyze the oxidation of hypoxanthine to xanthine in ischemic tissue, resulting in the excess accumulation of hypoxanthine. However, no additional conversion was observed until oxygen was re-introduced into the ischemic tissue. When blood flow is reperfused, XO converts hypoxanthine to xanthine in the presence of oxygen, with the generation of large amounts of a superoxide anion. This superoxide production sequentially leads to the generation of other types of oxygen radicals, thereby causing the tissue injury.

The same mechanism of free radical-mediated reperfusion injury is also important, even in other organs such as brain and heart that do not contain large amounts of XO in tissue homogenates. XO is immunohistochemically identified in the endothelial cells of many organs.[11] In vitro studies of anoxia and reoxygenation to rat pulmonary artery endothelial cell monolayers have demonstrated the occurrence of enzymatic conversion of XDH to XO during ischemia and injury at reoxygenation.[12] Moreover, this injury was prevented by allopurinol or superoxide dismutase. These results suggest that the XO-mediated superoxide generating system is also present in endothelial cells and that endothelial XO is also an important enzyme for generating superoxide anions.

ROLE OF NEUTROPHILS IN REPERFUSION INJURY

Accumulating evidence implies that neutrophils also play an important role in ischemia-reperfusion injury. Microscopic analyses of the tissues subjected to ischemia-reperfusion injury revealed massive adherence and emigration of neutrophils in postcapillary venules.[13] This neutrophil recruitment and activation in ischemic regions exacerbated tissue injury during the reperfusion period.[14,15] More direct proof was obtained in an experiment with neutropenic animals. Depletion of neutrophils using antineutrophil serum attenuated the reperfusion-induced vascular injury in the animals.[3] Furthermore, the prevention of neutrophil adherence with monoclonal antibodies against leukocyte adhesion molecules abolished reperfusion-induced vascular dysfunction as well as neutrophil infiltration in canine models.[16,17] All of these results suggest that polymorphonuclear leukocytes are important in the pathogenesis of reperfusion-induced injury.

The recruitment of neutrophils to the site of injury is dependent upon sequential events consisting of the multiple steps of interaction between leukocytes and endothelium. The primary transient interaction of leukocytes and endothelial cells is the tethering and rolling process.[18] This process is mediated by a class of adhesion molecules identified as selectins. L-selectin is expressed on all circulating leukocytes and is constitutively functional.[19] E-selectin is induced on vascular endothelial cells by lipopolysaccharide (LPS), interleukin-1 (IL-1) or tumor necrosis factor (TNF). P-selectin is stored in the endothelial cells, but rapidly expressed on the surface in response to thrombin or histamine. All selectins recognize sialylated carbohydrates as their counterreceptors. L-selectin recognizes the carbohydrates sialyl Lewis a and Lewis x as ligands. L-selectin and P-selectin also recognize O-linked mucine-like molecules which are serine- and threonine-rich proteins. These selectins mediate cooperatively both the attachment of leukocytes to endothelial cells in the vascular wall and leukocyte rolling in the direction of shear force.

Following the rolling process, the neutrophils are activated by chemoattractants and trigger activation of β2 integrins. Such an increase in number and affinity can occur in a few seconds and is mediated by G-protein coupled receptor. The types of chemoattractants determine the types of leukocytes involved in endothelial cell recognition. Once upregulated at this step, the integrins can bind to adhesion molecules, members of the immunoglobulin superfamily, on the endothelium, leading to the firm attachment of rolling leukocytes on endothelium. Leukocytes then transmigrate the endothelial lining of the blood vessel, following the directional gradient of the chemotactic factors.

The integrin family consists of several members of heterodimeric glycoproteins that are expressed on the surface of leukocytes. Each integrin contains α and β subunits, and three subfamilies can be distinguished by the characteristic β subunits such as β1 (CD29), β2 (CD18) and β3 (CD61). The β1 integrin subfamily binds to the extracellular matrix components such as fibronectin, laminin and collagen and is expressed on a variety of nonhematopoietic cells. Three β2 subfamilies consist of a common β chain and three variable α chains, resulting in the formation of CD11a/CD18 (LFA-1), CD11b/CD18 (Mac-1) and CD11c/CD18.[20] These three integrins are expressed only on leukocytes. The importance of these types of integrins has been unraveled by the discovery of patients with congenital leukocyte adhesion deficiency (LAD). Patients with LAD have mutations in the common β2 subunit genes, exhibit significant leukocytosis and suffer from recurrent bacterial infections.[21] Leukocytes from these patients fail to migrate in response to chemoattractants, so that they fail to form "pus" at the site of infection.

Intracellular adhesion molecule 1 (ICAM-1), a member of the immunoglobulin superfamily, is expressed on endothelial cells stimulated with LPS, IL-1 and TNF [22] and is an important counterreceptor for LFA-1 and Mac-1. LFA-1 can also interact with ICAM-2 and ICAM-3.[23] Chemoattractants stimulate strong, integrin-mediated adhesion of neutrophil to ICAM-1. Thus, neutrophils are arrested, spread and firmly adhere through the integrin-ICAM-1 interaction.

Monoclonal antibodies (mAbs) against various adhesion molecules have been used to define the role of these molecules in neutrophil adhesion in ischemia-reperfusion injury. A mAb against CD18 significantly diminished neutrophil adherence to endothelial cells and endothelial disruption by activated neutrophils in vitro.[24,25] Pretreatment with this mAb in vivo significantly reduced reperfusion-induced tissue injury after local ischemia in myocardium,[16] intestine[3] and central nervous system.[26] Anti-CD18 mAb was also effective in improving survival from hemorrhagic shock in rabbits.[27] MAbs to CD11a and CD11b could improve survival with less effectiveness than anti-CD18 mAb. Antibody against ICAM-1 was also effective in preventing reperfusion injury of liver.[28]

Activated neutrophils can damage endothelial cells and increase microvascular permeability through the production of reactive oxygen intermediates (ROI) including superoxide, hydrogen peroxide and hydroxyl radicals. Activated neutrophils produce these ROI through NADPH oxidase, which reduces oxygen to superoxide anion. In addition, they also secrete myeloperoxidase (MPO) that catalyzes the production of hypochlorous acid (HOCl). HOCl is a potent oxidizing agent and reacts rapidly with amines (RNH_2) to produce N-chloroamines, thereby causing cellular injury. In the reperfusion injury model of cat intestine, treatment with allopurinol significantly attenuated the ischemia reperfusion injury and reduced tissue accumulation of MPO activity. Since MPO levels can reflect the accumulation of neutrophils in the tissue, these observations suggest that neutrophil infiltration can correlate with reperfusion injury.[29] Furthermore, treatment of animals with catalase, anti-oxidants, the iron chelator deferoxamine or the OH· scavenger dimethylthiourea significantly inhibited the increase of vascular permeability and neutrophil accumulation in reperfusion injuries.[30] These results suggest the possibility that ROI initiate the production of chemotactic agents for neutrophils.

CHEMOTACTIC FACTORS IN ISCHEMIA REPERFUSION INJURY

Although numerous studies suggest that XO and ROI contribute to reperfusion-induced neutrophil recruitment, the exact nature of the factors involved in the recruitment has not been well understood until recently. Petrone et al[31] first reported the strong connection between the production of ROI in tissue following ischemia-reperfusion and the subsequent infiltration of neutrophils which generated additional ROI. The classic potent chemotactic factors, arachidonic acid products and complement fragments, have been reported to be an important key in neutrophil infiltration observed in reperfusion injury. High concentrations of breakdown products of arachidonic acid were found in plasma immediately after reperfusion of ischemic tissue. The ROI can interact with the cell membrane to activate phospholipase A2, which will subsequently result in production of powerful leukocyte chemotactic agents such as leukotriene B4 (LTB4) and platelet-activating factor (PAF).

LTB4 exhibits neutrophil chemotactic activity and is a potent stimulus for production of hydrogen peroxide and elastase from neutrophils. Inhibition of oxygen radicals with scavenging enzymes abrogated the generation of arachidonic acid metabolites following reperfusion.[32] A significant increase in mucosal LTB4 was observed in cat intestine during reperfusion.[33] Pretreatment with 5-lipoxygenase inhibitor or LTB4 receptor antagonist remarkably attenuated vascular injury and neutrophil accumulation.[33] These observations raised the possibility of LTB4 as a factor responsible for neutrophil infiltration and activation.

PAF, another potent chemotactic factor, upregulates leukocyte adhesion molecules (CD11b/CD18) and promotes neutrophil adhesion to endothelial cells.[34] Increased concentrations of PAF were also observed in reperfusion of the ischemic intestine.[35] Moreover, pretreatment of the experimental animals with two distinct PAF receptor antagonists significantly diminished emigration of neutrophils after reperfusion.[35] These observations suggest that PAF plays an important role in the neutrophil emigration observed in ischemia-reperfusion injury.

In ischemia-reperfusion injury, consumption of complement is increased as a result of activation of complement. Depletion of complement prevented the development of vascular injury and neutrophil accumulation in ischemia-reperfused tissue.[36] One of the ROI, H_2O_2, can cause the cleavage of C5, thus activating the complement pathway.[37,38]

None of these chemoattractants require de novo protein synthesis. Moreover, since they are unstable, their biological activities cannot persist for a long time in vivo.[39,40]

Isolation,[41] purification[42] and cDNA cloning[43] of a leukocyte chemotactic and activating factor, interleukin-8 (IL-8) has made a great impact on the field of chemotactic factors. Since IL-8 is resistant to inactivation by proteolysis and denaturation in vivo, its biological activities last much longer than other chemotactic factors such as LTB4, PAF and C5a. IL-8 production is observed in response to inflammatory stimuli such as lipopolysaccharide (LPS) and phytohemagglutinin (PHA), as well as by tumor necrosis factor (TNF) and interleukin-1β (IL-1β). IL-8 is produced by a wide variety of cell types including monocytes, endothelial cells and fibroblasts. IL-8 is a member of a chemokine family and exhibits cell type-specific leukocyte chemo-attraction. IL-8 directly binds its own specific receptors on neutrophils and stimulates a number of neutrophil functions including induction of shape change,[44] release of lysosomal enzymes such as myelo-peroxidase, α-mannosidase and β-gluconidase,[45] induction of respiratory burst,[46] adhesion of endothelium,[47] generation of superoxide and hydrogen peroxide[44] and generation of bioactive lipids.[48]

In vitro exposure of human blood monocytes to varying durations of anoxia before hyperoxia caused production of IL-8, in a manner dependent on the duration of anoxic exposure.[49] Moreover, induction of gene expression of IL-8 occurred, as revealed by Northern blotting analysis and nuclear tanscriptional assay, suggesting that exposure to oxidant stress augments tran-scriptional and translational levels of IL-8. In another experiment, exposure of human cndothelial cells only to hypoxia led to time-dependent release of IL-8 protein.[50] Increased IL-8 production was also observed at the transcriptional and translational level, as revealed by induction of IL-8 mRNA and by nuclear run-on assay.

Effect of neutrophil margination in pulmonary blood vessels was also examined in hypoxic condition in vivo. Exposure of mice to hypoxia caused leukocyte stagnation in pulmonary blood vessels, as demonstrated by increased myeloperoxidase activity in tissue homogenates. An IL-8 homolog in rat and mouse has not been identified so far;[51] murine C-X-C chemokines, cytokine induced neutrophil chemoattractants (CINC) (GRO homolog), are presumed to substitute for IL-8 in rodents. However, CINC was not detected in this condition. More interestingly, induction of the IL-8 related chemokine IP-10 was observed in hypoxic lung tissue. IP-10, with a molecular mass of about 10 kDa, was originally identified as an IFN-γ-inducible protein. IP-10 belongs to the C-X-C chemokine family, but is not active on neutrophils; it exhibits chemotaxis against monocytes and T cells. The biological significance of IP-10 in hypoxic conditions should be elucidated.

The pathways underlying IL-8 expression by endothelial cells in response to hypoxia have not yet been clarified. A previous report has indicated that ROI in-duce in vitro nuclear translocation of the transcription factor NF-κB.[52] For the transcription of the IL-8 gene, synergistic cooperation of the κB-site with either AP-1 or NF-IL6 binding sites is indispensable in any type of cells examined.[53] In a gel shift assay, NF-κB complexes appeared in nuclear protein extracted from endothelial cells exposed to hypoxia, but the mobility was different from authentic NF-κB. However, the anti-p50 or anti-p65 antibody failed to affect the complex formation, suggesting that species distinct from authentic NF-κB may not be involved in transcriptional activation in hypoxic culture.[50] The production of IL-8 in a hypoxic situation was also observed in human umbilical cord vein segment. Previous reports demonstrated that endothelial cells in a hypoxic situation could promote margination and migration of neutrophils.[54,55] From the results of experiments described above, this increased capacity of endothelial cells to bind neutrophils might be ascribed to the generation of the chemotactic polypeptide IL-8 in the ischemic site, causing the upregulation of the adhesion molecule CD11b/CD18.[47]

Hypoxia induced in vitro endothelial cells to increase the transcription of another chemokine, monocyte chemotactic and activating factor MCAF/MCP-1.[50] MCAF, a member of the C-C chemokines, was isolated and purified from culture supernatants of blood mononuclear cells or tumor cell lines.[56,57,58] The human MCAF cDNA encodes a 99 amino acid residue precursor protein with a 23 residue signal peptide and is cleaved to generate a mature protein consisting of 76 amino acids. MCAF can attract and activate monocytes in vitro. MCAF can induce generation and release of superoxide anion, mobilization of intracellular calcium and expression of β2-integrins CD11b/CD18 and CD11c/CD18.[59,60] MCAF can also attract basophils and induce histamine release in vitro.[61]

MCAF mRNA expression was demonstrated in vivo in rat ischemic cortex after focal stroke by occlusion of the middle cerebral artery.[62] Since almost no expres-

cerebral artery.[62] Since almost no expression of MCAF mRNA was found in the sham-operated contralateral cortex, MCAF may play an important role in monocyte infiltration into ischemic tissue injury. The precise pathophysiological role of MCAF in ischemic tissue awaits further elucidation.

DeForge et al[63] examined the involvement of ROI in IL-8 production by using the hydroxyl radical (OH·) scavenger dimethyl sulfoxide (DMSO). Direct addition of H_2O_2 to human whole blood stimulated IL-8 release in a dose-dependent manner. Moreover, DMSO dramatically inhibited IL-8 production in blood stimulated with lipopolysaccharide (LPS) or other agents such as tumor necrosis factor (TNF), interleukin-1β (IL-1β), phytohemagglutinin (PHA) and aggregated immune complex. This inhibition was also observed at pretranslational levels as revealed by Northern blotting analysis. Furthermore, other OH· scavenging agents such as dimethyl thiourea and thiourea had a similar inhibitory effect on LPS-stimulated IL-8 production. Collectively, endogeneously produced ROI may play an important role in the regulation of IL-8 production. These results were further confirmed by the same group's findings that oxidant stress from independently generated NADPH-oxidase is an important regulator of IL-8 gene expression.[64]

The most significant source of ROI in stimulated blood cells is NADPH-oxidase. In neutrophils from patients with inherited chronic granulomatous disease (CGD), the components of NADPH-oxidase are absent or impaired. Thus, the patients' neutrophils have an absent or markedly reduced ability to generate ROI.[65] In contrast to the assumption that NADPH-oxidase is a major enzyme responsible for production of ROI, leukoytes from CGD patients could produce IL-8 in response to a variety of stimulating agents. Moreover, this production was inhibited by DMSO and other antioxidants. Since the blood cells of CGD patients are unable to produce ROI, these results suggest the presence of several pathways of ROI production,[64] which

are independent of NADPH-oxidase and include mitochondrial electron transport and arachidonate metabolism. Moreover, in vitro, nonimmune cultured cells such as fibroblasts, Hep-G2 cells and pulmonary epithelial cells produce IL-8 in response to H_2O_2 in a dose-dependent manner.[64] Previous observations demonstrated that types of cells such as endothelial cells, fibroblasts and chondrocytes lacked NADPH-oxidase and could still produce a measurable amount of ROI in response to cytokine stimulation.[66,67,68] All of these observations imply that IL-8 production is regulated by endogeneously produced ROI not only in the immune-related leukocytes in CGD patients, but also in the resident and nonimmune cells that lack a classical NADPH-oxidase system. Therefore, in an ischemia-reperfused area, ROI may induce the production of IL-8, which then serves to recruit neutrophils to sites of inflammation.

IL-8 production in biological fluids has been reported in patients during acute myocardial infarction, and in those undergoing cardiopulmonary bypass operation.[69,70] However, the most direct evidence of the importance of IL-8 ischemia-reperfusion injury in vivo has been recently provided by two animal models, rabbit lung reperfusion injury[71] and ischemia-reperfusion canine myocardial injury.[72]

Lung reperfusion injury model in rabbits was established by clamping the left pulmonary hilus for 2 hours, followed by simultaneous declamping of the left hilus and clamping of the opposite hilus so that pulmonary blood was directed into the previously ischemic left lung. Reperfusion to ischemic lung for 3 hours significantly increased IL-8 content (Fig. 10.1). The number of neutrophils in bronchoalveolar lavage fluid (BALF) also increased, accompanied by a massive neutrophil infiltration in the interstitium and by destruction of pulmonary architecture, as well as severe pulmonary edema. Rabbit IL-8 was produced by bronchiolar ciliary cells and alveolar macrophages only 3 hours after reperfusion, but not during ischemia, as revealed by immunohistochemical

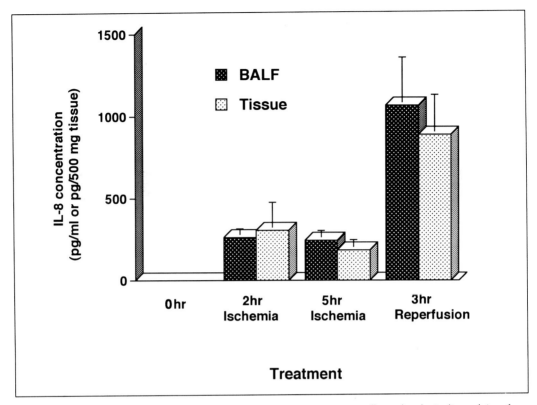

Fig. 10.1. IL-8 contents in BALF and in lung tissue homogenate. BALF was collected at the indicated time from the left lung with physiological saline. Lung tissue (500 mg) was homogenized with phosphate-buffered saline (PBS). After centrifugation of BALF and tissue homogenates, the supernatants were collected and IL-8 concentration measured by enzyme-linked immunosorbent assay (ELISA).

analyses. An anti-IL-8 monoclonal antibody inhibited neutrophil infiltration into lung tissue and the increase of neutrophils in BALF. Moreover, anti-IL-8 treatment inhibited the destruction of pulmonary architecture (Fig. 10.2).[71] These data demonstrated that IL-8 is a major and essential mediator responsible for neutrophil recruitment and neutrophil-dependent tissue damage observed in this reperfusion injury model. This is the first in vivo demonstration that IL-8 plays a crucial role in establishing the ischemia-reperfusion injury.

Another in vivo experiment which revealed the essential role of IL-8 in vivo was performed using a similar model in canine myocardium.[72] In this model, minimal induction of IL-8 mRNA was demonstrated after 3 or 4 hours of myocardium ischemia without reperfusion. However, IL-8 mRNA expression was markedly induced in the reperfused area after ischemia. In reperfused

models, IL-8 was immunohistochemically detected in the leukocytes infiltrated near the border between necrotic and viable myocardium. IL-8 was stained in the area where inflammatory infiltrates were observed, as well as in small veins in this area. On the other hand, IL-8 was rarely detected in the samples from 1 or 3 hours of ischemia without reperfusion. Since the detection limit of the protein in immunohistochemistry is quite high, IL-8 protein might be produced elsewhere during ischemia. All of these data suggest that IL-8 production is induced in reperfused, but not ischemic, myocardium. However, it remains to be elucidated whether or not the protection of myocardium in this model is obtained by inhibiting the action of IL-8.

A role for chemoattractants C5a and IL-8 in acute inflammation has not been extensively investigated. Ember et al[73]

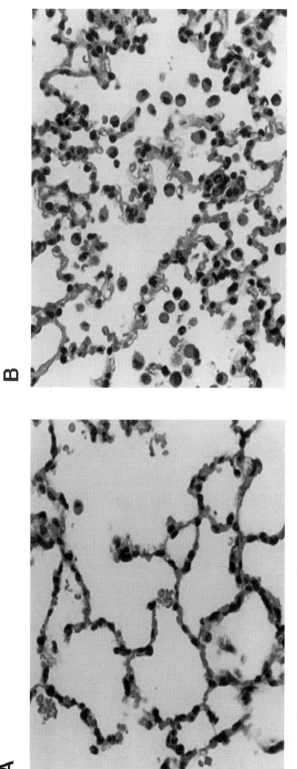

Fig. 10.2. Microscopic examination of effects of anti-IL-8 mAb (A) and control mAb (B) on the reperfused lung tissues. Anti-IL-8 mAb or control mAb was intravenously injected at the beginning of reperfusion. After 3 hours of reperfusion, lung tissues were collected for histological examination.

demonstrated that C5a induced both IL-8 synthesis and release from activated monocytes in vitro. Ivey et al suggested a similar result from in vivo experiments using rabbit myocardium models of ischemia-reperfusion.[74] In this model, immunoreactive C5a and IL-8 were detected in rabbit myocardial tissue only after reperfusion. However, the time courses for the production of these two factors were distinct from each other. C5a was detected within 5 minutes after the initiation of reperfusion and reached a plateau at 3-4.5 hours. In contrast, IL-8 production was detected only after 1.5 hours and reached a maximum at 4.5 hours after the reperfusion. Also in this model, neutrophils accumulated progressively, as evidenced by myeloperoxidase activity levels. Furthermore, depletion of neutrophils using mustine hydrochloride abolished IL-8, but not C5a, production in the reperfused area of ischemic myocardium. Ivey et al[74] expected that IL-8 production in this model was indirectly dependent on C5a production. They also raised the possibility that suppression of C5a could inhibit neutrophil accumulation more effectively than that of IL-8, although they did not provide any direct evidence.

Soluble complement receptor type 1 (sCR1) is a potent complement inhibitor which lacks transmembrane and cytoplasmic domains and is highly effective in suppressing both the classical and the alternative complement pathways.[75] Several independent groups reported that the administration of sCR1 could prevent myocardial contractile dysfunction and enhance recovery in an in vivo model of reperfusion injury of ischemic myocardium.[75,76] Thus, these results implied that complement activation is involved in ischemia-reperfusion injury in myocardium. However, sCR1 failed to inhibit neutrophil accumulation and adhesion to vascular endothelium. In addition, IL-8 production was not measured in these experiments, since they use rat as an animal model. Furthermore, no definitive report has been published on the role of the complement-derived leukocyte chemotactic factor C5a in animal experi-

mental models using anti-C5a antibody in reperfusion injury of ischemic tissue in vivo. This experiment might be essential to elucidate the role(s) of C5a in ischemia-reperfusion injury in vivo. For these reasons, it is premature to generalize that C5a plays a central role in neutrophil-dependent tissue injury in ischemic-reperfusion models at this moment.

Extrapulmonary organ failure, such as impaired hepatic function, transplantation and circulatory shock, can rapidly develop into a pulmonary insufficiency called adult respiratory distress syndrome (ARDS). Moreover, Matuschak et al[77] reported that the liver is a key organ for modulating the occurrence of ARDS. Colletti et al[78] demonstrated that severe hepatic ischemia-reperfusion injury elicited tumor necrosis factor-α (TNF-α) release by hepatic cells, followed by local and systemic tissue injuries. Without any evidence of endotoxin, TNF was detected in the plasma during reperfusion after 90 minutes of lobar hepatic ischemia in rat models. Reperfusion of ischemic hepatic tissue can advance into hepatic injury accompanied by substantial increases in hepatic enzymes. However, neutrophil recruitment into the liver was not observed until 6 hours of reperfusion, and the hepatic architecture remained intact until 24 hours of reperfusion. Moreover, in this model pulmonary dysfunction occurred as a result of hepatic insufficiency. Reperfusion of ischemic lobes in the liver initiated pulmonary neutrophil infiltration and edema as well as intra-alveolar hemorrhage in this model. Interestingly, anti-TNF antiserum treatment significantly reduced neutrophil-dependent damage as well as liver injury, as revealed by the reduction of serum glutamic pyruvic transaminase. These data suggest that ischemia and reperfusion of the liver induces TNF production, and that the produced TNF is indispensable for the liver and lung injury.

Further analyses of the involvement of chemokines were performed using the same model.[79] In this experiment, epithelial neutrophil activating protein-78 (ENA-78), a member of the C-X-C chemokine family, was detected biochemically in plasma and immunohistochemically in the alveolar-capillary membrane (ACM) in the lungs. Administration of anti-ENA-78 antiserum before hepatic ischemia significantly attenuated the lung permeability and neutrophil sequestration, suggesting that pulmonary derived ENA-78 is a major mediator of lung injury. Moreover, clinically, significantly high IL-8 levels in BALF were reported in patients at risk for ARDS. Furthermore, the patients with elevated IL-8 levels in BALF are more prone to develop ARDS than those who do not show any increase of IL-8 levels in BALF.[80] All of these results suggest that these C-X-C chemokines are important mediators for the recruitment of neutrophils causing lung injury in ARDS.

CONCLUDING REMARKS

There is a growing body of experimental evidence that ischemia-reperfusion injury is mediated both by the activation of neutrophils and the production of reactive oxygen metabolites. The involvement of chemokines, particularly IL-8, in the establishment of these conditions has also been proved in recent years. Moreover, chemokines are presumed to be involved in cell-mediated rejection of transplanted organs. The C-X-C chemokine ENA-78 and the C-C chemokine RANTES are expressed in biopsy specimens of cell-mediated organ rejections.[81,82] Although additional work is necessary to define the contributions of these mediators to the rejection, these observations shed new insights into molecular immunomodulation of organ transplantation and immune-mediated disease.

REFERENCES

1. Kurose I, Granger DN. Evidence implicating oxidase and neutrophils in reperfusion-indued microvascular dysfunction. Ann N Y Acad Sci 1994; 723:258-270.
2. Katz AM, Tada M. The "stone heart": a challenge to the biochemist. Am J Cardiol 1972; 29(4):578-580.
3. Hernandez LA, Grisham MB, Twohig B et al. Role of neutrophils in ischemia-reperfusion induced microvascular injury. Am J Physiol 1987; 253:H699-H703.
4. Adkins WK, Taylor AE. Role of xanthine oxidase and neutrophils in ischemia-reperfusion injury in rabbit lung. J Appl Physiol 1990; 69:2012-2018.
5. Oppenheim JJ, Zachariae COC, Mukaida N et al. Properties of the novel proinflammatory supergene "intercrine" ccytokine family. Ann Rev Immunol 1991; 9: 617-648.
6. Granger DN, Rutili G, McCord JM. Superoxide radicals in feline intestinal ischemia. Gastroenterology 1981; 81(1):22-29.
7. Parks DA, Bulkley GB, Granger DN et al. Ischemic injury in the cat small intestine: role of superoxide radicals. Gastroenterology 1982; 82(1):9-15.
8. Morris JB, Bulkley GB, Haglund U et al. The direct, real-time demonstration of oxygen free radical generation at reperfusion following ischemia in rat small intestine. Gastroenterology 1987; 92:A1541.
9. Parks DA, Granger DN. Ischemia-induced vascular changes: role of xanthine oxidase and hydroxyl radicals. Am J Physiol 1983; 245(2):G285-G289.
10. Granger DN. Role of xanthine oxidase and granulocytes in ischemia-reperfusion injury. Am J Physiol 1988; 255(6 Pt 2): H1269-1275.
11. Bruder G, Heid HW, Jarasch ED et al. Immunological identification and determination of xanthine oxidase in cells and tissues. Differentiation 1983; 23(3):218-225.
12. Ratych RE, Chuknyiska RS, Bulkley GB. The primary localization of free radical generation after anoxia/reoxygenation in isolated endothelial cells. Surgery 1987; 102(2): 122-131.
13. Oliver MG, Specian RD, Perry MA et al. Morphologic assessment of leukocyte-endothelial cell interactions in mesenteric venules subjected to ischemia and reperfusion. Inflammation 1991; 15(5):331-346.
14. Korthuis RJ, Grisham MB, Granger DN. Leukocyte depletion attenuates vascular injury in postischemic skeletal muscle. Am J Physiol 1988; 254:H823-H827.
15. Reynolds JM, McDonagh PF. Early in reperfusion, leukocytes alter perfused

coronary capillarity and vascular resistance. Am J Physiol 1989; 256:H982-H989.

16. Simpson PJ, Todd R, Fantone JC et al. Reduction of experimental canine myocardial reperfusion injury by a monoclonal antibody (anti-Mo1, anti-CD11b) that inhibits leukocyte adhesion. J Clin Invest 1988; 81(2):624-629.

17. Carden DL, Smith JK, Korthuis RJ. Neutrophil-mediated microvascular dysfunction in postischemic canine skeletal muscle. Role of granulocyte adherence. Circ Res 1990; 66(5):1436-1444.

18. Springer TA. Traffic signals for lymphocyte recirculation and leukocyte emigration: the multistep paradigm. Cell 1994; 76(2): 301-314.

19. von Andrian UH, Chambers JD, McEvoy LM et al. Two-step model of leukocyte-endothelial cell interaction in inflammation: distinct roles for LECAM-1 and the leukocyte beta 2 integrins in vivo. Proc Natl Acad Sci USA 1991; 88(17):7538-7542.

20. Springer TA. Adhesion receptors of the immune system. Nature 1990; 346(6283): 425-434.

21. Kishimoto TK, Larson RS, Corbi AL et al. The leukocyte integrins. Adv Immunol 1989; 46(149):149-182.

22. Dustin ML, Rothlein R, Bhan AK et al. Induction by IL 1 and interferon-gamma: tissue distribution, biochemistry, and function of a natural adherence molecule (ICAM-1). J Immunol 1986; 137(1): 245-254.

23. de Fougerolles A, Stacker SA, Schwarting R et al. Characterization of ICAM-2 and evidence for a third counter-receptor for LFA-1. J Exp Med 1991; 174(1):253-267.

24. Diener AM, Beatty PG, Ochs HD et al. The role of neutrophil membrane glycoprotein 150 (Gp-150) in neutrophil-mediated endothelial cell injury in vitro. J Immunol 1985; 135(1):537-543.

25. Harlan JM, Schwartz BR, Reidy MA et al. Activated neutrophils disrupt endothelial monolayer integrity by an oxygen radical-independent mechanism. Lab Invest 1985; 52(2):141-150.

26. Clark WM, Madden KP, Rothlein R et al. Reduction of central nervous system

ischemic injury in rabbits using leukocyte adhesion antibody treatment. Stroke 1991; 22(7):877-883.

27. Vedder NB, Winn RK, Rice CL et al. A monoclonal antibody to the adherence-promoting leukocyte glycoprotein, CD18, reduces organ injury and improves survival from hemorrhagic shock and resuscitation in rabbits. J Clin Invest 1988; 81(3): 939-944.

28. Farhood A, McGuire GM, Manning AM et al. Intercellular adhesion molecule 1 (ICAM-1) expression and its role in neutrophil-induced ischemia-reperfusion injury in rat liver. J Leukoc Biol 1995; 57(3):368-374.

29. Grisham MB, Hernandez LA, Granger DN. Xanthine oxidase and neutrophil infiltration in intestinal ischemia. Am J Physiol 1986; 251:G567-G574.

30. Zimmerman BJ, Grisham MB, Granger DN. Role of oxidants in ischemia/reperfusion-induced granulocyte infiltration. Am J Physiol 1990; 258:G185-G190.

31. Petrone WF, English DK, Wong K et al. Free radicals and inflammation: superoxide-dependent activation of a neutrophil chemotactic factor in plasma. Proc Natl Acad Sci USA 1980; 77(2):1159-1163.

32. Klausner JM, Paterson IS, Kobzik L et al. Oxygen free radicals mediate ischemia-induced lung injury. Surgery 1989; 105 (2 Pt 1):192-199.

33. Zimmerman BJ, Guillory DJ, Grisham MB et al. Role of leukotriene B4 in granulocyte infiltration into the postischemic feline intestine. Gastroenterology 1990; 99(5): 1358-1363.

34. Shappell SB, Toman C, Anderson DC et al. Mac-1 (CD11b/CD18) mediates adherence-dependent hydrogen peroxide production by human and canine neutrophils. J Immunol 1990; 144(7):2702-2711.

35. Kubes P, Suzuki M, Granger DN. Platelet-activating factor-induced microvascular dysfunction: role of adherent leukocytes. Am J Physiol 1990; 258(1 Pt 1):G158-G163.

36. Seekamp A, Ward PA. Ischemia-reperfusion injury. Agents Actions Suppl 1993; 41(137):137-152.

37. Shingu M, Nobunaga M. Chemotactic activity generated in human serum from the

fifth component of complement by hydrogen peroxide. Am J Pathol 1984; 117(2): 201-206.

38. von ZW, Hesse D, Nolte R et al. Generation of an activated form of human C5 (C5b-like C5) by oxygen radicals. Immunol Lett 1987; 14(3):209-215.

39. Colditz IG, Movat HZ. Kinetics of neutrophil accumulation in acute inflammatory lesions induced by chemotaxins and chemotaxinigens. J Immunol 1984; 133(4): 2169-2173.

40. Movat HZ, Rettl C, Burrowes CE et al. The in vivo effect of leukotriene B4 on polymorphonuclear leukocytes and the microcirculation. Comparison with activated complement (C5a des Arg) and enhancement by prostaglandin E2. Am J Pathol 1984; 115(2):233-244.

41. Yoshimura T, Matsushima K, Oppenheim JJ et al. Neutrophil chemotactic factor produced by lipopolysaccharide (LPS)-stimulated human blood mononuclear leukocytes: partial characterization and separation from interleukin 1 (IL 1). J Immunol 1987; 139:788-793.

42. Yoshimura T, Matsuhsima K, Tanaka S et al. Purification of a human monocyte-derived neutrophil chemotactic factor that has peptide sequence similarity to other host defense cytokines. Proc Natl Acad Sci USA 1987; 84:9233-9237.

43. Matsushima K, Morishita K, Yoshimura T et al. Molecular cloning of a human monocyte-derived neutrophil chemotactic factor (MDNCF) and the induction of MDNCF mRNA by interleukin 1 and tumor necrosis factor. J Exp Med 1988; 167:1883-1893.

44. Thelen M, Peveri P, Kernen P et al. Mechanism of neutrophil activation by NAF, a novel monocyte-derived peptide agonist. Faseb J 1988; 2(11):2702-2706.

45. Peveri P, Walz A, Dewald B et al. A novel neutrophil-activating factor produced by human mononuclear phagocytes. J Exp Med 1988; 167(5):1547-1559.

46. Schroder JM, Mrowietz U, Morita E et al. Purification and partial biochemical characterization of a human monocyte-derived, neutrophil-activating peptide that lacks interleukin 1 activity. J Immunol 1987; 139(10):3474-3483.

47. Detmers PA, Lo SK, Olsen EE et al. Neutrophil-activating protein 1/interleukin 8 stimulates the binding activity of the leukocyte adhesion receptor CD11b/CD18 on human neutrophils. J Exp Med 1990; 171(4):1155-1162.

48. Schroder JM. The monocyte-derived neutrophil activating peptide (NAP/interleukin 8) stimulates human neutrophil arachidonate-5-lipoxygenase, but not the release of cellular arachidonate. J Exp Med 1989; 170(3):847-863.

49. Metinko AP, Kunkel SL, Standiford TJ et al. Anoxia-hyperoxia induces monocyte-derived interleukin-8. J Clin Invest 1992; 90(3):791-798.

50. Karakurum M, Shreeniwas R, Chen J et al. Hypoxic induction of interleukin-8 gene expression in human endothelial cells. J Clin Invest 1994; 93(4):1564-1570.

51. Yoshimura T, Johnson DG. cDNA cloning and expression of guinea pig neutrophil attractant protein-1 (NAP-1). NAP-1 is highly conserved in guinea pig. J Immunol 1993; 151(11):6225-6236.

52. Schreck R, Rieber P, Baeuerle PA. Reactive oxygen intermediates as apparently widely used messengers in the activation of the NF-kappa B transcription factor and HIV-1. EMBO J 1991; 10(8):2247-2258.

53. Mukaida N, Mahe Y, Matsushima K. Cooperative interaction of nuclear factor-kappa B- and cis-regulatory enhancer binding protein-like factor binding elements in activating the interleukin-8 gene by pro-inflammatory cytokines. J Biol Chem 1990; 265(34):21128-21133.

54. Shreeniwas R, Koga S, Karakurum M et al. Hypoxia-mediated induction of endothelial cell interleukin-1 alpha. An autocrine mechanism promoting expression of leukocyte adhesion molecules on the vessel surface. J Clin Invest 1992; 90(6):2333-2339.

55. Yoshida N, Granger DN, Anderson DC et al. Anoxia/reoxygenation-induced neutrophil adherence to cultured endothelial cells. Am J Physiol 1992; 262(6 Pt 2):H1891-1898.

56. Matsushima K, Larsen CG, DuBois GC et al. Purification and characterization of a novel monocyte chemotactic and activating

factor produced by a human myelomonoytic cell line. J Exp Med 1989; 169:1485-1490.

57. Yoshimura T, Robinson EA, Tanaka S et al. Purification and amino acid analysis of two human monocyte chemoattractants produced by phytohemagglutinin-stimulated human blood mononuclear leukocytes. J Immunol 1989; 142:1956-1962.

58. Yoshimura T, Robinson EA, Tanaka S et al. Purification and amino acid analysis of two human glioma-derived monocyte chemoattractans. J Exp Med 1989; 169: 1449-1459.

59. Rollins BJ, Walz A, Baggiolini M. Recombinant human MCP-1/JE induces chemotaxis, calcium influx, and the respiratory burst in human monocytes. Blood 1991; 78:1112-1116.

60. Jiang Y, Beller DI, Frendl G et al. Monocyte chemoattractant protein-1 regulates adhesion molecule expression and cytokine production in human monocytes. J Immunol 1992; 148:2423-2428.

61. Kuna P, Redigari SR, Rucinski D et al. Monocyte chemotactic-activating factor is a potent histamine-releasing factor for human basophils. J Exp Med 1992; 175:489-493.

62. Wang X, Yue TL, Barone FC et al. Monocyte chemoattractant protein-1 messenger RNA expression in rat ischemic cortex. Stroke 1995; 26(4):661-665.

63. DeForge LE, Fantone JC, Kenney JS et al. Oxygen radical scavengers selectively inhibit interleukin 8 production in human whole blood. J Clin Invest 1992; 90(5):2123-2129.

64. DeForge LE, Preston AM, Takeuchi E et al. Regulation of interleukin 8 gene expression by oxidant stress. J Biol Chem 1993; 268(34):25568-25576.

65. Babior BM. The respiratory burst oxidase and the molecular basis of chronic granulomatous disease. Am J Hematol 1991; 37(4):263-266.

66. Bautista AP, Spitzer JJ. Superoxide anion generation by in situ perfused rat liver: effect of in vivo endotoxin. Am J Physiol 1990; 259(6 Pt 1):G907-G912.

67. Matsubara T, Ziff M. Increased superoxide anion release from human endothelial cells in response to cytokines. J Immunol 1986; 137(10):3295-3298.

68. Rosen GM, Freeman BA. Detection of superoxide generated by endothelial cells. Proc Natl Acad Sci USA 1984; 81(23): 7269-7273.

69. Abe Y, Kawakami M, Kuroki M et al. Transient rise in serum interleukin-8 concentration during acute myocardial infarction. Br Heart J 1993; 70(2):132-134.

70. Jorens PG, De JR, De BW et al. Interleukin-8 production in patients undergoing cardiopulmonary bypass. The influence of pretreatment with methylprednisolone. Am Rev Respir Dis 1993; 148(4 Pt 1):890-895.

71. Sekido N, Mukaida N, Harada A et al. Prevention of lung reperfusion injury in rabbits by a monoclonal antibody against interleukin-8. Nature 1993; 365(6447): 654-657.

72. Kukielka GL, Smith CW, LaRosa GJ et al. Interleukin-8 gene induction in the myocardium after ischemia and reperfusion in vivo. J Clin Invest 1995; 95(1):89-103.

73. Ember JA, Sanderson SD, Hugli TE et al. Induction of interleukin-8 synthesis from monocytes by human C5a anaphylatoxin. Am J Pathol 1994; 144(2):393-403.

74. Ivey CL, Williams FM, Collins PD et al. Neutrophil chemoattractants generated in two phases during reperfusion of ischemic myocardium in the rabbit. J Clin Invest 1995; 95:2720-2728.

75. Weisman HF, Bartow T, Leppo MK et al. Soluble human complement receptor type 1: in vivo inhibitor of complement suppressing postischemic myocardial inflammation and necrosis. Science 1990; 249(4965): 146-151.

76. Shandelya SM, Kuppusamy P, Herskowitz A et al. Soluble complement receptor type 1 inhibits the complement pathway and prevents contractile failure in the postischemic heart. Evidence that complement activation is required for neutrophil-mediated reperfusion injury. Circulation 1993; 88(6):2812-2826.

77. Matuschak GM, Rinaldo JE. Organ interaction in the adult respiratory distress syndrome during sepsis. Chest 1988; 94: 400-406.

78. Colletti LM, Remick DG, Burtch GD et al. Role of tumor necrosis factor-alpha in the

pathophysiologic alterations after hepatic ischemia/reperfusion injury in the rat. J Clin Invest 1990; 85(6):1936-1943.

79. Colletti LM, Kunkel SL, Walz A et al. Chemokine expression during hepatic ischemia/reperfusion-induced lung injury in the rat. The role of epithelial neutrophil activating protein. J Clin Invest 1995; 95(1):134-141.

80. Donnelly SC, Strieter RM, Kunkel SL et al. Interleukin-8 and development of adult respiratory distress syndrome in at-risk patient groups. Lancet 1993; 341(8846): 643-647.

81. Schmouder RL, Strieter RM, Walz A et al. Epithelial-derived neutrophil-activating factor-78 production in human renal tubule epithelial cells and in renal allograft rejection. Transplantation 1995; 59(1):118-124.

82. Pattison J, Nelson PJ, Huie P et al. RANTES chemokine expression in cell-mediated transplant rejection of the kidney. Lancet 1994; 343(8891):209-211.

CHAPTER 11

THE ROLE OF C-X-C CHEMOKINES IN REGULATION OF ANGIOGENESIS

Robert M. Strieter, Steven L. Kunkel, Armen B. Shanafelt,
Douglas A. Arenberg, Alisa E. Koch and Peter J. Polverini

SUMMARY

The regulation of angiogenesis is fundamental to a variety of physiological and pathological processes. While a number of factors have been identified that induce neovascularization, it is becoming increasingly apparent that endogenous angiostatic factors may play an important role in the regulation of angiogenesis during wound repair, chronic inflammation and growth of solid tumors. In this chapter, we will discuss evidence that the C-X-C chemokine family of cytokines displays disparate angiogenic activity depending upon the presence or absence of the ELR motif, a structural amino acid motif previously found to be important in receptor ligand binding on neutrophils. C-X-C chemokines containing the ELR motif are potent angiogenic factors, inducing both in vitro endothelial chemotaxis and in vivo corneal neovascularization. In contrast, the C-X-C chemokines that lack the ELR motif, PF4, IP-10 and MIG, not only fail to induce significant in vitro endothelial cell chemotaxis or in vivo corneal neovacularization, but are found to be potent angiostatic factors in the presence of C-X-C chemokines containing the ELR motif, as well as the unrelated angiogenic factor, basic fibroblast growth factor (bFGF). This suggests that the C-X-C chemokine family can display disparate angiogenic activity that depends upon the presence or absence of the ELR motif. Furthermore, these findings support the notion that the net biological balance in the magnitude of expression of angiogenic and angiostatic C-X-C chemokines at either the site of wound repair or during tumorigenesis may be important in the regulation of net angiogenesis.

Chemokines in Disease, edited by Alisa E. Koch and Robert M. Strieter.
© 1996 R.G. Landes Company.

INTRODUCTION

Angiogenesis is one of the most pervasive and essential biological events encountered in vertebrate animals.[1-5] A number of physiological and pathological processes, such as embryonic development, the formation of inflammatory granulation tissue during wound healing, chronic inflammation and the growth of malignant solid tumors, are strictly dependent upon neovascularization. Normally, physiologic angiogenesis occurs infrequently, yet can be rapidly induced in response to a number of diverse physiologic stimuli. Among the most extensively studied of these angiogenesis-dependent physiological processes is wound healing.[6] An important feature of wound-associated angiogenesis is that it is locally controlled and transient. The rate of normal capillary endothelial cell turnover in adults is typically measured in months or years.[7,8] However, when quiescent endothelial cells are stimulated, they will degrade basement membrane and proximal extracellular matrix, migrate directionally, divide and organize into new functioning capillaries invested by a new basal lamina all within a matter of days. This dramatic amplification of the microvasculature is nevertheless temporary. As rapidly as they are formed, they virtually disappear with similar swiftness, returning the tissue vasculature to a homeostatic environment. This demonstrates two key aspects of the angiogenic response: first, the formation of new microvasculature is rapid and controlled; and second, it is transient and characterized by regression to a physiologic steady-state level. The abrupt termination of angiogenesis that accompanies the resolution of the wound response suggests two possible mechanisms of control, neither of which are mutually exclusive. First, under circumstances not well understood, there is probably a marked reduction in the synthesis and/or elaboration of angiogenic mediators. Second, a simultaneous increase occurs in the levels of substances which inhibit new vessel growth.[9]

While angiogenesis under conditions of normal wound repair appears to be under strict control, during neoplastic transformation neovascularization is exaggerated. It appears that tumors are continually renewing and altering their vascular supply.[4] Interestingly, normal vascular mass of tissue is approximately 20%, whereas, during tumorigenesis, tumor vascular mass may be >50% of the total tumor.[4] These findings are consistent with the observations that angiogenic activity is both a marker of preneoplastic to neoplastic transformation as well as an event that perpetuates tumorigenesis. In addition, the magnitude of tumor-derived angiogenesis has been directly correlated with metastasis of melanoma, prostate cancer, breast cancer and non-small cell lung cancer (NSCLC).[4,10-15] Moreover, this would support the notion that tumor-associated angiogenesis is dysregulated in such a manner that a biological imbalance exists that favors either the over-expression of local angiogenic factors or the suppression of endogenous angiostatic factors.[4,10,16] While most investigations of angiogenesis have focused on the identification and mechanism of action of positive regulators of neovascularization, recent evidence suggests that inhibitory factors may play an equally important role in the control of blood vessel growth.[9,16-20]

A role for inhibitors in the control of angiogenesis was first suggested by Eisenstein and colleagues,[16] and Sorgente and associates,[17] who observed that hyaline cartilage was particularly resistant to vascular invasion. They reported that a heat labile guanidium chloride extract prepared from cartilage contained an inhibitor of neovascularization. Later, Brem and Folkman[18] and their co-workers Lee and Langer[19] showed that a similar or identical extract from rodent neonatal and shark cartilage was able to effectively block neovascularization and growth of tumors in vivo. Similar angiostatic factors have been reported for other cell and tissue extracts,[18-22] and for a variety of natural and artificial agents including: inhibitors of basement membrane biosynthesis,[23-26] placental ribonuclease inhibitor,[27] lymphotoxin,[28] interferons,[29] prostaglandin synthetase inhibitors,[30] heparin-binding fragments of fibronectin,[31] protamine,[32] angiostatic steroids,[33] several antineoplastic and anti-inflammatory agents,[34,35] platelet factor-4 (PF4),[36] interferon γ-inducible protein-10 (IP-10),[37-40] monokine induced by γ-interferon (MIG),[40] thrombospondin-1,[41-43] angiostatin,[44] and antagonists to $\alpha_v\beta_3$ integrins.[45] Although most inhibitors can act directly on the endothelial cell to block migration and/or mitogenesis in vitro, their effects in vivo may be considerably more complex, involving additional cells and their products.

Several lines of evidence suggest that an imbalance in the production of promoters and inhibitors of angiogenesis contributes to the pathogenesis of several angiogenesis-dependent disorders. For example, in rheumatoid arthritis the unrestrained proliferation of fibroblasts and capillary blood vessels leads to the formation of prolonged and persistent granulation tissue whose degradative enzymes contribute to profound destruction of joint spaces.[46] We have shown that a subpopulation of macrophages (MØ) isolated from rheumatoid synovium produce factors that are potentially angiogenic in vivo and chemotactic for capillary endothelial cells in vitro.[47,48] The inability of MØ to express appropriate angiogenic activity may also contribute to the pathogenesis of other diseases associated with defective angiogenesis.

Blood monocyte-derived MØ from patients with scleroderma fail to stimulate the expected angiogenesis when exposed to the activating agent lipopolysaccharide (LPS)[49] suggesting that a defect in MØ responsiveness to activating signals may contribute to the aberrant vascularization that is encountered in scleroderma. Psoriasis, a common genetic skin disease, is a well known angiogenesis-dependent disorder that is characterized by marked dermal neovascularization. We have recently reported that keratinocytes isolated from psoriatic plaques demonstrated a greater production of angiogenic activity, as compared to normal keratinocytes.[50] Interestingly, this aberrant phenotype is due, in

part, to a combined defect in the overproduction of the angiogenic cytokine IL-8, and a deficiency in the production of the angiogenesis inhibitor thrombospondin-1, resulting in a proangiogenic environment.[50] In rheumatoid arthritis, psoriasis or tumorigenesis, neovascularization is overinduced. In contrast, in chronic nonhealing wounds (ulcers), angiogenesis is impaired, ultimately leading to inadequate granulation tissue formation that fails to support re-epithelialization.[51] Although the complement of positive and negative regulators of angiogenesis may vary among different physiologic and pathologic settings, the recognition of this dual mechanism of control is necessary to gain a more thorough understanding of this complex process and its significance in regulating net angiogenesis.

THE ROLE OF C-X-C CHEMOKINES IN REGULATING ANGIOGENESIS

THE C-X-C CHEMOKINE FAMILY

The C-X-C chemokine family are cytokines which in their monomeric forms are all less than 10 kDa and are characteristically basic heparin-binding proteins. This family displays four highly conserved cysteine amino acid residues, with the first two cysteines separated by one nonconserved amino acid residue. In general, these cytokines appear to have specific chemotactic activity for neutrophils. Because of their chemotactic properties and the presence of the C-X-C cysteine motif, these cytokines have been designated the C-X-C chemokine family. These chemokines are all clustered on human chromosome 4, and exhibit between 20% to 50% homology on the amino acid level.[52-56]

Over the last decade, several human C-X-C chemokines have been identified (Table 11.1); they include PF4, NH₂-terminal truncated forms of platelet basic protein [PBP; connective tissue activating protein-III (CTAP-III), β-thromboglobulin (βTG) and neutrophil activating protein-2

Table 11.1. The C-X-C chemokines

Interleukin-8 (IL-8)
Epithelial neutrophil activating protein-78 (ENA-78)
Growth-related oncogene alpha (GROα)
Growth-related oncogene beta (GROβ)
Growth-related oncogene gamma (GROγ)
Granulocyte chemotactic protein-2 (GCP-2)
Platelet basic protein (PBP)
    Connective tissue activating protein-III (CTAP-III)
    Beta-thromboglobulin (βTG)
    Neutrophil activating protein-2 (NAP-2)
Platelet factor-4 (PF4)
Interferon-γ-inducible protein (IP-10)
Monokine induced by interferon-γ (MIG)

(NAP-2)], interleukin-8 (IL-8), growth-re-lated oncogene (GROα), GROβ, GROγ, IP-10, MIG, epithelial neutrophil activating protein-78 (ENA-78) and granulocyte chemotactic protein-2 (GCP-2).[52-59] The NH$_2$-terminal truncated forms of platelet basic protein are generated when platelet basic protein is released from platelet α-granules and undergoes proteolytic cleavage by monocyte-derived proteases.[60] PF4, the first member of the C-X-C chemokine family to be described, was originally identified for its ability to bind to heparin, leading to inactivation of heparin's anti-coagulation function.[61]

Both IP-10 and MIG are interferon-inducible chemokines.[57,62] Although IP-10 appears to be induced by all three interferons (IFN-α, IFN-β and IFN-γ), MIG is unique in that it appears to be expressed only in the presence of IFN-γ.[57] While IFN-γ induces the production of IP-10 and MIG, this cytokine attenuates the expression of IL-8, GROα and ENA-78.[63,64] These findings would suggest that members of the C-X-C chemokine family demonstrate disparate regulation in the presence of interferons. GROα, GROβ and GROγ are closely related C-X-C chemokines, with GROα originally described for its melanoma growth stimulatory activity.[65-67] IL-8, ENA-78 and GCP-2 were all initially identified on the basis of their ability to induce neutrophil activation and

chemotaxis.[52-59] These C-X-C chemokines have been found to be produced by an array of cells including monocytes, alveolar macrophages, neutrophils, platelets, keratinocytes, mesangial cells, epithelial cells, hepatocytes, fibroblasts and endothelial cells.[52-56,64,68-83] While numerous in vivo and in vitro investigations have shown the importance of C-X-C chemokines in acute inflammation as a chemotactic/activating factors for neutrophils, only recently has it become apparent that these C-X-C chemokines may be an important in the regulation of angiogenic activity.

The Role of IL-8 and PF4 in Regulation of Angiogenesis

Our laboratory and others have found that IL-8 is a potent angiogenic factor.[48,84,85] Recombinant IL-8 mediates both endothelial cell chemotactic and proliferative activity in vitro and angiogenic activity in vivo (corneal micropocket model in both rats and rabbits). We found that IL-8 induced similar angiogenic activity as bFGF.[48] Since monocytes/macrophages may represent a major source of angiogenic activity in wounds and other chronic diseases,[3] we extended our studies to determine whether IL-8 was a predominant angiogenic factor liberated by normal human monocytes activated in vitro or by synovial macrophages isolated from rheumatoid arthritis synovial tissues.[48] Conditioned media from both populations of mononuclear phagocytes induced significant chemotactic activity for endothelial cells. Furthermore, when these supernatants were exposed to neutralizing antibodies to IL-8, endothelial cell chemotaxis was markedly reduced.[37] Similar neutralization was seen utilizing the same conditioned media in the corneal micropocket model of angiogenesis.

To further demonstrate that the angiogenic effect was attributable to IL-8, we used an IL-8 antisense oligonucleotide strategy to inhibit the production of IL-8 at the pretranslational level.[48] Monocytes were stimulated with endotoxin in the presence of either an IL-8 antisense or sense oligonucleotides in concentrations >5 µM. The conditioned media from monocytes treated in the presence of IL-8 antisense inhibited endothelial cell chemotactic activity by 84%, as compared to the IL-8 sense oligonucleotide treated monocytes. Similar results were found in the in vivo corneal micropocket model of angiogenesis. These findings indicated that IL-8, at concentrations of approximately 10 nM, can function as a mediator of angiogenesis. This amount of IL-8 compares with amounts reported for the induction of corneal angiogenic activity by TNF-α, aFGF, bFGF, angiogenin, angiotropin and endothelial cell growth factor.[48]

Interestingly, another member of the C-X-C chemokine family, PF4, has been shown to have angiostatic properties,[36] and to attenuate the growth of tumors in vivo.[86] These studies had initially demonstrated that the angiostatic activity of PF4 was due to its heparin binding domain (within the COOH-terminus of the molecule).[36,86] However, studies have now shown that a PF4 mutant that lacks both the heparin-binding domain and functional heparin binding is equipotent in vivo to native PF4 for the attenuation of tumor growth.[87] The above findings would suggest that members of the C-X-C chemokine family can function as either angiogenic or angiostatic factors in regulating neovascularization.

Although it remained unclear whether the COOH-terminus of these chemokines dictated their biological role in regulating angiogenesis, the differences in C-X-C chemokine function could also be explained by other structural domains. Both Hébert[88] and Clark-Lewis[89] demonstrated a salient amino acid sequence in the primary structure of the C-X-C chemokine family that appears, in part, to account for the ability of these chemokines to function in neutrophil chemotaxis and activation. They demonstrated that the three amino acid residues that immediately preceded the first cysteine amino acid are critically important in binding and activating neutrophils. These amino acids are Glu-Leu-Arg, the

ELR motif, which is absent in certain members of the C-X-C chemokine family (PF4, IP-10 and MIG) that display markedly reduced potency in mediating neutrophil chemotaxis. Thus, these structural differences, in part, may explain the disparity of angiogenic activity of the C-X-C chemokine family.

THE C-X-C CHEMOKINE FAMILY DISPLAYS DISPARATE ANGIOGENIC ACTIVITY

We speculated that members of the C-X-C chemokine family may exert disparate effects in mediating angiogenesis as a function of the presence or absence of the ELR motif for primarily four reasons. First, members of the C-X-C chemokine family that display binding and activation of neutrophils share the highly conserved ELR motif that immediately precedes the first cysteine amino acid residue, whereas PF4, IP-10 and MIG lack this motif.[88,89] Second, IL-8 (contains ELR motif) mediates both endothelial cell chemotactic and proliferative activity in vitro and angiogenic activity in vivo.[40,48] In contrast, PF4 (lacking the ELR motif) has been shown to have angiostatic properties,[36] and attenuates growth of tumors in vivo.[86] Third, the interferons (IFN-α, IFN-β and IFN-γ) are all known inhibitors of wound repair, especially angiogenesis.[29,90-99] These cytokines, however, upregulate IP-10 and MIG from a number of cells, including keratinocytes, fibroblasts, endothelial cells and mononuclear phagocytes.[57,67] Finally, we and others have found that IFN-α, IFN-β and IFN-γ are potent inhibitors of the production of monocyte-derived IL-8, GROα and ENA-78,[63,64] supporting the notion that IFN-α, IFN-β and IFN-γ may shift the biological balance of ELR- and non-ELR-C-X-C chemokines toward a preponderance of angiostatic (non-ELR) C-X-C chemokines.

To evaluate whether C-X-C chemokines display disparate angiogenic activity, endothelial cell chemotaxis was performed in the presence or absence of IL-8, ENA-78, PF4 and IP-10 at concentrations of 50 pM to 50 nM. We found that both IL-8 and ENA-78 demonstrated a dose-dependent increase in endothelial migration that was significantly greater than control at concentrations equal to or above 0.1 nM and 1 nM, respectively.[40] In contrast, neither PF4 nor IP-10 induced significant endothelial cell chemotaxis.[40] Other C-X-C chemokines were tested for their ability to induce endothelial cell chemotaxis, including ELR-C-X-C chemokines IL-8, ENA-78, GCP-2, GROα, GROβ, GROγ, PBP, CTAP-III and NAP-2, or the non-ELR C-X-C chemokines IP-10, PF4 and MIG. In a similar fashion to IL-8 or ENA-78, all of the ELR-C-X-C chemokines tested demonstrated significant endothelial cell chemotactic activity over the background control, whereas the endothelial cell chemotactic activity induced by MIG was either similar to background control or to the endothelial cell chemotactic activity seen with either PF4 or IP-10.[40] These findings suggested that C-X-C chemokines could be divided into two groups with defined biological activities, one which contains the ELR motif and is chemotactic for endothelial cells and the other which lacks the ELR motif and does not induce endothelial chemotaxis.

PF4, IP-10 OR MIG INHIBIT IL-8-, ENA-78- OR bFGF-INDUCED ANGIOGENIC ACTIVITY

The above studies suggested that PF4, IP-10 and MIG were not significant chemotactic factors for endothelial cells, and suggested that these C-X-C chemokines may be potent inhibitors of angiogenesis. To test this hypothesis, endo-

thelial cell chemotaxis was performed in the presence or absence of IL-8 (10 nM), ENA-78 (10 nM) or bFGF (5 nM) with or without varying concentrations of PF4, IP-10 or MIG from 0-10 nM. Endothelial cell migration in response to either IL-8, ENA-78 or bFGF was significantly inhibited by PF4, IP-10 or MIG in a dose-dependent manner.[40] PF4 and IP-10 in a concentration of 50 pM inhibited either IL-8- or ENA-78-induced endothelial chemotaxis by 50%, whereas, PF4 and IP-10 in a concentration of 1nM attenuated the response to bFGF by 50%. MIG at a concentration of 1nM, 5nM, 1nM inhibited the endothelial cell chemotactic response to IL-8, ENA-78 and bFGF, respectively, by 50% (Table 11.2). Interestingly, while IP-10 and MIG inhibited IL-8-induced endothelial cell chemotactic activity, neither IP-10 nor MIG were effective in attenuating IL-8-induced neutrophil chemotactic activity.

The rat corneal micropocket model of neovascularization was used to determine whether IP-10 or MIG could inhibit the angiogenic activity of either the ELR containing C-X-C chemokines or bFGF in vivo. Hydron pellets alone, pellets containing IL-8, ENA-78, GROα, GCP-2, IP-10, MIG or bFGF in a concentration of 10nM, or pellets containing combinations of 10nM each of IL-8 + IP-10, ENA-78 + IP-10, GROα + IP-10, GCP-2 + IP-10, IL-8 + MIG, ENA-78 + MIG, bFGF + IP-10 or bFGF + MIG, were embedded into the normally avascular rat cornea and assessed for a neovascular response. The C-X-C chemokines (IL-8, ENA-78, GROα or GCP-2) or bFGF induced positive corneal angiogenic responses without evidence for

Table 11.2. The IC_{50} of PF4, IP-10, and MIG for the inhibition of the agonists IL-8, ENA-78, and bFGF

Agonist	IL-8 (10nM)	ENA-78 (10nM)	bFGF (5nM)
Inhibitor (IC_{50})			
PF4	5×10^{-11} M	5×10^{-11} M	1×10^{-9} M
IP-10	5×10^{-11} M	5×10^{-11} M	1×10^{-9} M
MIG	5×10^{-10} M	5×10^{-9} M	1×10^{-9} M

significant leukocyte infiltration. In contrast, hydron pellets alone, or pellets containing either IP-10 or MIG (10nM) did not induce a neovascular response in the cornea. When IP-10 was added in combination with the ELR-C-X-C chemokines (IL-8, ENA-78, GROα or GCP-2) or bFGF, IP-10 significantly abrogated the ELR-C-X-C chemokine and bFGF-induced angiogenic activity. In addition, MIG inhibited IL-8, ENA-78 and bFGF-induced corneal angiogenic activity in a similar manner to IP-10.

C-X-C Chemokines: The Role of the Amino Acid ELR Motif in the Regulation of Angiogenesis

To establish whether the ELR motif is the critical molecular domain that dictates angiogenic activity for members of the C-X-C chemokine family, our laboratories constructed muteins of IL-8 lacking the ELR motif and a mutant of MIG containing the ELR motif. The ELR motif in wild type IL-8 was mutated to either TVR (TVR-IL-8; corresponding IP-10 sequence) or DLQ (DLQ-IL-8; corresponding to PF4 sequence) by site-directed mutagenesis, and expressed in *E. coli*. TVR-IL-8 and DLQ-IL-8 alone failed to induce endothelial cell chemotactic activity, yet these muteins in-

hibited the maximal endothelial chemotactic activity of wild type IL-8 by 83% and 88%, respectively.[40] Neither TVR-IL-8 nor DLQ-IL-8 induced neutrophil chemotaxis, nor were they effective in attenuating neutrophil chemotaxis in response to IL-8.

Using the in vivo rat cornea micropocket model of neovascularization, TVR-IL-8 (10 nM) alone did not induce a positive neovascular response. However, TVR-IL-8 (10 nM) in combination with either IL-8 (10 nM) or ENA-78 (10 nM) resulted in a significant reduction in the ability of either IL-8 or ENA-78 to induce cornea neovascularization.[40] Moreover, the angiostatic activity of the IL-8 muteins was not only unique to inhibition of ELR-C-X-C chemokine-induced angiogenic activity, as TVR-IL-8 (10 nM) inhibited both bFGF-induced (10 nM) maximal endothelial cell chemotaxis and corneal neovascularization. In addition, ELR-MIG (10 nM) induced significant angiogenic responses as compared to wild type MIG.[40] Interestingly, MIG (10nM) inhibited the angiogenic response of ELR-MIG in both endothelial migration and cornea neovascularization assays. These data further support the importance of the ELR motif as a domain for mediating angiogenic activity (Table 11.3).

Table 11.3. The C-X-C chemokines that display disparate angiogenic activity

Angiogenic C-X-C chemokines containing the ELR motif
    Interleukin-8 (IL-8)
    Epithelial neutrophil activating protein-78 (ENA-78)
    Growth-related oncogene alpha (GROα)
    Growth-related oncogene beta (GROβ)
    Growth-related oncogene gamma (GROγ)
    Granulocyte chemotactic protein-2 (GCP-2)
    Platelet basic protein (PBP)
    Connective tissue activating protein-III (CTAP-III)
    Beta-thromboglobulin (βTG)
    Neutrophil activating protein-2 (NAP-2)

Angiostatic C-X-C chemokines that lack the ELR motif
    Platelet factor-4 (PF4)
    Interferon-γ-inducible protein (IP-10)
    Monokine induced by interferon-γ (MIG)

C-X-C Chemokine Receptors on Endothelial Cells

The finding that IP-10 is angiostatic has also been substantiated by other investigators. Angiolillo and associates[38] have determined that IP-10 can inhibit bFGF-induced angiogenesis in vivo. In addition, Luster and colleagues have found that IP-10 binds to a specific cell surface site on endothelial cells that is shared by PF4 and appears to be a heparan sulfate proteoglycan receptor.[39] This binding site is specific for IP-10 and PF4, as neither ELR containing C-X-C chemokines nor various C-C chemokines compete for this binding site on endothelial cells. Furthermore, these investigators demonstrated that binding of IP-10 to endothelial cells resulted in an inhibition of proliferation that was independent of calcium flux and apoptosis, and dependent on reversible cell cycle arrest. These findings suggest that IP-10, PF4 and potentially MIG are unique members of the C-X-C chemokine family that share a heparan sulfate proteoglycan receptor that accounts for their binding to endothelial cells and subsequent angiostatic activity.

In contrast to the recently described specific proteoglycan receptor for IP-10 and PF4 on endothelial cells, a specific endothelial receptor(s) has not been established for the activity of ELR-C-X-C chemokine-induced neovascularization. However, indirect evidence would suggest that the endothelial receptor for ELR-C-X-C chemokines is the IL-8 receptor B (IL-8RB). In support of this contention are the following findings:

(a) while endothelial cells have recently been found to express IL-8 receptor A mRNA by RT-PCR, this study found that both IL-8 and NAP-2 could compete for binding on endothelial cells that was inhibited by heparin and heparan sulfate.[100] However, only IL-8, not NAP-2, can bind to IL-8RA.[101]

(b) IL-8RB on neutrophils binds all ELR-C-X-C chemokines with high affinity,[58,101,102] and all ELR-C-X-C chemokines are angiogenic.[40]

(c) while the Duffy antigen receptor for chemokines has been identified on postcapillary venule endothelial cells,[103] this receptor binds not only ELR-C-X-C chemokines, but also C-C chemokines, monocyte chemoattractant protein-1 (MCP-1) and regulated on activation normal T cell expressed and secreted (RANTES).[104] We have found that these latter two C-C chemokines are not chemotactic for endothelial cells.

(d) human burn tissue 2 to 12 days after injury has been found to express IL-8RB associated with capillary endothelial cells in areas of neovascularization.[105] Nevertheless, further studies will be required to delineate the specific endothelial cell receptor(s) for the angiogenic activities of the ELR-C-X-C chemokines.

THE ROLE OF C-X-C CHEMOKINES IN THE REGULATION OF ANGIOGENESIS IN NON-SMALL CELL LUNG CANCER (NSCLC)

The evidence that C-X-C chemokines could function as either angiogenic or angiostatic factors depending upon the presence of the ELR motif led to our investigation of whether C-X-C chemokines were present in natural human NSCLC, and whether they contributed to overall NSCLC tumor-derived angiogenic activity. IL-8, ENA-78 and GROα have been found in 4-, 3- and 2.5-fold excess, respectively, in tumor tissue as compared to normal lung tissue. We have found similar elevations of IL-8 and ENA-78 from both adenocarcinomas and squamous cell carcinomas, whereas GROα was found to be especially elevated in squamous cell carcinomas. In contrast, PF4 levels have been found in the carcinoma tissue homogenates to be equivalent to normal lung tissue. Although IP-10 levels tend toward being greater in tumors than in normal lung tissue homogenates, we have found that IP-10 is significantly lower in adenocarcinomas than in normal lung tissue. Importantly, these specific findings may be reflected in the different clinical behaviors of squamous cell carcinoma and adenocarcinoma NSCLCs. The more aggressive course of adenocarcinomas could be related to their capacity to generate a greater angiogenic as compared to angiostatic C-X-C chemokine signal.

Since it was apparent that NSCLC was associated with significantly elevated levels of IL-8, we next determined whether IL-8 contributed to overall tumor-derived angiogenic activity. Using neutralizing antibodies to IL-8, we found that IL-8 accounted for 42% to 80% of the angiogenic activity for each of the tumor specimens, as determined by bioassays of angiogenesis.[106] While IL-8-dependent angiogenic activity represented a significant proportion of overall NSCLC-derived angiogenesis, we wanted to compare the relative contribution of IL-8 to other known angiogenic factors in NSCLC. Neutralizing antibodies to IL-8 resulted in a significant reduction of endothelial cell chemotactic activity in response to NSCLC tissue, with a decline to 75%, 39% and 61% of the standard bioactivity, respectively, for adenocarcinoma, squamous cell carcinoma and A549 (adenocarcinoma) samples.[106] In contrast, anti-bFGF antibodies had no significant effect on the endothelial cell chemotaxis in response to samples of A549 cells/tissue or squamous cell carcinoma tissue; however, neutralizing anti-bFGF antibodies reduced the endothelial cell chemotactic activity from adenocarcinoma tissue by 35% of the standard bioactivity.[106] Interestingly, the neutralization of TGF-α had no significant effect on the chemotaxis in response to adenocarcinoma or to the A549 cell/tissue. However, these antibodies resulted in a significant reduction (45%) in the endothelial cell chemotactic response to squamous cell carcinoma tissue.[106] Although bFGF and TGF-α have been previously described as potential angiogenic factors involved in tumor angiogenesis, our studies were the first to demonstrate that a primary angiogenic signal for NSCLC neovascularization was directly mediated by tumor-associated IL-8.

To further substantiate that IP-10 may be acting as an endogenous angiostatic C-X-C chemokine to balance the effect of angiogenic factors in the context of NSCLC, we assessed squamous cell carcinoma tissue homogenates for angiogenesis in the presence of neutralizing IP-10 or control antibodies. Using either endothelial cell chemotaxis or corneal micropocket model of neovascularization, we found that neutralizing IP-10 antibodies significantly augmented tumor-derived angiogenic activity by 2-fold. These findings support the presence of an imbalance in ELR-C-X-C, as compared to non-ELR C-X-C chemokines, with the balance favoring a greater presence of angiogenic C-X-C chemokines in NSCLC tumors.

To extend these studies to an in vivo model of human tumorigenesis, we employed a human NSCLC/SCID mouse chimera by injecting the human NSCLC cell lines A549 (adenocarcinoma) and Calu 1 (squamous cell carcinoma) into the flanks of SCID mice. We found that tumor-derived IL-8 production directly correlated with the rate of growth of the two human NSCLC cells lines in vivo. IL-8 was not found to behave as an autocrine growth factor for the proliferation of NSCLC cells. Moreover, when IL-8 was depleted in vivo by a strategy of passive immunization with neutralizing antibodies, tumorigenesis was markedly reduced via a reduction in tumor-derived angiogenic activity. These findings support the contention that IL-8 mediated angiogenesis is critical to tumorigenesis.

These findings support the contention that members of the C-X-C chemokine family may exert disparate effects in the regulation of angiogenesis, and that the ELR motif is the putative domain that dictates the angiogenic activity of this family. The magnitude of the expression of either angiogenic and angiostatic C-X-C chemokines during neovascularization may significantly contribute to the regulation of net angiogenesis during tumorigenesis (Fig. 11.1).

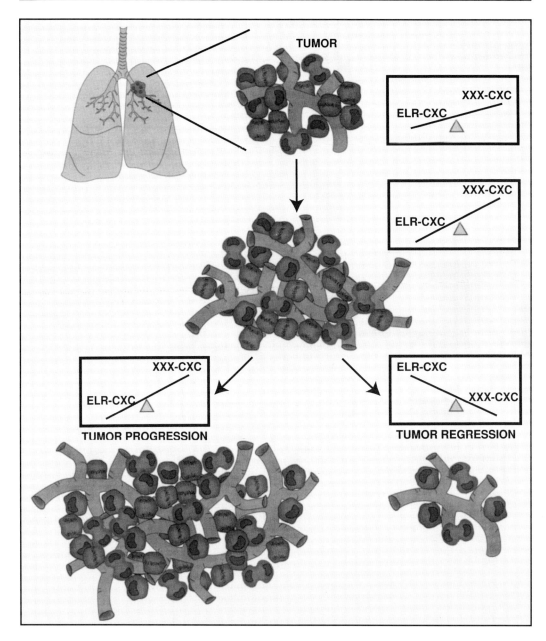

Fig. 11.1. The role of C-X-C chemokines in mediating angiogenesis in the context of tumorgenesis. ELR = chemokines containing the ELR motif that have angiogenic activity. XXX = chemokines that lack the ELR motif that have angiostatic activity.

ACKNOWLEDGMENTS

This work was supported, in part, by: NIH grants HL50057, CA66180 and 1P50HL46487 (R.M.S.), HL39926 (P.J.P.), AR30692 and AR41492 (A.E.K.) and HL31693 and HL35276 (S.L.K.). We would like to acknowledge Robin G. Kunkel for her outstanding artwork.

REFERENCES

1. Folkman J, Cotran R. Relation of vascular proliferation to tumor growth. Int Rev Exp Pathol 1978; 16:207.

2. Auerbach R. Angiogenesis-inducing factors: a review. In: Lymphokines 69. New York: Academic Press, 1981.

3. Polverini, PJ. Macrophage-induced angiogenesis: a review. In: Cytokines. Basel: Karger, 1989:54-73.

4. Folkman J. Tumor angiogenesis. Adv Cancer Res 1985; 43:175-203.

5. Folkman J, Klagsbrun M. Angiogenic factors. Science 1987; 235:442-47.

6. Leibovich SJ, Weisman DM. Macrophages, wound repair and angiogenesis. Prog Clin Biol Res 1988; 266:131-45.

7. Engerman RL, Pfaffenenbach D, Davis MD. Cell turnover of capillaries. Lab Invest 1967; 17:738-43.

8. Tannock IF, Hayashi S. The proliferation of capillary and endothelial cells. Cancer Res 1972; 32:77-82.

9. Bouck N. Tumor angiogenesis: oncogenes and tumor suppresser genes. Cancer Cells 1990; 2:179-85.

10. Folkman J, Watson K, Ingber D, Hanahan D. Induction of angiogenesis during the transition from hyperplasia to neoplasia. Nature 1989; 339:58-61.

11. Maiorana A, Gullino PM. Acquisition of angiogenic capacity and neoplastic transformation in the rat mammary gland. Cancer Res 1978; 38:4409-14.

12. Herlyn M, Clark WH, Rodeck U, Mancianti ML, Jambrosic J, Koprowski H. Biology of tumor progression in human melanocytes. Lab Invest 1987; 56:461-74.

13. Weidner N, Semple JP, Welch WR, Folkman J. Tumor angiogenesis and metastasis-correlation in invasive breast carcinoma. N Eng J Med 1991; 324:1-8.

14. Weidner N, Carroll PR, Flax J, Blumenfeld W, Folkman J. Tumor angiogenesis correlates with metastasis in invasive prostate carcinoma. Am J Pathol 1993; 143:401-09.

15. Macchiarini P, Fontanini G, Hardin MJ, Squartini F, Angeletti CA. Relation of neovascularization to metastasis of non-small cell lung cancer. Lancet 1992; 340:145-46.

16. Eisenstein R, Kuettner KE, Neopolitan C, Sobel LW, Sorgente N. The resistance of certain tissues to invasion III. Cartilage extracts inhibit the growth of fibroblasts and endothelial cells in culture. Am J Pathol 1975; 81:337-47.

17. Sorgente N, Kuettner KE, Soble LW, Eisenstein R. The resistance of certain tissues to invasion. II. Evidence for extractable factors in cartilage which inhibit invasion by vascularized mesenchyme. Lab Invest 1975; 32:217-22.

18. Brem H, Folkman J. Inhibition of tumor angiogenesis mediated by cartilage. J Exp Med 1975; 141:427-39.

19. Lee A, Langer R. Shark cartilage contains inhibitors of tumor angiogenesis. Science 1983; 221:1185-87.

20. Langer R, Conn H, Vacanti J, Haudenschild CC, Folkman J. Control of tumor growth in animals by infusion of an antiangiogenesis inhibitor. Proc Natl Acad Sci USA 1980; 77:4331-35.

21. Brem S, Preis I, Langer R, Brem H, Folkman J, Patz A. Inhibition of neovascularization by an extract derived from vitreous. Am J Ophthalmol 1977; 84:323-28.

22. Lutty GA, Thompson DC, Gallup JY, Mello RJ, Fenselau A. Vitreous: an inhibitor of retinal extract-induced neovascularization. Inv Opthalmol Vis Sci 1983; 24:52-56.

23. Madri JA, Pratt BM, Tucker AM. Phenotypic modulation of endothelial cells by transforming growth factor-beta depends upon the composition and organization of the extracellular matrix. J Cell Biol 1988; 106:1375-84.

24. Ingber DE, Madri JA, Folkman J. A possible mechanism for inhibition of angiogenesis by angiostatic steroids: Induction of capillary basement membrane dissolution. Endocrinology 1986; 119:1768-75.

25. Ingber DE, Folkman J. Inhibition of

angiogenesis through modulation of collagen metabolism. Lab Invest 1988; 59:44-51.

26. Maragoudakis ME, Sarmonika M, Panoutscaopoulou M. Inhibition of basement membrane biosynthesis prevents angiogenesis. J Pharmacol Exp Therapy 1988; 244:729-33.

27. Shapiro R, Vallee BL. Human placental ribonuclease inhibitor abolishes both angiogenic and ribonucleolytic activities of angiogenin. Proc Natl Acad Sci USA 1987; 84:2238.

28. Sato N, Fukuda K, Nariuchi H, Sagara N. Tumor necrosis factor inhibits angiogenesis in vitro. JNCI 1987; 79:1383.

29. Sidky YA, Borden EC. Inhibition of angiogenesis by interferons: effects on tumor- and lymphocyte-induced vascular responses. Cancer Res 1987; 47:5155-61.

30. Peterson, H-I. Tumor angiogenesis inhibition by prostaglandin synthetase inhibitors. Anticancer Res 1986; 6:251-54.

31. Homandberg GA, Kramer-Bjerke J, Grant D, Christianson G, Eisenstein R. Heparin-binding fragments of fibronectin are potent inhibitors of endothelial cell growth: structure and function correlates. Biochem Biophys Acta 1986; 874:61.

32. Taylor S, Folkman J. Protamine is an inhibitor of angiogenesis. Nature 1982; 297:307-12.

33. Crum R, Szabo S, Folkman J. A new class of steroids inhibits angiogenesis in the presence of heparin or a heparin fragment. Science 1985; 230:1375-78.

34. Polverini PJ, Novak RF. Inhibition of angiogenesis by the antineoplastic agents mitoxantrone and bisantrene. Biochem Biophys Res Comm 1986; 140:901-07.

35. Lee K, Erturk E, Mayer R, Cockett ATK. Efficacy of antitumor chemotherapy in C3H mice enhanced by the antiangiogenesis steroid, cortisone acetate. Cancer Res 1987; 47:5021.

36. Maione TE, Gray GS, Petro J, Hunt AJ, Donner AL, Bauer SI, Carson HF, Sharpe RJ. Inhibition of angiogenesis by recombinant human platelet factor-4. Science 1990; 247:77-79.

37. Strieter RM, Kunkel SL, Arenberg DA, Burdick MD, Polverini PJ. Interferon γ-inducible protein 10 (IP-10) a member of the C-X-C chemokine family is an inhibitor of angiogenesis. Biochem Biophysiol Res Comm 1995; 210:51-57.

38. Angiolillo AL, Sgadari C, Taub DD, Liao F, Farber JM, Maheshwari S, Kleinman HK, Reaman GH, Tosato G. Human interferon-inducible protein 10 is a potent inhibitor of angiogenesis in vivo. J Exp Med 1995; 182:155-62.

39. Luster AD, Greenberg SM, Leder P. The IP-10 chemokine binds to a specific cell surface heparan sulfate site shared with platelet factor 4 and inhibits endothelial cell proliferation. J Exp Med 1995; 182:219-31.

40. Strieter RM, Polverini PJ, Kunkel SL, Arenberg DA, Burdick MD, Kasper J, Dzuiba J, VanDamme J, Walz A, Marriott D, Chan S-Y, Roczniak S, Shanafelt AB. The functional role of the ELR motif in C-X-C chemokine-mediated angiogenesis. J Biol Chem 1995; 270:27348-57.

41. Rastinejad F, Polverini PJ, Bouck NP. Regulation of the activity of a new inhibitor of angiogenesis by a cancer suppresser gene. Cell 1989; 56:345-55.

42. Good DJ, Polverini PJ, Rastinejad F, LeBeau MM, Lemons RS, Frazier WA, Bouck NP. A tumor suppresser-dependent inhibitor of angiogenesis is immunologically and functionally indistinguishable from a fragment of thrombospondin. Proc Natl Acad Sci USA 1990; 87:6624-28.

43. Tolsma SS, Volpert OV, Good DJ, Frazier WA, Polverini PJ, Bouck N. Peptides derived from two separate domains of the matrix protein thrombospondin-1 have antiangiogenic activity. J Cell Biol 1993; 122:497-511.

44. O'Reilly MS, Holmgren L, Shing Y, Chen C, Rosenthal RA, Moses M, Lane WS, Cao Y, Sage EH, Folkman J. Angiostatin: a novel angiogenesis inhibitor that mediates the suppression of metastases by Lewis lung cancer carcinoma. Cell 1994; 79:315-28.

45. Brooks PC, Montgomery AMP, Rosenfeld M, Reisfeld RA, Hu T, Klier G, Cheresh DA. Integrin avb3 antagonists promote tumor regression by inducing apoptosis of angiogenic vessels. Cell 1994; 79:1157-64.

46. Harris ED Jr. Recent insights into the

pathogenesis of the proliferative lesion in rheumatoid arthritis. Arthritis Rheum 1976; 19:68.

47. Koch AE, Polverini PJ, Leibovich SJ. Stimulation of neovascularization by human rheumatoid synovial tissue macrophages. Arthritis Rheum 1986; 29:471-79.

48. Koch AE, Polverini PJ, Kunkel SL, Harlow LA, DiPietro LA, Elner VM, Elner SG, Strieter RM. Interleukin-8 (IL-8) as a macrophage-derived mediator of angiogenesis. Science 1992; 258:1798-1801.

49. Koch AE, Litvak MA, Burrows JC, Polverini PJ. Decreased monocyte-mediated angiogenesis in scleroderma. Clin Immunol Immunopath 1992; 64:153-60.

50. Nickoloff BJ, Mitra RS, Varani J, Dixit VM, Polverini PJ. Aberrant production of interleukin-8 and thrombospondin-1 by psoriatic keratinocytes. Am J Pathol 1994; 144:820-28.

51. Davidson JM. Wound repair. In: Gallin JI, Goldstein IM, Snyderman R, eds. Inflammation: Basic Principles and Clinical Correlates. New York: Raven Press Ltd, 1992.

52. Baggiolini M, Dewald B, Walz A. Interleukin-8 and related chemotactic cytokines. In: Gallin JI, Goldstein IM, Snyderman R, eds. Inflammation: Basic Principles and Clinical Correlates. New York: Raven Press Ltd, 1992.

53. Baggiolini M, Walz A, Kunkel SL. Neutrophil-activating peptide-1/interleukin 8, a novel cytokine that activates neutrophils. J Clin Invest 1989; 84:1045-49.

54. Matsushima K, Oppenheim JJ. Interleukin 8 and MCAF: Novel inflammatory cytokines inducible by IL-1 and TNF. Cytokine 1989; 1:2-13.

55. Oppenheim JJ, Zachariae OC, Mukaida N, Matsushima K. Properties of the novel proinflammatory supergene "intercrine" cytokine family. Annu Rev Immunol 1991; 9:617-48.

56. Miller MD, Krangel MS. Biology and biochemistry of the chemokines: a family of chemotactic and inflammatory cytokines. Crit Rev Immunol 1992; 12:17-46.

57. Farber JM. HuMIG: a new member of the chemokine family of cytokines. Biochem Biophys Res Comm 1993; 192:223-30.

58. Proost P, De Wolf-Peeters C, Conings R, Opdenakker G, Billiau A, Van Damme J. Identification of a novel granulocyte chemotactic protein (GCP-1) from human tumor cells: in vitro and in vivo comparison with natural forms of GROα, IP-10, and IL-8. J Immunol 1993; 150:1000-10.

59. Walz A, Burgener R, Car B, Baggiolini M, Kunkel SL, Strieter RM. Structure and neutrophil-activating properties of a novel inflammatory peptide (ENA-78) with homology to IL-8. J Exp Med 1991; 174:1355-62.

60. Walz A, Baggiolini M. Generation of the neutrophil-activating peptide NAP-2 from platelet basic protein or connective tissue-activating peptide III through monocyte proteases. J Exp Med 1990; 171:449-54.

61. Deutsch E, Kain W. Studies on platelet factor 4. In: Jonson SA, Monto RW, Rebuck JW et al, eds. Blood Platelets. Boston: Little, Brown, 1961:337.

62. Kaplan G, Luster AD, Hancock G, Cohn Z. The expression of a γ interferon-induced protein (IP-10) in delayed immune responses in human skin. J Exp Med 1987; 166:1098-1108.

63. Gusella GL, Musso T, Bosco MC, Espinoza-Delgado I, Matsushima K, Varesio L. IL-2 upregulates but IFN-γ suppresses IL-8 expression in human monocytes. J Immunol 1993; 151:2725-32.

64. Schnyder-Candrian S, Strieter RM, Kunkel SL, Walz A. Interferon-α and interferon-γ downregulate the production of interleukin-8 and ENA-78 in human monocytes. J Leuk Biol 1995; 57:929-35.

65. Ansiowicz A, Zajchowski D, Stenman G, Sager R. Functional diversity of gro gene expression in human fibroblasts and mammary epithelial cells. Proc Natl Acad Sci USA 1988; 85:9645-49.

66. Ansiowicz A, Bardwell L, Sager R. Constitutive overexpression of a growth-regulated gene in transformed Chinese hamster and human cells. Proc Natl Acad Sci USA 1987; 84:7188-92.

67. Richmond A, Thomas HG. Melanoma growth stimulatory activity: isolation from human melanoma tumors and characterization of tissue distribution. J Cell Biochem 1988; 36:185-98.

68. Yoshimura T, Matsushima K, Oppenheim JJ, Leonard EJ. Neutrophil chemotactic factor produced by LPS-stimulated human blood mononuclear leukocytes: Partial characterization and separation from interleukin-1. J Immunol 1987; 139:788-94.

69. Matsushima K, Morishita K, Yoshimura T, Lavu S, Obayashi Y, Lew W, Appella E, Kung HF, Leonard EJ, Oppenheim JJ. Molecular cloning of a human monocyte-derived neutrophil chemotactic factor (MDNCF) and the induction of MDNCF mRNA by interleukin-1 and tumor necrosis factor. J Exp Med 1988; 167:1883-93.

70. Strieter RM, Kunkel SL, Showell HJ, Marks RM. Monokine-induced gene expression of human endothelial cell-derived neutrophil chemotactic factor. Biochem Biophys Res Commun 1988; 156:1340-45.

71. Strieter RM, Kunkel SL, Showell H, Remick DG, Phan SH, Ward PA, Marks RM. Endothelial cell gene expression of a neutrophil chemotactic factor by TNF-α, LPS, and IL-1β. Science 1989; 243:1467-69.

72. Strieter RM, Phan SH, Showell HJ, Remick DG, Lynch JP, Genard M, Raiford C, Eskandari M, Marks RM, Kunkel SL. Monokine-induced neutrophil chemotactic factor gene expression in human fibroblasts. J Biol Chem 1989; 264:10621-26.

73. Thornton AJ, Strieter RM, Lindley I, Baggiolini M, Kunkel SL. Cytokine-induced gene expression of a neutrophil chemotactic factor/interleukin-8 by human hepatocytes. J Immunol 1990; 144:2609-13.

74. Elner VM, Strieter RM, Elner SG, Baggiolini M, Lindley I, Kunkel SL. Neutrophil chemotactic factor (IL-8) gene expression by cytokine-treated retinal pigment epithelial cells. Am J Path 1990; 136:745-50.

75. Strieter RM, Chensue SW, Basha MA, Standiford TJ, Lynch JP, Kunkel SL. Human alveolar macrophage gene expression of interleukin-8 by TNF-α, LPS and IL-1β. Am J Respir Cell Mol Biol 1990; 2:321-26.

76. Standiford TJ, Kunkel SL, Basha MA, Chensue SW, Lynch JP, Toews GB, Strieter RM. Interleukin-8 gene expression by a pulmonary epithelial cell line: A model for cytokine networks in the lung. J Clin In-

vest 1990; 86:1945-53.

77. Strieter RM, Kasahara K, Allen R, Showell HJ, Standiford TJ, Kunkel SL. Human neutrophils exhibit disparate chemotactic factor gene expression. Biochem Biophys Res Comm 1990; 173(2):725-30.

78. Brown Z, Strieter RM, Chensue SW, Ceska P, Lindley I, Nield GH, Kunkel SL, Westwick J. Cytokine activated human mesangial cells generate the neutrophil chemoattractant—interleukin 8. Kidney International 1991; 40:86-90.

79. Rolfe MW, Kunkel SL, Standiford TJ, Chensue SW, Allen RM, Evanoff HL, Phan SH, Strieter RM. Pulmonary fibroblast expression of interleukin-8: a model for alveolar macrophage-derived cytokine networking. Am J Respir Cell Mol Biol 1991; 5:493-501.

80. Nickoloff BJ, Karabin GD, Barker JNWN, Giffiths CEM, Sarma V, Mitra RS, Elder JT, Kunkel SL, Dixit VM. Cellular localization of interleukin-8 and its inducer, tumor necrosis factor-alpha in psoriasis. Am J Pathol 1991; 138:129-40.

81. Strieter RM, Kasahara K, Allen RM, Standiford TJ, Rolfe MW, Becker FS, Chensue SW, Kunkel SL. Cytokine-induced neutrophil-derived interleukin-8. Am J Pathol 1992; 141:397-407.

82. Koch AE, Kunkel SL, Harlow LA, Mazarakis DD, Haines GK, Burdick MD, Pope RM, Walz A, Strieter RM. Epithelial neutrophil activating peptide-78: A novel chemotactic cytokine for neutrophils in arthritis. J Clin Invest 1994; 94:1012-18.

83. Koch AE, Kunkel SL, Shah MR, Hosaka S, Halloran MM, Haines GK, Burdick MD, Pope RM, Strieter RM. Growth related gene product α: a chemotactic cytokine for neutrophils in rheumatoid arthritis. J Immunol 1995; 155:3660-66.

84. Strieter RM, Kunkel SL, Elner VM, Martonyl CL, Koch AE, Polverini PJ, Elner SG. Interleukin-8: A corneal factor that induces neovascularization. Am J Pathol 1992; 141:1279-84.

85. Hu DE, Hori Y, Fan TPD. Interleukin-8 stimulates angiogenesis in rats. Inflammation 1993; 17:135-43.

86. Sharpe RJ, Byers HR, Scott CF, Bauer SI,

Maione TE. Growth inhibition of murine melanoma and human colon carcinoma by recombinant human platelet factor 4. J Natl Cancer Inst 1990; 82:848-53.

87. Maione TE, Gray GS, Hunt AJ, Sharpe RJ. Inhibition of tumor growth in mice by an analogue of platelet factor 4 that lacks affinity for heparin and retains potent angiostatic activity. Cancer Res 1991; 51:2077-83.

88. Hebert CA, Vitangcol RV, Baker JB. Scanning mutagenesis of interleukin-8 identifies a cluster of residues required for receptor binding. J Biol Chem 1991; 266: 18989-94.

89. Clark-Lewis I, Dewald B, Geiser T, Moser B, Baggiolini M. Platelet factor 4 binds to interleukin 8 receptors and activates neutrophils when its N terminus is modified with Glu-Leu-Arg. Proc Natl Acad Sci USA 1993; 90:3574-77.

90. Nickoloff BJ. The cytokine network in psoriasis. Arch Dermatol 1991; 127:871-84.

91. McKay IA, Leigh IM. Epidermal cytokines and their role in cutaneous wound healing. Br J Dermatol 1991; 124:513-18.

92. Symington FW. Lymphotoxin, tumor necrosis factor and gamma interferon are cytostatic for normal human keratinocytes. J Invest Dermatol 1989; 92:798-805.

93. Yaar M, Karassik RL, Schipper LE, Gilchrest BA. Effect of alpha and beta interferon on cultured human keratinocytes. J Invest Dermatol 1985; 85:70-74.

94. Nickoloff BJ, Varani J, Mitra S. Modulation of keratinocyte biology by gamma interferon: relevance to cutaneous wound healing. In: Clinical Experimental Approaches to Dermal and Epidermal Repair: Normal and Chronic Wounds. Wiley-Liss Inc., 1991:141-154.

95. Nickoloff BJ, Mitra RS. Inhibition of 125I-epidermal growth factor binding to cultured keratinocytes by antiproliferative molecules gamma interferon, cyclosporine A, and transforming growth factor-beta. J Invest Dermatol 1989; 93:799-803.

96. Klagsbrun M, D'Amore M. Regulators of angiogenesis. Annu Rev Physiol 1991; 53:217-39.

97. Pober JS, Cotran RS. Cytokines and endothelial cell biology. Pathol Rev 1990; 70:427-51.

98. Stout AJ, Gresser I, Thompson D. Inhibition of wound healing in mice by local interferon α/β injection. Int J Exp Path 1993; 74:79-85.

99. Demaeyer E, Demaeyer-Guignard J. Interferons and other regulatory cytokines. New York: Wiley, 1988.

100. Schonbeck U, Brandt E, Peterson F, Hans-Dieter F, Loppnow H. IL-8 specifically binds to endothelial but not to smooth muscle cells. J Immunol 1995; 154:2374-83.

101. Lee J, Horuk R, Rice GC, Bennett GL, Camerato T, Wood WI. Characterization of two high affinity human interleukin-8 receptors. J Biol Chem 1992; 267:16283-87.

102. Taub DD, Oppenheim JJ. Chemokines, inflammation and immune system. Therapeutic Immunol 1994; 1:229-46.

103. Hadley TJ, Lu ZH, Wasniowska K, Martin AW, Pieper SC, Hesselgesser J, Horuk R. Postcapillary venule endothelial cells in kidney express a multispecific chemokine receptor that is structurally and functionally identical to the erythroid isoform, which is the Duffy blood group antigen. J Clin Invest 1994; 94:985-91.

104. Neote K, Darbonne W, Ogez J, Horuk R, Schall T. Identification of a promiscuous inflammatory peptide receptor on the surface of red blood cells. J Biol Chem 1993; 268:12247-49.

105. Nanney LB, Mueller SG, Bueno R, Peiper SC, Richmond A. Distributions of melanoma growth stimulatory activity or growth-regulated gene and the interleukin-8 receptor B in human wound repair. Am J Pathol 1995; 147:1248-60.

106. Smith DR, Polverini PJ, Kunkel SL, Orringer MB, Whyte RI, Burdick MD, Wilke CA, Strieter RM. Inhibition of Interleukin 8 attenuates angiogenesis in bronchogenic carcinoma. J Exp Med 1994; 179:1409-15.

INDEX

Items in italics denote figures (f) and tables (t).